T0226503

Penile and Urethral Cancer

Guest Editor

JACK H. MYDLO, MD, FACS

UROLOGIC CLINICS OF NORTH AMERICA

www.urologic.theclinics.com

August 2010 • Volume 37 • Number 3

SAUNDERS an imprint of ELSEVIER, Inc.

W.B. SAUNDERS COMPANY
A Division of Elsevier Inc.

1600 John F. Kennedy Blvd. • Suite 1800 • Philadelphia, PA 19103-2899

http://www.theclinics.com

UROLOGIC CLINICS OF NORTH AMERICA Volume 37, Number 3
August 2010 ISSN 0094-0143, ISBN-13: 978-1-4377-2534-6

Editor: Kerry Holland
Developmental Editor: Donald Mumford

Urologic Clinics of North America (ISSN 0094-0143) is published quarterly by Elsevier Inc., 360 Park Avenue South, New York, NY 10010-1710. Months of issue are February, May, August, and November. Business and Editorial Offices: 1600 John F. Kennedy Blvd., Suite 1800, Philadelphia, PA 19103-2899. Periodicals postage paid at New York, NY and additional mailing offices. Subscription prices are $291.00 per year (US individuals), $463.00 per year (US institutions), $333.00 per year (Canadian individuals), $568.00 per year (Canadian institutions), $414.00 per year (foreign individuals), and $568.00 per year (foreign institutions). Foreign air speed delivery is included in all *Clinics* subscription prices. All prices are subject to change without notice. **POSTMASTER:** Send address changes to *Urologic Clinics of North America*, Elsevier Health Sciences Division, Subscription Customer Service, 3251 Riverport Lane, Maryland Heights, MO 63043. Customer Service: 1-800-654-2452 (US). From outside the United States, call 1-314-447-8871. Fax: 1-314-447-8029. E-mail: JournalsCustomerServiceusa@elsevier.com (for print support) and JournalsOnlineSupport-usa@elsevier.com (for online support).

Reprints. For copies of 100 or more, of articles in this publication, please contact the Commercial Reprints Department, Elsevier Inc., 360 Park Avenue South, New York, New York 10010-1710. Tel.: 212-633-3813; Fax: 212-462-1935; E-mail: reprints@elsevier.com.

Urologic Clinics of North America is covered in MEDLINE/PubMed (*Index Medicus*), *Excerpta Medica, Current Contents/ Clinical Medicine, Science Citation Index,* and *ISI/BIOMED.*

Printed and bound by CPI Group (UK) Ltd, Croydon, CRO 4YY
Transferred to Digital Print 2011

Contributors

GUEST EDITOR

JACK H. MYDLO, MD, FACS
Professor and Chair, Department of Urology,
Temple University School of Medicine,
Philadelphia, Pennsylvania

AUTHORS

KENNETH W. ANGERMEIER, MD
Associate Professor, Cleveland Clinic,
Glickman Urological and Kidney Institute,
Center for Genitourinary Reconstruction,
Cleveland, Ohio

DANIEL A. BAROCAS, MD, MPH
Assistant Professor, Department of Urologic
Surgery, Center for Surgical Quality and
Outcomes Research, Vanderbilt University
Medical Center, Nashville, Tennessee

RODNEY H. BREAU, MD, FRCSC
Instructor, Department of Urology, Mayo Clinic,
Rochester, Minnesota

SAM S. CHANG, MD
Associate Professor, Department of Urologic
Surgery, Vanderbilt University Medical Center,
Nashville, Tennessee

PAUL L. CRISPEN, MD
Assistant Professor of Surgery, Division of
Urology, Department of Surgery, University of
Kentucky, Lexington, Kentucky

JUANITA CROOK, MD, FRCPC
Professor of Radiation Oncology, British
Columbia Cancer Agency, Cancer Center for
the Southern Interior, Department of Radiation
Oncology, Kelowna, British Columbia, Canada

C.P. DINNEY, MD
Professor and Chairman, Departments of
Urology and Cancer Biology, The University
of Texas MD Anderson Cancer Center,
Houston, Texas

MOIRA DWYER, MD
Department of Urology, Mayo Clinic
Rochester, Rochester, Minnesota

RICHARD E. GREENBERG, MD, FACS
Chief, Division of Urologic Oncology, Fox
Chase Cancer Center; Professor of Urology,
Temple University School of Medicine,
Philadelphia, Pennsylvania

P.K. HEGARTY, MD
Department of Urology, Guy's and
St Thomas' NHS Foundation Trust, London,
United Kingdom

PIET HOEBEKE, MD, PhD
Diensthoofd Urologie, Kinderurologie
and Urogenitale Reconstructie, Department
of Urology, Ghent University Hospital, Ghent,
Belgium

JEAN HOFFMAN-CENSITS, MD
Assistant Professor, Department of Medical
Oncology, Kimmel Cancer Center, Thomas
Jefferson University, Philadelphia,
Pennsylvania

BRANT A. INMAN, MD
Assistant Professor of Surgery, Division of
Urology, Department of Surgery, Duke
University Medical Center, Durham,
North Carolina

R. JEFFREY KARNES, MD, FACS
Assistant Professor, Department of Urology,
Mayo Clinic, Rochester, Minnesota

BRIDGET F. KOONTZ, MD
Assistant Professor, Department of Radiation Oncology, Duke University Medical Center, Durham, North Carolina

RICHARD A. LEDER, MD
Assistant Professor of Radiology, Department of Radiology, Duke University Medical Center, Durham, North Carolina

W. ROBERT LEE, MD, MS, MEd
Professor, Department of Radiation Oncology, Duke University Medical Center, Durham, North Carolina

DEBORAH J. LIGHTNER, MD
Associate Professor, Department of Urology, Mayo Clinic, Rochester, Minnesota

NICOLAAS LUMEN, MD
Department of Urology, Ghent University Hospital, Ghent, Belgium

S. BRUCE MALKOWICZ, MD
Thomas Stichter Memorial Professor of Urological Research, Co-Director of Urologic Oncology, Professor of Urology, Division of Urology, Department of Surgery, University of Pennsylvania School of Medicine, University of Pennsylvania Health System, Philadelphia, Pennsylvania

SAMIR MARDINI, MD
Division of Plastic Surgery, Mayo Clinic, Rochester, Rochester, Minnesota

VITALY MARGULIS, MD
Assistant Professor, Department of Urology, The University of Texas Southwestern Medical Center, Dallas, Texas

STAN MONSTREY, MD, PhD
Department of Plastic Surgery, Ghent University Hospital, Ghent, Belgium

JACK H. MYDLO, MD, FACS
Professor and Chair, Department of Urology, Temple University School of Medicine, Philadelphia, Pennsylvania

C.A. PETTAWAY, MD
Departments of Urology and Cancer Biology, The University of Texas MD Anderson Cancer Center, Houston, Texas

ARTHUR I. SAGALOWSKY, MD
Professor, Department of Urology, The University of Texas Southwestern Medical Center, Dallas, Texas

CHRISTOPHER J. SALGADO, MD
Associate Professor of Surgery/Plastic Surgery, University of Miami Miller School of Medicine, Miami, Florida

SUZANNE BIEHN STEWART, MD
Division of Urology, Department of Surgery, Duke University Medical Center, Durham, North Carolina

R. STAN TAYLOR, MD
Professor, Department of Dermatology, University of Texas Southwestern, Dallas, Texas

EDOUARD J. TRABULSI, MD
Associate Professor, Department of Urology, Kimmel Cancer Center, Thomas Jefferson University, Philadelphia, Pennsylvania

MICHAEL J. WELLS, MD
Associate Professor, Department of Dermatology, Texas Tech University Health Sciences Center, Lubbock, Texas

SHAWN E. WHITE, MD
Instructor in Surgery, Division of Urology, Department of Surgery, University of Pennsylvania School of Medicine, University of Pennsylvania Health System, Philadelphia, Pennsylvania

HADLEY M. WOOD, MD
Associate Staff, Cleveland Clinic, Glickman Urological and Kidney Institute, Center for Genitourinary Reconstruction, Cleveland, Ohio

Contents

This article reviews anatomic considerations in penile and urethral surgery, with a particular emphasis on lymphatic anatomy. The historical evolution of techniques to reduce the unnecessary use and operative morbidity of inguinofemoral lymph node dissection are reviewed, with an emphasis on sentinel node (SN) biopsy and dynamic SN biopsy techniques.

Invasive penile cancer is an aggressive malignancy that often requires partial or complete penile amputation. Premalignant penile lesions, such as penile intraepithelial neoplasia, will have been present prior to the development of invasive disease in a substantial percentage of patients. Early detection and treatment of premalignant penile lesions may prevent malignant progression while avoiding penile amputation. This review focuses on premalignant penile lesions and the associations of these lesions with the development of invasive penile cancer.

Penile cancer is an uncommon malignancy in developed countries, with an estimated 1290 new cases of invasive penile cancer and 290 deaths among men in the United States in 2009, but is much more common in the developing countries of Asia, Africa, and South America. This disease can result in loss of function, disfigurement, and death. Thus, recognizing penile cancer early in the clinical setting and accurately diagnosing the patients is critical. Because the management and prognosis varies by the extent of local disease, lymph node status, and other factors, accurate staging of penile cancer is of utmost importance. This article focuses on the presentation, diagnosis, and staging of invasive squamous cell carcinoma of the penis. The authors highlight the recent changes to the American Joint Committee on Cancer's staging system for penile carcinoma and discuss other prognostic factors and predictive models.

In penile and urethral cancers, imaging has come to play a crucial role in enhancing the precision of clinical staging and facilitating optimal surgical planning. Over the years, great improvements have occurred in imaging. High-resolution magnetic resonance imaging (MRI) now represents the gold standard for evaluating the primary tumor and its local extension. Lymphotropic nanoparticle-enhanced MRI, dynamic sentinel lymph node biopsy, and ultrasonography with fine-needle aspiration seem to be the superior modalities for detecting malignant regional lymph nodes. Positron emission tomography combined with computed tomography has shown great promise as a whole body screen for the detection of distant metastases. Ultimately, the ability of imaging to augment clinical evaluation and enhance the accuracy of staging penile and urethral cancers will translate into improved surgical decision making and overall superior patient outcomes.

The potential devastating impact of curative traditional surgery on the patient's quality of life should always be a consideration even as urologic oncologists attempt to cure this potentially life-threatening malignancy. The development of penile-preserving surgical techniques will reduce the negative impact of amputations on functional and cosmetic outcomes only if oncologists continue to place oncologic objectives first and foremost for patients.

This article describes penile reconstruction after surgery. Patient considerations in reconstruction, reconstruction of varied urethral defects, general principles of urethroplasty, surgical techniques of urethral reconstruction, reconstruction of scrotal and testicular defects, reconstruction of the penile shaft, and timing of reconstruction are discussed. The use of local pedicled flaps in penile reconstruction, distant free tissue transfer in penile reconstruction, varied forms of prostheses, management of complications following penile reconstruction, postoperative care in penile reconstruction patient, and penile transplantation are described.

Mohs micrographic surgery (MMS) has been shown to reduce recurrence rates when used to excise many different mucocutaneous neoplasms, especially of the head and neck. The low recurrence rates are due to careful microscopic evaluation of the horizontal and vertical surgical margins. This article discusses the utility and limitations of MMS in controlling neoplasia of the male genitalia. Specific penoscrotal neoplasias discussed in this article include invasive and in situ squamous cell carcinoma, basal cell carcinoma, extramammary Paget disease, and granular cell tumor.

Presence and magnitude of the inguinal nodal metastases are the most important determinants of oncologic outcome in patients with squamous carcinoma of the penis (SCP). Surgical removal of the inguinal lymph nodes provides an important staging and therapeutic benefit to SCP patients, while the methodology of appropriate patient selection for lymph node dissection continues to evolve. Compliant, motivated, and reliable patients with low risk of harboring metastatic inguinal lymph nodes can be managed with careful inguinal surveillance. In SCP patients whose primary tumors demonstrate pathologic features of aggressive disease, modified bilateral inguinal lymph node dissection should be performed and converted to classic ilioinguinal lymph node dissection if metastatic disease is confirmed on frozen sections. Patients with bulky inguinal metastases are unlikely to be cured by surgery alone. Integration of systemic therapy, especially in a presurgical setting, is an attractive strategy for management of patients with advanced SCP, and is currently being studied prospectively.

Patients with penile cancer who are proven to have negative inguinal lymph nodes have an excellent prognosis. Furthermore, patients with small-volume inguinal node involvement can often be cured by surgery alone. Lymphadenectomy has clear survival benefits for patients when applied to those with lymph node metastasis. However, the current morbidity of the standard technique of lymphadenectomy is an impediment to its universal application, and innovative strategies to reduce the morbidity of staging/treatment that do not compromise oncologic control must be developed and standardized. The optimal integration of multimodality therapy to improve survival in advanced disease will occur only through collaborative studies between centers with significant patient volume, which would be facilitated through the development of regional referral centers.

Radiotherapy, in the form of external beam radiotherapy or interstitial brachytherapy, provides an effective penile-sparing option for localized squamous cell carcinoma of the penis. Interstitial brachytherapy is completed in 4 to 5 days and provides 5-year penile preservation rates of 70% to 88%, and at 10 years, 67% to 72%. Surgery provides effective salvage for local failures, maintaining cause-specific survival at 84% to 92% at 10 years. Ideal tumors for brachytherapy should be less than 4 cm without extension onto the shaft. More advanced cases can be considered for external radiotherapy.

Primary urethral cancers represent less than 1% of genitourinary malignancy. Given this is an uncommon disease, there are limited data to guide diagnostic and treatment strategies. Surgical extirpation remains the standard for most patients, with the addition of chemotherapy and radiation therapy in select patients. The surgical approach to urethral cancer depends largely on the location and extent of the tumor.

Urethral cancer is a rare but aggressive neoplasm. Early-stage distal lesions can be successfully treated with a single modality. Results for definitive radiotherapy using either or both external beam radiation therapy and brachytherapy have shown excellent cure rates in men and women. The primary advantage of radiotherapy is organ preservation. Advanced tumors, however, have poor outcomes with single modality treatment. Results have been improved using a combination of radiotherapy and chemotherapy, chiefly 5-fluorouracil and mitomycin C. Although literature is limited to case reports because of the rarity of the disease, the markedly improved results compared with older results of surgery with or without radiation warrant consideration.

Although surgery is the mainstay of curative treatment of carcinomas of the penis and urethra, there is a role for systemic cytotoxic chemotherapy for locally advanced, unresectable, or metastatic tumors. Although this field is limited by a paucity of clinical trials or prospective data, the available single institutional retrospective reviews indicate that multi-agent cisplatin-based combination chemotherapy regimens have significant activity and may allow curative surgery for patients with otherwise unresectable tumors. Toxicity remains a concern in this typically older patient population, and clearly new regimens are necessary. This article reviews the available literature on chemotherapy for carcinoma of the penis and urethra in the neoadjuvant, adjuvant, and metastatic setting.

Approximately 70,000 new cases of bladder cancer are diagnosed yearly, of which 52,000 are male patients. In 2009 there were approximately 14,000 deaths attributed to bladder cancer, 10,000 of which were men. Approximately 40% to 45% of all cases are high-grade tumors with half of these being muscle-invasive tumors at the time of diagnosis. With the preponderance of men in this population, there is a need for clear management strategies regarding the retained urethra in those men undergoing radical cystectomy. This article reviews the incidence of urothelial carcinoma in the retained urethra, risk factors for the development of urethral urothelial carcinoma, surveillance strategies, treatment modalities, and outcomes following intervention.

GOAL STATEMENT

The goal of *Urologic Clinics of North America* is to keep practicing urologists and urology residents up to date with current clinical practice in urology by providing timely articles reviewing the state of the art in patient care.

ACCREDITATION

The *Urologic Clinics of North America* is planned and implemented in accordance with the Essential Areas and Policies of the Accreditation Council for Continuing Medical Education (ACCME) through the joint sponsorship of the University of Virginia School of Medicine and Elsevier. The University of Virginia School of Medicine is accredited by the ACCME to provide continuing medical education for physicians.

The University of Virginia School of Medicine designates this educational activity for a maximum of 15 *AMA PRA Category 1 Credits*™ for each issue, 60 credits per year. Physicians should only claim credit commensurate with the extent of their participation in the activity.

The American Medical Association has determined that physicians not licensed in the US who participate in this CME activity are eligible for a maximum of 15 *AMA PRA Category 1 Credits*™ for each issue, 60 credits per year.

Credit can be earned by reading the text material, taking the CME examination online at http://www.theclinics.com/home/cme, and completing the evaluation. After taking the test, you will be required to review any and all incorrect answers. Following completion of the test and evaluation, your credit will be awarded and you may print your certificate.

FACULTY DISCLOSURE/CONFLICT OF INTEREST

The University of Virginia School of Medicine, as an ACCME accredited provider, endorses and strives to comply with the Accreditation Council for Continuing Medical Education (ACCME) Standards of Commercial Support, Commonwealth of Virginia statutes, University of Virginia policies and procedures, and associated federal and private regulations and guidelines on the need for disclosure and monitoring of proprietary and financial interests that may affect the scientific integrity and balance of content delivered in continuing medical education activities under our auspices.

The University of Virginia School of Medicine requires that all CME activities accredited through this institution be developed independently and be scientifically rigorous, balanced and objective in the presentation/discussion of its content, theories and practices.

All authors/editors participating in an accredited CME activity are expected to disclose to the readers relevant financial relationships with commercial entities occurring within the past 12 months (such as grants or research support, employee, consultant, stock holder, member of speakers bureau, etc.). The University of Virginia School of Medicine will employ appropriate mechanisms to resolve potential conflicts of interest to maintain the standards of fair and balanced education to the reader. Questions about specific strategies can be directed to the Office of Continuing Medical Education, University of Virginia School of Medicine, Charlottesville, Virginia.

The faculty and staff of the University of Virginia Office of Continuing Medical Education have no financial affiliations to disclose.

The authors/editors listed below have identified no professional or financial affiliations for themselves or their spouse/partner:
Daniel A. Barocas, MD, MPH; Rodney H. Breau, MD, FRCSC; Paul L. Crispen, MD; Juanita Crook, MD, FRCPC; Moira Dwyer, MD; P. K. Hegarty, MD; Piet Hoebeke, MD, PhD; Kerry K. Holland (Acquisitions Editor); Brant A. Inman, MD; R. Jeffrey Karnes, MD; Bridget F. Koontz, MD; Richard A. Leder, MD; W. Robert Lee, MD, MS, MEd; Deborah J. Lightner, MD; Nicolaas Lumen, MD; Samir Mardini, MD; Vitaly Margulis, MD; Stan Monstrey, MD, PhD; C. A. Pettaway, MD; Christopher J. Salgado, MD; Suzanne Biehn Stewart, MD; R. Stan Taylor, MD; Michael J. Wells, MD; Shawn E. White, MD; and Hadley M. Wood, MD.

The authors/editors listed below identified the following professional or financial affiliations for themselves or their spouse/partner:
Kenneth W. Angermeier, MD is a consultant for American Medical Systems, Inc.
Sam S. Chang, MD is a consultant for Sanofi Aventis, Endo, Allergan and Centocor Ortho Biotech.
C. P. Dinney, MD receives research support from NCI; is a consultant for Schering-Plough; is conducting scientific study for Astrazeneca; and is a lecturer/meeting participant for Abbott/Vyvsis.
Richard E. Greenberg, MD is a consultant for Best Doctors and Imedecs; on the Speakers' Bureau for Endo Pharma; and is on the Advisory Committee/Board for Parexel Corporation.
Jean Hoffman-Censits, MD owns stock in GSK, Novartis, and Sanofi Aventis.
S. Bruce Malkowicz, MD is an industry funded research/investigator, is a consultant, and is on the Speakers' Bureau for GTx; is on the Speakers' Bureau for Endo Pharmaceuticals and Firmagon; and is a consultant for Tenigon.
Jack H. Mydlo, MD, FACS (Guest Editor) is a consultant for MOL Laboratories.
Arthur I. Sagalowsky, MD is a member of the Data Monitoring Committee for Bioniche.
William Steers, MD (Test Author) is employed by the American Urologic Association, is a reviewer and consultant for NIH, and is an investigator for Allergan.
Edouard J. Trabulsi, MD is an industry funded research/investigator for Lantheus Medical Imaging and Bostwick Laboratory, and is a consultant for Intuitive Surgical Corp.

Disclosure of Discussion of Non-FDA Approved Uses for Pharmaceutical Products and/or Medical Devices.
The University of Virginia School of Medicine, as an ACCME provider, requires that all faculty presenters identify and disclose any off-label uses for pharmaceutical and medical device products. The University of Virginia School of Medicine recommends that each physician fully review all the available data on new products or procedures prior to clinical use.

TO ENROLL

To enroll in the Urologic Clinics of North America Continuing Medical Education program, call customer service at 1-800-654-2452 or visit us online at http://www.theclinics.com/home/cme. The CME program is available to subscribers for an additional fee of $207.00.

Urologic Clinics of North America

THE CLINICS ARE NOW AVAILABLE ONLINE!

Access your subscription at:
www.theclinics.com

Preface

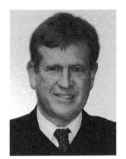

Jack H. Mydlo, MD, FACS
Guest Editor

Penile and urethral cancers are not common entities. Due to the limited number of cases seen in any one institution or experienced in one career, it is not a familiar encounter. Although the techniques for diagnosis have been well established, sometimes the direction of treatment has been on a pendulum.

After American Urological Association in-service and American Board of Urology examinations, it is not uncommon to have residents and even faculty members remember the specific penile/urethral cancer questions, which are then brought up at the next day of conference for an open discussion. Clearly, the exposure of residents and practicing urologists to these diseases is limited, and updates are necessary to keep abreast of the most recent treatment modalities.

Urologists have always been up to date on the latest advances in their chosen field. In this issue of the *Urologic Clinics of North America*, a compilation of experts has delineated the imaging techniques for these lesions and outlined the surgical, radiation, and chemotherapy treatments of the disease. They have also addressed controversies involving the management of lymph node dissections, microsurgery, and reconstruction. This issue provides a strong, comprehensive, contemporary summary of penile and urethral cancers and should be an important part of any urologist's library.

Jack H. Mydlo, MD, FACS
Temple University Hospital
3401 North Broad Street, Suite 340
Philadelphia, PA 19140, USA

E-mail address:
jmydlo@temple.edu

Urol Clin N Am 37 (2010) xi
doi:10.1016/j.ucl.2010.05.002
0094-0143/10/$ – see front matter

Anatomic Considerations of the Penis, Lymphatic Drainage, and Biopsy of the Sentinel Node

Hadley M. Wood, MD*, Kenneth W. Angermeier, MD

KEYWORDS

- Anatomy • Penis • Urethra • Lymphatics
- Sentinel node • Cancer

Although penile and male urethral cancers are 2 of the least common urologic malignancies, they are important for the urologist to identify and diagnose promptly and treat adequately for several reasons. First, diagnosis is often delayed because of embarrassment on behalf of the patient in seeking treatment or delayed diagnosis on account of the treating physician because they are rare and can manifest with a wide array of presentations and symptoms. Second, complete surgical excision is the only therapy that is potentially curative, even in the case of node-positive disease.[1] These 2 cancers are often accompanied by substantial local symptoms that can prove difficult to control if the disease is allowed to progress without surgical intervention.

The crux of the penile cancer dilemma for the urologist is that diagnostic modalities for identifying nodal disease must demonstrate near-perfect sensitivity. This demonstration is difficult because clinical examination is notoriously inaccurate, with 11% to 62% of negative examinations demonstrating micrometastatic disease at the time of inguinofemoral lymph node (LN) dissection (IFLND).[2] Moreover, preemptive IFLND has been shown to demonstrate a survival advantage over delayed IFLND in T2N0M0 disease or T1 tumors with unfavorable characteristics (high grade, lymphovascular invasion),[3] suggesting that missing an early diagnosis of micrometastatic disease may result in a lost opportunity for cure. Failed detection and treatment of microscopic node-positive disease has been demonstrated to result in only 35% survival at 3 years.[4] Therefore, in the case of patients with intermediate- or high-risk disease and nonpalpable nodes, the ultimate goal would be to develop a diagnostic tool that will identify patients with micrometastatic disease to the groins with high sensitivity and low morbidity.

Although historical treatment of primary urethral cancer has been primarily surgical, emerging data suggest that multimodal therapy may be a reasonable alternative for some patients with invasive urethral cancer.[5–7] Unlike penile cancer, prophylactic IFLND has not resulted in a survival benefit for patients with metastatic urethral cancer.

This article reviews the anatomy relevant to the diagnosis and management of penile and urethral cancer, as well as the historical development of diagnostic modalities for the assessment of inguinal nodes.

ANATOMIC CONSIDERATIONS: PENIS, BLOOD VESSELS, AND INTEGUMENTS

Anatomically, the penis is divided into the root, the body, and the glans, and is structurally composed

Financial disclosures: Research funding, American Medical Systems, Inc (H.M.W); Consultant, American Medical Systems, Inc (K.W.A).

Cleveland Clinic, Glickman Urological and Kidney Institute, Center for Genitourinary Reconstruction, 9500 Euclid Avenue, Mail Code Q10, Cleveland, OH 44195, USA

* Corresponding author.

E-mail address: woodh@ccf.org

Urol Clin N Am 37 (2010) 327–334

doi:10.1016/j.ucl.2010.04.013

of 2 smooth muscle-containing erectile bodies and the surrounding integuments (**Fig. 1**). The erectile bodies are distinct proximally, where they course inferior to the pubic rami, and distally, where they separate to form 2 distinct corporal tips that terminate in the glans. However, along the length of the body of the penis, these 2 structures freely communicate through a shared, perforated midline septum. The urethra is similarly divided into the posterior (prostatic-membranous) and anterior (bulbar-pendulous-glanular) urethra. The bulbar and pendulous urethra is surrounded by a third erectile body, the corpus spongiosum.

Distally, the corpus spongiosum fuses to form the glans.[8]

The posterior urethra is believed to develop from the urogenital sinus, the anterior separation of the cloaca after descent of the urorectal septum at a gestational age of approximately 5 weeks. Although anterior urethral development remains controversial, most investigators agree that the anterior urethra is derived by medial migration of mesodermal pilings that develop lateral to the cloacal membrane as it extends toward the genital tubercle.[9] These structures develop into the penile and proximal glanular urethra.[10] Complete

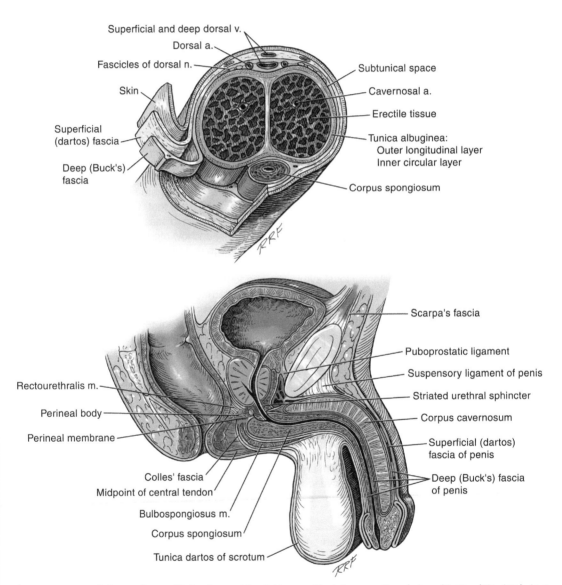

Fig. 1. Anatomy of the penis: erectile bodies and fascial layers. (*Top*) Cross-sectional view. (*Bottom*) Sagittal view. (*From* Jordan GH, Schlossberg SM. Chapter 33: surgery of the penis and urethra. In: Wein AJ, Kavoussi LR, Novick AC, et al, editors. Campbell-Walsh urology. 9th edition. Philadelphia: Saunders/Elsevier; 2007. p. 1029; with permission).

development of the distal urethra, frenulum, and circumferential prepuce depends on ventral migration of the urethral and preputial folds. The distally located lacunar folds fuse to form the distal one-third of the glanular urethra, which is lined only by ectoderm.[11] All these infoldings occur in a carefully orchestrated sequence in a proximal-to-distal fashion. Development of the corpora cavernosa occurs via coalescence of the mesoderm that flanks the urethral groove dorsolaterally and is thought to be secondary to urethral development, possibly acting as an inductive force on development of the erectile bodies.[12] Although the exact mechanism that drives penile (corporal and urethral) elongation has not been elucidated, paracrine testosterone production plays an important role in this process.

The penis is enveloped in 2 layers of fascia. The superficial fascia is continuous with the dartos fascia and connected to the underlying structures by loose areolar tissues, making this the plane that separates easily for penile degloving. The deep fascia (Buck's fascia and the tunica albuginea of the corpus cavernosae) comprises the dense fibrous layer that surrounds the erectile chambers and allows for expansion in length and girth with stimulation to the elastic limit of the tissues, thus providing rigidity for erections. The deep fascia of the root of the penis is continuous with the external oblique fascia and fascia of the urogenital diaphragm.[8]

Arterial supply to the penis is well described, and anatomic variability is often present. The main blood supply, the common penile artery, arises from the internal pudendal artery, a branch of the internal iliac artery. The paired common penile arteries trifurcate into the paired bulbourethral arteries, cavernosal arteries, and dorsal penile arteries. The bulbourethral arteries enter the bulbar urethra posteriorly, near the upturn of the most dependent portion of the bulbar corpus spongiosum. The cavernosal arteries course through the middle of the corpora cavernosa and are responsible for arterial inflow during initiation of erections. The dorsal penile arteries course under Buck's fascia to feed the corpus spongiosum in a retrograde fashion via the glans. The arteries also send off circumflex branches to the corpora spongiosum and corpora cavernosa.[13] Together, intact bulbourethral and dorsal penile arterial supply guarantee redundant blood supply to the anterior urethra, allowing transection of the urethra and reanastomosis. The most common and surgically relevant variation to arterial blood supply is the possible presence of accessory pudendal arteries. These arteries occur approximately 30% of the time and are most often branches either of the obturator (84%) or other iliac branches.[14,15]

The skin of the penis is supplied by branches of the external pudendal arteries, which are branches of the proximal femoral arteries.

Penile and urethral venous drainage consists of the superficial, intermediate, and deep systems. The superficial drainage system comprises multiple veins that run in a dorsolateral fashion between Colles' fascia and Buck's fascia. These superficial branches coalesce into a single or paired superficial dorsal vein that subsequently drains into one or both saphenous veins.[16] The intermediate system originates as emissary veins from the glans to form the retrocoronal plexus, which subsequently drain into the deep dorsal vein. Along the way, circumflex veins (arising from the corpus spongiosum) and distal emissary veins (arising from the corpus cavernosum) further contribute to the deep dorsal vein. The deep dorsal vein may be single or multiple and subsequently courses between the limbs of the suspensory ligament to contribute to the dorsal vein complex of the prostate.[16] The deep venous system consists of the cavernous and crural veins. The cavernous veins run along the dorsum of the urethral bulb under the crus of the penis and drain into the internal pudendal system. There are multiple connections between this system and the periprostatic plexus. The crural veins emerge from the dorsolateral surface of the penis and drain into the internal pudendal veins.[16]

The major sensory and somatic supply to the penis is derived from the pudendal nerve (S2–4). After passing through the Alcocky's canal, the pudendal nerve sends a dorsal branch to the penis as the dorsal nerve of the penis. This branch is believed to be responsible for the penile and glanular sensory apparatus. The dorsal nerve pierces the transversus perinei muscle and travels along the dorsum of the penis toward the glans, lateral to the dorsal arteries. The nerve's course is relatively invariable.[16] After leaving the pudendal canal, the pudendal nerve terminates as 2 branches: the inferior rectal and perineal branches. The inferior rectal nerve courses posteriorly to the external anal sphincter. The perineal nerve has been demonstrated to provide motor function to the bulbospongiosus muscle and then pierce this muscle along its midline raphe to innervate the corpus spongiosum. These perineal nerve branches course along the urethra laterally and intermingle with branches of the dorsal nerve of the penis distally.[17] The cavernous nerves are a network of fine fibers that emanate from the corpora cavernosa and course along with the cavernous artery and vein, deep to the dorsal vein complex of the prostate and along the prostatic capsule as part of the prostatic neurovascular bundle.[16]

ANATOMIC CONSIDERATIONS: LYMPHATIC DRAINAGE
Penile Lymphatics

Penile lymphatic drainage parallels venous drainage, with a superficial system that drains the skin and a deeper system that drains the glans and corporal bodies (**Fig. 2**). The lymphocapillary networks originate in the skin, in the mucous membrane and submucosa of the urethra, in the septum of the glans, in the tunica albuginea of the corpora cavernosa, and in the fascia.[18] The skin of the glans is composed of a bilayered network located in the stratum papillare and the stratum reticulare, and there is free communication between the 2 networks. The networks running parallel to the skin are oriented radially from the urethral meatus. All these radially oriented branches coalesce to form a single network at the corona, occupying the papillary and reticular layers of the skin, and course through the inner and outer prepuce.[18] The skin of the penile shaft is more segregated, with distinct layers of lymphatics coursing in the papillary and reticular layers of the skin. A separate lymphatic system is seen in the fascia of the penis and tunica albuginea.[18]

Cadaver dissections of the inguinal regions suggest that the superficial lymphatic basin for the penis is bounded superiorly by a line 1 cm above and parallel to the inguinal ligament, beginning medially just above the pubic tubercle (over the adductor canal) and coursing for a length of 12 cm. The inferior boundary is marked by a perpendicular line dropped 20 cm from the lateral extent of this line and 15 cm from the medial extent.[19] The superficial inguinal nodes were divided by Rouviere[20] into 5 zones (superomedial, superolateral, inferomedial, inferolateral, and central) (**Figs. 3** and **4**). This area contains 4 to 25 LNs (mean = 8.25).[19] The deep inguinal lymphatic basin is smaller in size and is located primarily along the medial aspect of the femoral vessels deep to the fascia lata (**Fig. 5**).[19]

Cabanas[21] described the lymphoangiographic patterns demonstrated in a large series of patients with penile cancers (N = 80) and benign diseases of the penis (N = 10). Injection into the lymphatics of the dorsal penile vessels consistently drained to

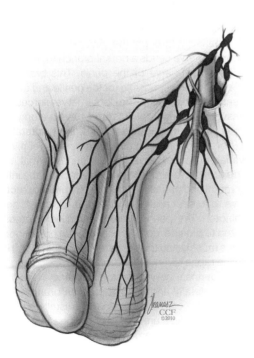

Fig. 2. Penile lymphatic drainage to the inguinal region. (*Courtesy of* Cleveland Clinic Foundation, Inc., Cleveland, OH.)

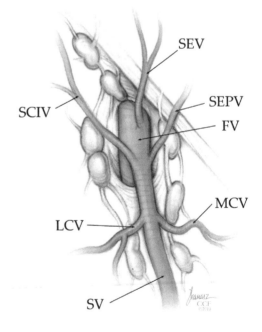

Fig. 3. Major branches of the femoral vein (FV) and their relationship with the surrounding superficial inguinal LNs. LCV, lateral cutaneous vein; MCV, medial cutaneous vein; SCIV, superficial circumflex iliac vein; SEPV, superficial external pudendal vein; SEV, superficial epigastric vein; SV, saphenous vein. (*Courtesy of* Cleveland Clinic Foundation, Inc., Cleveland, OH.)

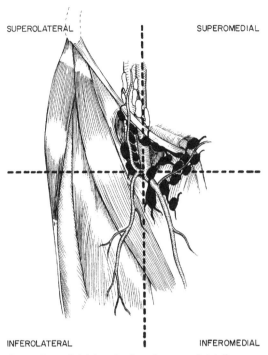

SUPEROLATERAL

SUPEROMEDIAL

INFEROLATERAL

INFEROMEDIAL

Fig. 4. Superficial inguinal nodes were initially organized by Rouviere into 5 zones (superomedial, superolateral, inferomedial, inferolateral, and central). The central zone is not pictured. (*From* Colberg JW, Andriole GL, Catalona WJ. Penectomy and inguinal lymphadenectomy for carcinoma of the penis. In: Marshall FF, editor. Textbook of operative urology. 1st edition. Philadelphia: WB Saunders; 1996. p. 639, Chapter 76; with permission.)

a LN located anterior or medial to the superficial epigastric vein and superomedial to the epigastric-saphenous junction, with subsequent drainage into the deep inguinal and iliac chains. All patients in this study who subsequently went on to have IFLND and who were found to have metastatic disease demonstrated involvement of this sentinel node (SN). No prepubic LNs were identified. However, subsequent investigators have challenged these findings, reporting that the location of or drainage to the SN was not as consistent as that reported initially by Cabanas.[22–24] Although inguinal drainage patterns still remain somewhat contested, it is almost universally accepted that penile lymphatics drain to the inguinal nodes before draining into the iliac nodes.[25] Anecdotal observations of patients with positive iliac metastases in the setting of negative inguinal dissections have been reported.[26] Such a presence is likely caused by undersampling of the inguinal nodes either at the time of dissection or at the time of pathologic assessment.

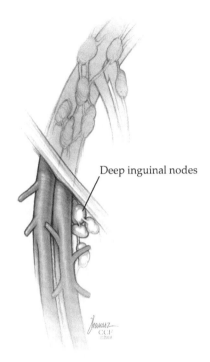

Deep inguinal nodes

Fig. 5. Deep inguinal LNs. (Courtesy of Cleveland Clinic Foundation, Inc., Cleveland, OH.)

Urethral Lymphatics

Urethral lymphatic drainage rests in a double-layered lymphocapillary network that runs parallel to the urethra, is situated partially in the mucous membrane and partially in the submucosa, and undulates with the folds of the urethral wall.[18] This network is particularly dense in the region of the fossa navicularis. These smaller branches coalesce into 4 main collecting trunks. Distally, these lymphatics traverse the urethra at the level of the frenulum and join the penile lymphatics of the glans at the prepuce. The penile urethral lymphatics course laterally around the corpora cavernosae and join the lymphatic trunks from the glans. Bulbar urethral drainage is more variable with some lymphatics coursing along the bulbar artery, some terminating in the medial retrofemoral node, and others coursing superiorly under the pubis along the dorsum of the prostate toward the anterior bladder wall, terminating in the retrofemoral nodes and medial external iliac nodes. The lymphatic drainage of the prostatic urethra corresponds to lymphatic drainage of the prostate.[20]

SENTINEL NODE BIOPSY

Metastatic penile cancer remains a highly lethal disease and one for which cure has only been demonstrated with complete removal of involved LNs. Chemotherapy and radiation have not been demonstrated to provide curative benefit in the setting of metastatic penile cancer. Given that lymphatic drainage is often bilateral,[25] complete bilateral IFLND provides the best hope for cure in patients with nodal disease. However, this approach can prove to be costly to the patient, with substantial risk of perioperative and long-term morbidity in the form of flap loss, seromas, vascular thrombosis or injury, and wound problems, as well as potentially disabling lower extremity edema.[27–29] Routine radical IFLND for all patients overstages up to 80% of the patients, needlessly subjecting these patients to the attendant side effects of surgery.[4] Therefore, a variety of staging methodologies have been proposed to most effectively select patients for radical IFLND.

The first such methodology was popularized by Cabanas.[21] In his landmark study, he demonstrated positivity in all SNs for patients with penile cancer who subsequently had metastatic disease demonstrated on IFLND. Further, he demonstrated that the SN was positive in 4% of cases where the LNs were not deemed clinically suspicious and therefore concluded that routine SN biopsy could identify patients with micrometastatic disease earlier than the standard approach of waiting for LN enlargement prior to IFLND. After publication of this methodology, several reports suggested that this approach was unreliable.[22–24] Srinivas and colleagues[24] postulated multiple reasons for the discrepancy between the high specificity seen by Cabanas and the multiple reports that followed suggesting this approach resulted in an unacceptable false-negative rate: selection of the wrong node, improper pathologic sectioning of the specimen such that microfoci would be missed, and a long time-lapse between SN dissection and groin dissection that allowed arborization of lymphatics along alternative channels. In an effort to reduce wrong node selection, "extended SN dissection" was introduced to improve diagnostic accuracy. However, false-negative rates for this approach were still substantial (25%), and this approach has subsequently lost favor.[30]

Senthil Kumar and colleagues[31] proposed an alternative SN for penile cancer, a node they referred to as the medial inguinal node (MIN). This node lies lateral to the pubic tubercle and is the most medial of the nodes of the horizontal chain. To test the accuracy of clinical examination, 3 tests—fine-needle aspiration (FNA), SN biopsy, and MIN biopsy—were performed on 28 consecutive patients with penile cancer before formal IFLND. Clinical examination performed the poorest, with 74% and 61% sensitivity and specificity,

respectively. The remaining tests all demonstrated 100% specificity; only FNA demonstrated 100% sensitivity for the detection of metastatic disease. MIN biopsy demonstrated 91% sensitivity, and SN biopsy demonstrated 78% sensitivity. It is important that because FNA is only applicable in the setting of clinically palpable nodes, the accuracy demonstrated for this methodology was only for this subset of patients. The most important aspect of SN biopsy and MIN biopsy is that both demonstrate false-negative rates that are unacceptably high (22% and 8.7% in this study) for a disease that is only curable by surgical excision of all involved LNs.

The controversy over the Cabanas approach and subsequent refinement of intraoperative lymphoscintigraphy for breast and melanoma staging has led to a push for dynamic SN biopsy in penile cancer.[32] The procedure starts the day before surgery with the intradermal injection of technetium-99m nanocolloid at 3 or 4 sites around the primary tumor. Dynamic anterior lymphoscintigraphy is subsequently performed at defined intervals. The location of the SN is marked on the skin. Shortly before surgery, 1 mL of patent blue dye is injected around the tumor in a similar fashion. The SN is harvested after dissection of blue lymphatic vessels and intraoperative detection of radioactivity by use of a γ-ray detection probe. Valdes Olmos and colleagues[33] validated the use of preoperative lymphoscintigraphy in 74 consecutive patients that met these criteria. Patients who demonstrated positive SN using their methodology (22%) underwent formal LND. At a median of 28-month follow-up, 2 patients with negative SNs developed LN metastases for a calculated sensitivity of 89% and a negative predictive value of 96%. Subsequent series of comparable cases have demonstrated almost identical sensitivity of this technique with minimal attendant comorbidity.[34–38] Other studies have suggested that this technique still offers unacceptable false-negative rates, particularly in cases where patients with enlarged LNs are included and/or demonstrate high-risk disease in their primary tumor, with sensitivities in the range of 63% to 71%.[34,35,39–42] However, more recent amendments to this algorithm with the addition of routine inguinal exploration in the absence of radiotracer visualization, intraoperative palpation of the wound for abnormal nodes, and extended pathologic analysis of excised nodes as means of decreasing the number of false-negative biopsy results have demonstrated promising outcomes, with false-negative rates as low as 5% and a low rate of complications.[36] The divergence in outcomes between centers likely relates to the technical difficulty in using this technique, resulting in a substantial learning curve, as well as the addition of more refined selection criteria to best select patients who will be adequately staged using this technique. As a result of the low overall incidence of penile cancer, particularly in the Western world, optimization of dynamic SN biopsy techniques are likely to be achieved only in referral centers of excellence.

The newest development on the horizon for the evaluation of LN status in penile cancer is lymphotropic nanoparticle-enhanced magnetic resonance (MR) imaging. Using this technology, Tabatabaei and colleagues[43] demonstrated sensitivity and specificity for detection of node-positive disease of 100% and 97%, respectively, in a small group of patients with squamous cell carcinoma of the penis (N = 7). Although this diagnostic modality shows early promise, it is still under investigation.

SUMMARY

Penile and urethral cancers remain therapeutically distinct entities in that penile cancer affords hope for cure with complete surgical excision of disease that is advanced to the level of the locoregional LNs. Urethral cancer does not offer such an opportunity at present. Even so, surgical excision, transurethral resection (for T1 and Tis urethral cancer only), partial penectomy, or total penectomy remains the mainstay of treatment for local control of the primary tumor for penile and urethral cancer. IFLND offers no therapeutic benefit for metastatic urethral cancer but may increase survival or provide a cure for some patients with invasive penile cancer. For both entities, IFLND may help control and palliate local symptoms that develop when groin LNs become enlarged. Despite more than 40 years of searching for less invasive methods to assess which patients may benefit from extended IFLND in penile cancer, techniques for identification of micrometastatic disease to the LNs continue to evolve. Lymphotropic nanoparticle-enhanced MR imaging currently may hold the greatest promise, although accuracy of this technique remains to be demonstrated outside of small pilot studies.

REFERENCES

1. Solsana E, Algaba F, Horenblas S, et al. EAU Guidelines on penile cancer. Eur Urol 2004;46:1–8.
2. Feldman AS, McDougal WS. Inguinal node dissection for penile carcinoma. AUA Update Series 2008;27(7):58–63.
3. McDougal WS. Carcinoma of the penis: improved survival by early regional lymphadenectomy based on the histological grade and depth of invasion of the primary lesion. J Urol 1995;154:1364.
4. Kroon BK, Horenblas S, Lont AP, et al. Patients with penile carcinoma benefit from immediate resection of clinically occult lymph node metastases. J Urol 2005;173:816–9.
5. Licht MR, Klein EA, Bukowski R, et al. Combination radiation and chemotherapy for the treatment of squamous cell carcinoma of the male and female urethra. J Urol 1995;153(6):1918–20.
6. Dalbagni G, Zhang ZF, Lacombe L, et al. Male urethral carcinoma: analysis of treatment outcome. Urology 1999;53(6):1126–32.
7. Cohen MS, Triaca V, Billmeyer B, et al. Coordinated chemoradiation therapy with genital preservation for the treatment of primary invasive carcinoma of the male urethra. J Urol 2008;179(2):536–41.
8. Devine CJ, Angermeier KW. Anatomy of the penis and male perineum: part I. AUA Update Series 1994;13(2):10–5.
9. Hynes PJ, Fraher JP. The development of the male genitourinary system. I the origin of the urorectal septum and the formation of the perineum. Br J Plast Surg 2004;57(1):27–36.
10. Hynes PJ, Fraher JP. The development of the male genitourinary system II. The origin and formation of the urethral plate. Br J Plast Surg 2004;57:112–21.
11. Hynes PJ, Fraher JP. The development of the male genitourinary system. III the formation of the spongiose and glandular urethra. Br J Plast Surg 2004; 57:203–14.
12. Baskin LS, Lee YT, Cunha GR. Neuroanatomical ontogeny of the human fetal penis. Br J Urol 1997; 79:628–40.
13. Juskiewenski S, Vaysse PH, Moscovici J, et al. A study of arterial blood supply of the penis. Anat Clin 1982;4:101–7.
14. Park BJ, Sung DJ, Kim MJ, et al. The incidence and anatomy of accessory pudendal arteries as depicted on multidetector-row CT angiography: clinical implications of preoperative evaluation for laparoscopic and robot-assisted radical prostatectomy. Korean J Radiol 2009;10(6):587–95.
15. Secin FP, Touijer K, Mulhall J, et al. Anatomy and preservation of accessory pudendal arteries in laparoscopic radical prostatectomy. Eur Urol 2007;51(5):1229–35.
16. Breza J, Aboseif SR, Orvis BR, et al. Detailed anatomy of the penile neurovascular structures: surgical significance. J Urol 1989;141:437–43.
17. Yucel S, Baskin LS. Neuroanatomy of the male urethra and perineum. BJU Int 2003;92:624–30.
18. Spirin BA. Internal lymphatic system of the penis. Arkhiv Anatomii, Gistologii I Embriologii 1963;44(3): T159–67.
19. Daseler EH, Anson BJ, Reimann AF. Radical excision of the inguinal and iliac lymph glands: a study based upon 450 anatomical dissections and upon

supportive clinical observations. Surg Gynecol Obstet 1948;87(6):679–94.

20. Rouviere H. Anatomy of the human lymphatic system. Ann Arbor (MI): Edwards Brothers Inc; 1938. p. 215–7.

21. Cabanas RM. An approach for the treatment of penile carcinoma. Cancer 1977;39:456–66.

22. Perinetti E, Crane CB, Catalona WJ. Unreliability of sentinel lymph node biopsy for staging penile carcinoma. J Urol 1980;124:734–5.

23. Wespes E, Simon J, Schulman CC. Cabanas approach: is sentinel node biopsy reliable for staging penile carcinoma? Urology 1986;28(4): 278–9.

24. Srinivas V, Joshi A, Agarwal B, et al. Penile cancer— the sentinel lymph node controversy. Urol Int 1991; 47:108–9.

25. Riveros M, Garcia R, Cabanas R. Lymphadenography of the dorsal lymphatics of the penis. Cancer 1967;20:2026–31.

26. Lopes A, Bezerra ALR, Serrano SV, et al. Iliac nodal metastases from carcinoma of the penis treated surgically. BJU Int 2000;86:690–3.

27. Bevan-Thomas R, Slaton JW, Pettaway CA. Contemporary morbidity from lymphadenectomy for penile squamous cell carcinoma: The M.D. Anderson Cancer Center experience. J Urol 2002; 167:1638–42.

28. Bouchot O, Rigaud J, Maillet F, et al. Morbidity of inguinal lymphadenectomy for invasive penile carcinoma. Eur Urol 2004;45:761–5.

29. Nelson BA, Cookson MS, Smith JA Jr, et al. Complications of inguinal and pelvic lymphadenectomy for squamous cell carcinoma of the penis: a contemporary series. J Urol 2004;172:494–7.

30. Pettaway CA, Pisters LL, Colin PN, et al. Sentinel lymph node dissection for penile carcinoma: the M.D. Anderson Cancer Center experience. J Urol 1995;154:1999–2003.

31. Senthil Kumar MP, Ananthakrishnan N, Prema V. Predicting regional lymph node metastasis in carcinoma of the penis: a comparison between fine-needle aspiration cytology, sentinel lymph node biopsy and medial inguinal lymph node biopsy. Br J Urol 1998; 81:453–7.

32. Horenblas S, Jansen L, Meinhardt W, et al. Detection of occult metastasis in squamous cell carcinoma of the penis using a dynamic sentinel node procedure. J Urol 2000;163:100–4.

33. Valdes Olmos RA, Tanis PJ, Hoefnagel CA, et al. Penile lymphoscintigraphy for sentinel node identification. Eur J Nucl Med 2001;28(5):581–5.

34. Kroon BK, Horenbas S, Meinhardt W, et al. Dynamic sentinel node biopsy in penile carcinoma: evaluation of 10 years experience. Eur Urol 2005;47:601–6.

35. Tanis PJ, Lont AP, Meinhardt W, et al. Dynamic sentinel node biopsy for penile cancer: reliability of a staging technique. J Urol 2002;168:76–80.

36. Leijte JA, Kroon BK, Valdes Olmos RA, et al. Reliability and safety of current dynamic sentinel node biopsy for penile carcinoma. Eur Urol 2007;52:170–7.

37. Hadway P, Smith Y, Corbishley C, et al. Evaluation of dynamic lymphoscintigraphy and sentinel lymphnode biopsy for detecting occult metastases in patients with penile squamous cell carcinoma. BJU Int 2007;100:561–5.

38. Jensen BJ, Jensen KME, Ulhoi BP, et al. Sentinel lymph-node biopsy in patients with squamous cell carcinoma of the penis. BJU Int 2009;103:1199–203.

39. Ferreira U, Ribeiro MAV, Reis LO, et al. Sentinel lymph node biopsy in penile cancer: a comparative study using modified inguinal dissection. Int Braz J Urol 2008;34(6):725–33.

40. Hungerbuber E, Schlenker B, Frimberger D, et al. Lymphoscintigraphy in penile cancer: limited value of sentinel node biopsy in patients with clinically suspicious lymph nodes. World J Urol 2006;24:319–24.

41. Spiess PE, Izawa JI, Bassett R, et al. Lymphoscintigraphy and dynamic sentinel node biopsy for staging penile cancer: results with pathological correlation. J Urol 2007;177:2157–61.

42. Heyns CF, Theron PD. Evaluation of dynamic sentinel lymph node biopsy in patients with squamous cell carcinoma of the penis and palpable inguinal nodes. BJU Int 2008;102:305–9.

43. Tabatabaei S, Harisihghani M, McDougal WS. Regional lymph node staging using lymphotrophic nanoparticle enhanced magnetic resonance imaging with ferumoxtran-10 in patients with penile cancer. J Urol 2005;174:923.

Penile Intraepithelial Neoplasia and Other Premalignant Lesions of the Penis

Paul L. Crispen, MD[a],*, Jack H. Mydlo, MD, FACS[b]

KEYWORDS

- Penile intraepithelial neoplasia • Human papilloma virus
- Lichen sclerosis • Penile cancer

Penile cancer is a rare disease whose incidence varies geographically throughout the world. In the United States it is estimated that approximately 1300 new cases will be diagnosed and 300 men will die of penile cancer in 2009. Although penile cancer only accounts for 1% of malignancies diagnosed in United State males, the rate is much greater in parts of Asia, South America, and Africa, where it approaches 10%.[1] There are several known risk factors for the development of invasive cancer, including human papilloma virus (HPV) infection and premalignant penile lesions.[2] The presence of prior or concomitant penile lesions and/or symptoms with cases of invasive penile cancer is reported in up to 42% of cases, which suggests an opportunity for intervention prior to the development of invasive and/or metastatic disease.[3] In addition, it has been noted that approximately 25% of dysplastic or neoplastic penile lesions will have been incorrectly diagnosed as being benign by another practitioner, leading to delayed treatment.[4] With prompt diagnosis and treatment of premalignant penile lesions, malignant progression may be evaded while avoiding the need for partial or complete penile amputation, which is often required for the treatment of invasive disease. This review discusses the role of HPV in the development of penile intraepithelial neoplasia (PIN), the malignant potential and recommended treatment of PIN, and potential strategies to prevent PIN. Additional premalignant penile lesions including lichen sclerosus (LS), pseudo-epitheliomatous keratotic and micaceous balanitis (PKMB), and penile cutaneous horn are discussed briefly.

HUMAN PAPILLOMA VIRUS

HPV is the most common sexually transmitted viral infection in the developed world, with a prevalence of approximately 5% in healthy males and a peak incidence occurring between the ages 16 and 35 years.[5–7] While a large proportion of HPV infections will spontaneously regress, a number of patients will have persistent infection with a risk of developing PIN and, rarely, invasive penile cancer. Risk factors for contracting the virus include multiple sexual partners and the lack of barrier protection use. Infection with HPV is clinically variable and can be classified as latent, subclinical, and clinical.[8] Latent HPV infection is defined by the presence of detectable HPV DNA, but without evidence of microscopic or macroscopic disease. Subclinical HPV infection is defined by the presence of detectable HPV DNA and microscopic disease, but without evidence of macroscopic infection. Clinical HPV infection is defined by the presence of macroscopic lesions. HPV types can be classified as low- and high-risk based on their association with premalignant and malignant lesions. High-risk HPV types (16, 18, 31, 33, 35, 39, 45, 51,

a Division of Urology, Department of Surgery, University of Kentucky, MS 235A, 800 Rose Street, Lexington, KY 40536, USA
b Temple University Hospital, 3401 North Broad Street, Suite 340, Philadelphia, PA 19140, USA
* Corresponding author.
E-mail address: crispen.paul@uky.edu

Urol Clin N Am 37 (2010) 335–342
doi:10.1016/j.ucl.2010.04.003

52, 54, 56, 58, 59, 66, 68, 69) have been associated with several premalignant and malignant conditions including PIN, vulvar intraepithelial neoplasia, carcinoma in situ of cervix, and invasive carcinoma of the cervix.[8] The most common and recognizable clinical manifestation of infection with HPV is the development of condyloma acuminatum, or genital warts. The most common sites of genital infection in males include the prepuce and glans in uncircumcised males and the penile shaft and glans in circumcised males. Lesions are typically multifocal, ranging from 1 to 10 mm in size. Genital warts resulting from HPV infection are frequently benign, with 90% being associated with HPV types 6 or 11. However, coinfection with high-risk HPV types may be present in 19% to 44% of patients.[8]

Although the growth of most genital warts is limited, some may continue to grow to a much larger size and are then classified as giant condyloma. Giant condylomas have also been referred to as Buschke-Lowenstein tumors. Giant condylomas are thought to grow slowly and be related to poor hygiene.[9] Although associated with the low-risk HPV types 6 and 11, giant condylomas can grow to involve underlying and surrounding structures such as the dermis, subcutaneous fat, urethra, corpora, and rectum. Even though giant condylomas can be locally destructive, they are not associated with the development of metastatic disease.[10] During pathologic evaluation, care must be taken to differentiate giant condyloma from verrucous carcinoma. While histologic examination can often characterize giant condyloma, HPV typing is sometimes useful to differentiate it from verrucous carcinoma, the latter not being associated with HPV infection.[8]

The prevalence of HPV infection associated with penile cancer ranges from 15% to 100%.[11] The wide range in association reported is likely attributed to the method of HPV detection in cancer specimens.[12] The most common type of HPV associated with penile cancer is HPV 16, being noted in 65% of HPV-associated penile cancers.[11] The association with HPV and penile cancer also varies by subtype of penile cancer. Whereas HPV is commonly noted in basaloid and warty penile cancer (80%–100%), the association is much lower in keratinizing and verrucous penile carcinomas (0%–35%).[12] The noted association between HPV and invasive penile carcinoma is more similar to that in vulvar intraepithelial neoplasia (VIN) (50%) and cervical intraepithelial neoplasia (CIN) (100%). Although a suggested association between age of onset of penile cancer and HPV infection has been made, this finding has not been noted in all series.[13,14]

Flat penile lesions associated with HPV are commonly located on the glans and prepuce. Histologically, flat penile lesions demonstrate squamous hyperplasia and features of low-grade PIN. The occurrence of flat penile lesions in men is strongly associated with CIN in female sexual partners, with 50% to 70% of affected men having CIN-positive female partners compared with 10% to 20% of men whose sexual partners are CIN negative.[11] The majority of flat penile lesion will regress in 1 to 2 years; however, a small percentage may persist. The natural history of persistent flat penile lesions associated with HPV is currently unknown, but these lesions may potentially progress to high-grade PIN and/or invasive penile cancer.

PENILE INTRAEPITHELIAL NEOPLASIA

PIN is characterized by epithelial dysplasia equal to that of squamous cell carcinoma in situ, and includes erythroplasia of Queyrat (EQ), Bowen disease (BD), and bowenoid papulosis (BP).[15] The differential diagnosis when considering PIN is presented in **Box 1**. PIN can be characterized in several ways based on clinicopathologic features, including the degree of dysplasia, location, age of onset, and morphologic features. When categorizing PIN according to the degree of dysplasia, mild dysplasia is equivalent PIN I,

---

Box 1
Differential diagnosis of PIN

Benign Conditions

Benign pigmented warts

Lichen sclerosus

Seborrheic keratosis

Melanocytic nevi

Angiokeratoma

Lichen planus

Psoriasis

Balanitis

Eczema

Contact dermatitis

Malignant Conditions

Malignant melanoma

Paget disease

Basal cell carcinoma

Kaposi sarcoma

moderate dysplasia is equivalent to PIN II, and severe dysplasia is categorized as PIN III. When comparing the PIN I, II, and III classification system with categories of PIN based on other clinicopathologic features, PIN II is synonymous with BP, and PIN III is synonymous with EQ and BD.[16] EQ, BD, and BP can be further distinguished based on clinical features (**Table 1**).[15]

When comparing types of PIN, BP is more common in young men and is known to spontaneously regress. The mean duration of disease is approximately 2 years, with the majority (73%) of lesions regressing or not recurring after excision.[12] However, the lesions can also recur, progress to EQ or BD, and become malignant.[11] BP has also been noted to have a strong relationship with the occurrence of CIN in female sexual partners.[12] Suspected risk factors for malignant progression of BP include smoking, immune suppression, high-risk HPV types, and genetics. In contrast to BP, EQ and BD are more commonly detected in older men. In addition, the malignant progression rate of EQ and BD is considerably higher, being noted in up to 10% to 20% of cases.[12] A series by Malek and colleagues[17] evaluating the natural history of PIN, with follow-up ranging from 3 to 19 years, noted an 89% rate of progression to invasive penile cancer. The estimated time for malignant progression for cases of low-grade PIN may be up to 20 years.[5] This estimate is based on series that show a mean onset age of PIN I to II lesions as 35.8 years, PIN III lesions as 56.1 years, and invasive penile cancer of 65.3 years.[17,18] The association between PIN and invasive penile cancer was also noted in a series by Cubilla and colleagues.[19] In this series the occurrence of associated epithelial lesions with invasive penile cancer

was examined in 288 cases of invasive penile cancer. The presence of squamous hyperplasia, low-grade PIN, and high-grade PIN were present in 89%, 59%, and 44% of cases, respectively. The observed association with squamous hyperplasia was more common with keratinizing and verrucous carcinomas than with basaloid and warty penile carcinoma. However, the association with high-grade PIN was stronger with basaloid and warty penile cancer than with keratinizing and verrucous penile carcinoma.

HPV infection has been associated with all types of PIN, and the rate HPV infection in PIN ranges from 70% to 100%.[5] In addition, a history of having anogenital warts was noted to be a significant risk factor for the development of PIN and penile cancer, with an odds ratio of 7.01 (95% confidence interval: 2.48–19.8).[20] HPV types 16 and 18 have been associated with PIN in several series, and it is not uncommon for PIN lesions to be associated with more than one type of HPV.[8] Concurrent infection with HPV 8, 16, 39, and 51 have been noted in EQ.[21] In a report by Wieland and colleagues,[21] all patients with EQ demonstrated HPV 8 DNA, 88% demonstrated HPV 16 DNA, and 50% demonstrated HPV 39 or 51 DNA. Further evidence linking HPV and PIN is provided by series that evaluate the relationship between HPV-related genital lesions in sexual partners. The rate of PIN in males whose female partner has CIN is 33% compared with 1.4% in men whose female partner has condyloma.[22] In addition, similar lesions (VIN and CIN) have been noted in the sexual partners of men with PIN.[12]

Malignant potential of PIN is known to be dependent on the type of PIN with BP rarely progressing to invasive squamous cell carcinoma

Table 1
Clinical characteristics of PIN

	Bowenoid Papulosis	Erythroplasia of Queyrat	Bowen Disease
Age at diagnosis	<40 years	>40 years	>40 years
Location	Penile shaft, glans, or prepuce	Glans and prepuce	Follicle-bearing skin of the genitals
Size	2–10 mm	10–15 mm	10–15 mm
Gross appearance	Multiple small well-demarcated smooth brown, red, or pink papillomatous papules or patches	One or more moist velvety shiny red patches	Single scaly red or slightly pigmented plaque
Malignant progression	<1%	10%–20%%	10%–20%

(SCC), while EQ and BD have been clearly documented as precursors of invasive penile carcinoma. Despite the association between high-risk HPV infection and PIN and PIN being an established precursor of invasive penile carcinoma, there is a disconnect with regard to the number HPV-positive cases of invasive penile cancer. The percentage of HPV-positive PIN cases, 70% to 100%, has been noted to be significantly higher than the percentage of HPV-positive invasive penile carcinoma cases, 54%.[20] Several theories for this apparent disconnect between high-risk HPV infection and the development of invasive penile cancer have been made,[6] the first of which is based on discrepancies in the methods used in detecting HPV infection, including the assays used and the methods of tissue preparation. The second theory is based on the potential clearance of HPV during progression from PIN to invasive penile carcinoma. The third and most likely explanation involves 2 separate pathways for the development of penile cancer: an HPV-dependent and an HPV-independent pathway.[23] The observed disconnect between high-risk HPV infection and invasive penile cancer also raises the question of whether another unknown precursor of invasive penile cancer exists that has yet to be identified.

The current understanding of the tumorigenesis of penile cancer speculates that 2 different pathways may lead to invasive penile cancer, with one leading to basaloid and warty penile cancer and the other leading to keratinizing and verrucous penile cancer. Keratinizing is the most common type of penile cancer, accounting for approximately 50% of cases. Basaloid, warty, verrucous, and warty-basaloid account for 4%, 6%, 8%, and 17% of penile cancer, respectively. The remaining cases comprise papillary, SCC mixed, and sarcomatoid carcinomas of the penis. With its known associations with HPV infections it is believed that PIN is a precursor lesion of basaloid and warty penile cancer, while the precursor lesions of keratinizing and verrucous carcinoma remain unknown. The strongest association between HPV infection and development of penile cancer is seen in basaloid penile cancer, with 70% to 100% of basaloid carcinomas being HPV positive while 47% of basaloid and/or warty, 11% of keratinizing, and 0% of verrucous penile carcinoma are associated with HPV infection.[11,24]

TREATMENT OF PENILE INTRAEPITHELIAL NEOPLASIA

The goals of treatment in PIN should be to eradicate disease while limiting penile mutilation. Due to the small numbers of PIN diagnosed each year, treatment recommendations based on level I evidence are not available. In addition, treatment response is typically based on clinical response as opposed to pathologic response determined via a posttreatment biopsy.[3]

Although most treating physicians would recommend ablative therapy, topical therapy with 5-fluorouracil (5-FU) and imiquimod have been reported. Topical treatment with 5-FU as a 5% cream is an attractive alternative to excisional therapy; however, there is a dearth of evidence to support its routine use as front-line agent for PIN.[3] Alternating topical 5-FU and corticosteroids is another option, with patients switching application between the 2 medications based on irritating symptoms secondary to 5-FU.[25] Topical imiquimod is also being investigated for efficacy in the treatment of PIN; however, literature supporting its use is largely in the form of case reports.[26,27]

Ablative treatments of PIN include cyrosurgery, electrosurgery, and laser vaporization. Cryosurgery is not recommended because of lack of consistent depth of treatment.[5,28] Electrosurgery, although effective, is not currently recommended as first-line treatment for PIN because of the risk of disfigurement.[3,29] However, laser vaporization allows for adequate destruction of the PIN lesion while limiting depth of penetration and unnecessary destruction of healthy tissue. Experience with several different types of laser has been described, and selection of laser source seems largely user dependent.[3] Recurrence rates following laser vaporization ranges from 0% to 33%.[4,30–32] Excisional therapy remains the gold standard for treatment of PIN, with reported recurrence rates of 13% to 33%.[3,33] Although excisional therapy offers excellent disease control rates, the resultant cosmesis presents a potential drawback. Mohs micrographic surgery may offer all of the benefits of excisional therapy while limiting excision of uninvolved tissue and disfigurement.[34] For more extensive and recalcitrant cases of PIN involving the glans, total glans resurfacing may present an efficacious alternative to more radical excisions. In a report of 10 patients with recurrent or persistent EQ, total glans resurfacing was performed by removing the epithelium and subepithelium from the glans and subcoronal areas, followed by covering the areas with extragenital skin.[35] Short-term follow-up of these initial 10 patients revealed no recurrent disease and excellent cosmetic results at a median of 30 months.

A posttreatment biopsy of the involved area is recommended to document adequate treatment response. Following pathologic confirmation of disease clearance, a follow-up visit at 3 months should be scheduled to evaluate for persistent and/or recurrent disease. While further recommendations for the frequency and duration of follow-up are not available, patients should be encouraged to return for evaluation as soon as suspicious lesions reappear.[3]

ROLE OF HUMAN PAPILLOMA VIRUS IN THE MOLECULAR PATHOGENESIS OF PENILE CANCER

The underlying tumorigenesis of penile cancer seems to be dependent on the presence or absence of HPV infection. This assumption is apparent when considering the rate of HPV infections associated with the histologic variants of penile cancer (keratinizing, verrucous, basaloid, and warty). Whereas the late molecular events in the pathogenesis of penile cancer appear similar in HPV- and non-HPV–dependent penile cancer, the early molecular events appear to be triggered differently.[36] The key differences appear in the mechanisms by which the p53 and Rb pathways are altered.[11] In HPV-associated penile cancers, tumorigenesis is believed to be driven by the E6 and E7 HPV oncoproteins. The E6 and E7 oncoproteins bind and inactivate the p53 and Rb tumor suppressor gene products, leading to alterations in the control of cell division and apoptosis. Although the p53 and Rb pathways are involved in the tumorigenesis of non-HPV–dependent penile cancer, the mechanisms by which these pathways are altered differs compared with HPV-dependent penile cancer. In non-HPV–dependent penile cancer hypermethylation of the p16 promoter sequence and overexpression of BMI-1 are believed to disrupt the Rb pathway, while somatic mutations of the p53 gene, increased expression of MDM2, and p14 mutations are believed to alter the p53 pathway.[11,37,38]

LICHEN SCLEROSUS

LS of the male genitalia, also known as balanitis xerotica obliterans, can be diagnosed as early as the first decade of life, but the majority of cases are diagnosed in the third to fifth decades of life.[39,40] The etiology of LS is currently unknown; however, the disease has been attributed to several causes including chronic irritation, trauma, autoimmune disease, infection, hormonal influence, and genetic factors.[40] In addition, the exact incidence of LS in men is unknown due to inconsistent presentation, misdiagnosis, and number of specialists treating the condition. Presenting symptoms may include dysuria, decreased stream

of urination, itching, and pain. Proper diagnosis and treatment can prevent further urologic conditions including urethral stricture and phimosis. LS lesions are typically located on the glans, urethral meatus, and/or prepuce, and appear as plaques or papules. LS has also been reported to affect the anterior and membranous urethra.[41] LS lesions typically appear as ivory-white atrophic and sclerotic plaques; however, telangiectasia and hemorrhagic petechiae can be seen as well.[42] A biopsy is required to definitively differentiate LS from other disease entities. Differential diagnosis includes EQ, lichen planus, leukoplakia, and scleroderma. The histologic appearance of LS consists of hyperkeratosis, hydropic degeneration of the basal cells, sclerosis of the subepithelial collagen, dermal lymphocytic infiltration, atrophic epidermis with loss of rete pegs, homogenization of the underlying stroma, and a dense zone of lymphocytes and histiocytes beneath the homogenized collagen.[39] Treatment ranges from topical pharmacotherapy to surgical excision, depending on the site and extent of disease. Topical treatment with steroid creams is recommended. In males with phimosis related to LS, circumcision should be considered.

Unlike the association between LS and vulvar carcinoma, the relationship between LS and penile cancer has not been clearly defined or accepted.[43] In women with LS of vulva the risk of SCC ranges from 4% to 5%. Based on this and the greater than 300 times risk of SCC of the vulva compared with women without LS noted in longitudinal case-controlled series, routine follow-up for SCC is recommended in all women with LS.[9,43] However, despite a similar observed rate of SCC in men with a history of LS, no standardized follow-up is currently accepted or recommended. The incidence of penile carcinoma in patients with LS has been reported as between 0% and 8.4%,[25,44–47] and LS has been noted in up to 28% to 50% of patients with penile cancer.[48,49] In a report by Pietrzak and colleagues,[48] 44 patients were noted to have LS in association with penile cancer. LS was diagnosed at the time of penile carcinoma presentation in the majority of patients, 87% (39 of 44). Only 3 patients were known to have a long-standing history of LS prior to the diagnosis of penile cancer. Compared with penile cancer patients with and without associated LS, there was no significant difference with regard to age or tumor stage at the time of presentation. In a report of 86 LS patients by Nasca and colleagues,[44] 5.8% (5 of 86) were noted to develop penile carcinoma. The average time from diagnosis of LS to the diagnosis of penile cancer in this series was 17 years, with a range of 10 to 23 years. The long duration between the diagnosis of LS and development of penile cancer was noted to be similar in a report by Barbagli and colleagues,[47] with a mean interval of 12 years. Although most cases of penile carcinoma that have been associated with LS have been SCC, cases of verrucous and adenosquamous carcinoma of the penis have also been reported.[50,51]

PSEUDO-EPITHELIOMATOUS KERATOTIC AND MICACEOUS BALANITIS

PKMB is an extremely rare premalignant penile condition detected in elderly males.[9,10] Although once considered benign, it appears that progression to SCC is common in PKMB.[52] PKMB presents clinically as a single, raised, well-demarcated thick scaly lesion on the glans. These lesions should not be merely observed but should be treated promptly and followed closely for recurrence.[10] Treatment options include topical application of 5-FU and Mohs micrographic surgery.[52]

CUTANEOUS HORN

Penile cutaneous horn represents a wart-like growth with excessive keratosis.[9] The development of the lesion has been associated with benign, premalignant, and malignant conditions.[53] Of note, up to 37% of penile cutaneous horns have been associated with a malignant process.[54,55] As with other penile lesions, an association with HPV 16 infection and penile cutaneous horn has been made. Surgical excision is recommended, with follow-up depending on the presence or absence of underlying malignancy. The prognosis of SCC associated with a penile cutaneous horn is typically favorable, as most lesions are low grade.[55]

PREVENTION OF PREMALIGNANT LESIONS AND PENILE CANCER

Several strategies to prevent penile cancer have been described. Such strategies aim to decrease inflammation/irritation of the penis and HPV infection. Given the association with the intact prepuce and increased malignancy, Malek[16] refers to the foreskin as the "cocoon of carcinogenesis." Circumcision has been associated with a decreased rate of penile cancer; this is thought to be the product of several events including improved hygiene, decreased incidence of LS, and a decreased rate of HPV infections compared with noncircumcised males. While these are known benefits associated with neonatal circumcision, it is not known whether circumcision in adulthood significantly reduces the risk of penile cancer, as many of the risk factors may have already been acquired, if not necessitating

the circumcision.[11] In addition to circumcision, HPV infection can be reduced with barrier protection during sexual encounters and potentially with HPV vaccination. Condom use is known to be an effective measure in reducing HPV infections and has been associated with a decreased rate of HPV-associated genital lesions.[56,57] Further evidence supporting condom use in an attempt to decrease premalignant and malignant penile lesions was reported by Madsen and colleagues.[20] In a population-based case-control study of Danish men, the lack of condom use was an independent risk factor for the diagnosis of PIN and penile cancer following multivariate analysis.

Prevention of HPV infection through vaccination has been proven in women through efforts to decrease the rate of cervical cancer. At present, there are 2 Food and Drug Administration–approved HPV vaccines available, Gardasil (Sanofi Pasteur) and Cervarix (GlaxoSmithKline). Gardasil is a quadrivalent vaccine against HPV 16/18/6/11 while Cervarix is a bivalent vaccine against HPV 16/18. The vaccines have been proven to be safe and effective in decreasing the rate of high-grade cervical lesions in HPV-negative women.[58,59] With the documented success of HPV vaccination in women and the results of a randomized clinical trial in men, Gardasil was approved for males ages 9 to 26 years in the United States in the fall of 2009. In a randomized trial of 4065 males aged 16 to 26 years, vaccination with Gardasil was approximately 90% successful in preventing genital warts caused by HPV 16/18/6/11, this was a significant reduction compared with placebo.[60] Although the indication of the vaccination in males is not as preventive against premalignant and malignant lesions as it is in women, the approval and use in males is a step that will hopefully decrease the incidence of HPV and in turn decrease the occurrence of premalignant penile lesions.

SUMMARY

Premalignant penile lesions represent a diverse group of conditions with variable malignant potential. Although most cases of HPV are benign and self limited, HPV infection is associated with several premalignant penile lesions including PIN. PIN is represented by BP, EQ, and BD, all of which can demonstrate malignant progression to invasive penile carcinoma. Based on the existing data on the natural history of PIN, 2 pathways in the development of penile carcinoma have been described, the HPV-dependent and HPV-independent pathways. Continued efforts on decreasing the incidence of HPV infection, via condom use and HPV vaccination, may prove beneficial in decreasing the occurrence of PIN and invasive penile carcinoma.

REFERENCES

1. American Cancer Society. Facts and figures 2009. Available at: http://www.cancer.org/downloads/STT/500809web.pdf. Accessed January 30, 2010.
2. Dillner J, von Krogh G, Horenblas S, et al. Etiology of squamous cell carcinoma of the penis. Scand J Urol Nephrol Suppl 2000;(205):189–93.
3. von Krogh G, Horenblas S. The management and prevention of premalignant penile lesions. Scand J Urol Nephrol Suppl 2000;(205):220–9.
4. Tietjen DN, Malek RS. Laser therapy of squamous cell dysplasia and carcinoma of the penis. Urology 1998;52(4):559–65.
5. Horenblas S, von Krogh G, Cubilla AL, et al. Squamous cell carcinoma of the penis: premalignant lesions. Scand J Urol Nephrol Suppl 2000;(205):187–8.
6. Dillner J, Meijer CJ, von Krogh G, et al. Epidemiology of human papillomavirus infection. Scand J Urol Nephrol Suppl 2000;(205):194–200.
7. Grussendorf-Conen EI, de Villiers EM, Gissmann L. Human papillomavirus genomes in penile smears of healthy men. Lancet 1986;2(8515):1092.
8. Gross G, Pfister H. Role of human papillomavirus in penile cancer, penile intraepithelial squamous cell neoplasias and in genital warts. Med Microbiol Immunol 2004;193(1):35–44.
9. von Krogh G, Horenblas S. Diagnosis and clinical presentation of premalignant lesions of the penis. Scand J Urol Nephrol Suppl 2000;(205):201–14.
10. Grossman HB. Premalignant and early carcinomas of the penis and scrotum. Urol Clin North Am 1992;19(2):221–6.
11. Bleeker MC, Heideman DA, Snijders PJ, et al. Penile cancer: epidemiology, pathogenesis and prevention. World J Urol 2009;27(2):141–50.
12. Obalek S, Jablonska S, Beaudenon S, et al. Bowenoid papulosis of the male and female genitalia: risk of cervical neoplasia. J Am Acad Dermatol 1986;14(3):433–44.
13. Lont AP, Kroon BK, Horenblas S, et al. Presence of high-risk human papillomavirus DNA in penile carcinoma predicts favorable outcome in survival. Int J Cancer 2006;119(5):1078–81.
14. Cubilla AL, Reuter VE, Gregoire L, et al. Basaloid squamous cell carcinoma: a distinctive human papilloma virus-related penile neoplasm: a report of 20 cases. Am J Surg Pathol 1998;22(6):755–61.
15. Porter WM, Francis N, Hawkins D, et al. Penile intraepithelial neoplasia: clinical spectrum and treatment of 35 cases. Br J Dermatol 2002;147(6):1159–65.
16. Malek RS. Update Series. Human papillomavirus and carcinoma of the penis: modern concepts in pathogenesis and their impact on management of penile lesions, vol. XIX. Houston (TX): AUA; 1999. p. 1–7, Lesson 1.
17. Malek RS, Goellner JR, Smith TF, et al. Human papillomavirus infection and intraepithelial, in situ, and invasive carcinoma of penis. Urology 1993;42(2):159–70.
18. Aynaud O, Ionesco M, Barrasso R. Penile intraepithelial neoplasia. Specific clinical features correlate with histologic and virologic findings. Cancer 1994;74(6):1762–7.
19. Cubilla AL, Velazquez EF, Young RH. Epithelial lesions associated with invasive penile squamous cell carcinoma: a pathologic study of 288 cases. Int J Surg Pathol 2004;12(4):351–64.
20. Madsen BS, van den Brule AJ, Jensen HL, et al. Risk factors for squamous cell carcinoma of the penis—population-based case-control study in Denmark. Cancer Epidemiol Biomarkers Prev 2008;17(10):2683–91.
21. Wieland U, Jurk S, Weissenborn S, et al. Erythroplasia of Queyrat: coinfection with cutaneous carcinogenic human papillomavirus type 8 and genital papillomaviruses in a carcinoma in situ. J Invest Dermatol 2000;115(3):396–401.
22. Barrasso R, De Brux J, Croissant O, et al. High prevalence of papillomavirus-associated penile intraepithelial neoplasia in sexual partners of women with cervical intraepithelial neoplasia. N Engl J Med 1987;317(15):916–23.
23. Cubilla AL, Meijer CJ, Young RH. Morphological features of epithelial abnormalities and precancerous lesions of the penis. Scand J Urol Nephrol Suppl 2000;(205):215–9.
24. Gregoire L, Cubilla AL, Reuter VE, et al. Preferential association of human papillomavirus with high-grade histologic variants of penile-invasive squamous cell carcinoma. J Natl Cancer Inst 1995;87(22):1705–9.
25. Singh S, Bunker C. Male genital dermatoses in old age. Age Ageing 2008;37(5):500–4.
26. Micali G, Nasca MR, De Pasquale R. Erythroplasia of Queyrat treated with imiquimod 5% cream. J Am Acad Dermatol 2006;55(5):901–3.
27. Taliaferro SJ, Cohen GF. Bowen's disease of the penis treated with topical imiquimod 5% cream. J Drugs Dermatol 2008;7(5):483–5.
28. Simmons PD, Langlet F, Thin RN. Cryotherapy versus electrocautery in the treatment of genital warts. Br J Vener Dis 1981;57(4):273–4.
29. Veien SK, Veien NK, Hattel T, et al. [Results of treatment of non-melanoma skin cancer in a dermatologic practice. A prospective study]. Ugeskr Laeger 1996;158(50):7213–5 [in Danish].
30. Gerber GS. Carcinoma in situ of the penis. J Urol 1994;151(4):829–33.
31. Malloy TR, Wein AJ, Carpiniello VL. Carcinoma of penis treated with neodymium YAG laser. Urology 1988;31(1):26–9.

32. Schlenker B, Gratzke C, Seitz M, et al. Fluorescence-guided laser therapy for penile carcinoma and precancerous lesions: long-term follow-up. Urol Oncol 2009. [Epub ahead of print].

33. Bissada NK. Conservative extirpative treatment of cancer of the penis. Urol Clin North Am 1992; 19(2):283–90.

34. Mohs FE, Snow SN, Larson PO. Mohs micrographic surgery for penile tumors. Urol Clin North Am 1992; 19(2):291–304.

35. Hadway P, Corbishley CM, Watkin NA. Total glans resurfacing for premalignant lesions of the penis: initial outcome data. BJU Int 2006;98(3):532–6.

36. Kayes O, Ahmed HU, Arya M, et al. Molecular and genetic pathways in penile cancer. Lancet Oncol 2007;8(5):420–9.

37. Cubilla AL, Velazquez EF, Young RH. Pseudohyperplastic squamous cell carcinoma of the penis associated with lichen sclerosus. An extremely well-differentiated, nonverruciform neoplasm that preferentially affects the foreskin and is frequently misdiagnosed: a report of 10 cases of a distinctive clinicopathologic entity. Am J Surg Pathol 2004; 28(7):895–900.

38. Soufir N, Queille S, Liboutet M, et al. Inactivation of the CDKN2A and the p53 tumour suppressor genes in external genital carcinomas and their precursors. Br J Dermatol 2007;156(3):448–53.

39. Das S, Tunuguntla HS. Balanitis xerotica obliterans—a review. World J Urol 2000;18(6):382–7.

40. Pugliese JM, Morey AF, Peterson AC. Lichen sclerosus: review of the literature and current recommendations for management. J Urol 2007;178(6): 2268–76.

41. Garat JM, Chechile G, Algaba F, et al. Balanitis xerotica obliterans in children. J Urol 1986;136(2):436–7.

42. Jebakumar SP, Woolley PD. Balanitis xerotica obliterans. Int J STD AIDS 1995;6(2):81–3.

43. Scurry J. Does lichen sclerosus play a central role in the pathogenesis of human papillomavirus negative vulvar squamous cell carcinoma? The itch-scratch-lichen sclerosus hypothesis. Int J Gynecol Cancer 1999;9(2):89–97.

44. Nasca MR, Innocenzi D, Micali G. Penile cancer among patients with genital lichen sclerosus. J Am Acad Dermatol 1999;41(6):911–4.

45. Depasquale I, Park AJ, Bracka A. The treatment of balanitis xerotica obliterans. BJU Int 2000;86(4): 459–65.

46. Wallace HJ. Lichen sclerosus et atrophicus. Trans St Johns Hosp Dermatol Soc 1971;57(1):9–30.

47. Barbagli G, Palminteri E, Mirri F, et al. Penile carcinoma in patients with genital lichen sclerosus: a multicenter survey. J Urol 2006;175(4):1359–63.

48. Pietrzak P, Hadway P, Corbishley CM, et al. Is the association between balanitis xerotica obliterans and penile carcinoma underestimated? BJU Int 2006;98(1):74–6.

49. Powell J, Robson A, Cranston D, et al. High incidence of lichen sclerosus in patients with squamous cell carcinoma of the penis. Br J Dermatol 2001;145(1):85–9.

50. Weber P, Rabinovitz H, Garland L. Verrucous carcinoma in penile lichen sclerosus et atrophicus. J Dermatol Surg Oncol 1987;13(5):529–32.

51. Jamieson NV, Bullock KN, Barker TH. Adenosquamous carcinoma of the penis associated with balanitis xerotica obliterans. Br J Urol 1986;58(6):730–1.

52. Ganem JP, Steele BW, Creager AJ, et al. Pseudo-epitheliomatous keratotic and micaceous balanitis. J Urol 1999;161(1):217–8.

53. Nayyar R, Singh P, Seth A. Penile cutaneous horn over long standing radiation dermatitis. J Postgrad Med 2009;55(4):287.

54. Mastrolorenzo A, Tiradritti L, Locunto U, et al. Incidental finding: a penile cutaneous horn. Acta Derm Venereol 2005;85(3):283–4.

55. Raghavaiah NV, Soloway MS, Murphy WM. Malignant penile horn. J Urol 1977;118(6):1068–9.

56. Bleeker MC, Hogewoning CJ, Voorhorst FJ, et al. Condom use promotes regression of human papillomavirus-associated penile lesions in male sexual partners of women with cervical intraepithelial neoplasia. Int J Cancer 2003;107(5):804–10.

57. Hogewoning CJ, Bleeker MC, van den Brule AJ, et al. Condom use promotes regression of cervical intraepithelial neoplasia and clearance of human papillomavirus: a randomized clinical trial. Int J Cancer 2003;107(5):811–6.

58. Harper DM, Franco EL, Wheeler CM, et al. Sustained efficacy up to 4.5 years of a bivalent L1 virus-like particle vaccine against human papillomavirus types 16 and 18: follow-up from a randomised control trial. Lancet 2006;367(9518):1247–55.

59. Villa LL, Costa RL, Petta CA, et al. Prophylactic quadrivalent human papillomavirus (types 6, 11, 16, and 18) L1 virus-like particle vaccine in young women: a randomised double-blind placebo-controlled multicentre phase II efficacy trial. Lancet Oncol 2005;6(5):271–8.

60. Hsueh PR. Human papillomavirus, genital warts, and vaccines. J Microbiol Immunol Infect 2009; 42(2):101–6.

Penile Cancer: Clinical Presentation, Diagnosis, and Staging

Daniel A. Barocas, MD, MPH, Sam S. Chang, MD*

KEYWORDS

• Penile cancer • Presentation • Diagnosis • Staging

Penile cancer is an uncommon malignancy in developed countries, with an estimated 1290 new cases of invasive penile cancer and 290 deaths among men in the United States in 2009, but is much more common in the developing countries of Asia, Africa, and South America.[1] Between 1998 and 2001, invasive squamous cell penile cancer accounted for 0.1% of all invasive tumors diagnosed among men in the United States, whereas this figure is reportedly was high as 10% to 20% of cancers among men in some countries.[2–4] This disease can result in loss of function, disfigurement, and death.[1,5] The 5-year survival for all patients is approximately 50%; it ranges from 66% for patients with negative lymph nodes to 25% to 30% for those with positive inguinal lymph nodes and approaches 0% for those with pelvic lymph node metastases.[6–10] Thus, recognizing penile cancer early in the clinical setting and accurately diagnosing the patients is critical. Because the management and prognosis varies by the extent of local disease, lymph node status, and other factors, accurate staging of penile cancer is of utmost importance.

Other articles in this issue have described the premalignant and early carcinomas of the penis as well as imaging for penile cancer and management of the lymph nodes. This article focuses on the presentation, diagnosis, and staging of invasive squamous cell carcinoma of the penis. The authors highlight the recent changes to the staging system of the American Joint Committee on Cancer (AJCC) for penile carcinoma, and discuss other prognostic factors and predictive models.

RISK FACTORS

Penile cancer can occur in any male patient, but certain risk factors have been identified.[11] Although up to 15% of cases occur in men younger than 50 years, penile cancer is a disease of older men, with a median age at diagnosis in the United States of 68 years and with an increased risk as the age advances beyond 50 years.[2] Penile cancer is far more common among uncircumcised men than those who were circumcised early in life.[12,13] Phimosis is strongly associated with the risk for penile cancer and hampers surveillance of the glans, inner preputial layer, and coronal sulcus, which are the areas of high incidence.[14–16] Human papilloma virus (HPV) infection is identified in about half of the men with penile cancer[17] and some HPV subtypes (such as HPV-16 and HPV-18) have been associated with malignant transformation of condyloma acuminata.[18–20] Sexual behaviors such as high number of lifetime partners also confer additional risk of penile cancer.[11,12] Human immunodeficiency virus (HIV) is associated with an 8-fold increased risk of penile cancer, but this may be mediated to an extent by the higher incidence of HPV among men with HIV.[21] Cigarette smokers are 3 to 4.5 times more likely to develop penile carcinoma than nonsmokers,[12,22] and users of other tobacco products are also at increased risk.[23] Psoralen-UV-A photochemotherapy for psoriasis has also been shown to be a risk factor for penile cancer.[14,24] Lichen sclerosus (balanitis xerotica obliterans) is associated with a 3% to

Department of Urologic Surgery, Vanderbilt University Medical Center, A-1302 Medical Center North, Nashville, TN 37232, USA
* Corresponding author.
E-mail address: sam.chang@vanderbilt.edu

Urol Clin N Am 37 (2010) 343–352
doi:10.1016/j.ucl.2010.04.002

9% risk of development of penile cancer over long-term follow-up,[25,26] and other premalignant lesions are also, by definition, risk factors.

PRESENTATION

Approximately two-thirds of men with penile carcinoma present with localized disease.[2] Penile carcinoma most often presents with a visible or palpable lesion on the penis. The lesion may arise de novo as invasive carcinoma, or may have progressed from a premalignant lesion or carcinoma in situ. The appearance varies from an ulceration with heaped-up edges to areas of induration or erythema to a warty, exophytic appearance. In a review of more than 3500 published cases from 1908 to 1984, Huben and Sufrin[15] found that the most common lesion was described as a mass, lump, or nodule in 47% of cases, a sore or ulcer in 35%, an inflammatory lesion in 17%, and an incidental diagnosis on evaluation of a circumcision specimen in 0.7%. The lesion may be hidden by the foreskin, particularly in patients with phimosis, which has been reported to be as high as 60% among patients with penile cancer in Brazil.[27] The lesion may also be obscured by associated inflammatory conditions such as balanitis or lichen sclerosis.

Penile carcinoma can be associated with penile pain, discharge, bleeding, or foul odor. These secondary signs may be particularly important components of the presentation in patients with phimosis.

The most common locations for penile cancer are the glans penis, prepuce, and coronal sulcus. A recent study of almost 5000 cases of invasive carcinoma of the penis among men in the United States showed that the primary site of disease was the glans penis in 34.5% of cases, prepuce in 13.2%, shaft in 5.3%, overlapping in 4.5%, and unspecified in 42.5%.[2] Thus, of those cases with a specified site, only 11.2% had the disease confined to the shaft. These results corroborate earlier data compiled by Huben and Sufrin,[15] who found that the lesions were confined to the glans in 48% of patients, only on the prepuce in 21%, glans or prepuce with extension to the shaft in 14%, both glans and prepuce in 9%, coronal sulcus in 6%, and isolated carcinomas on the shaft in less than 2%.

The patients may also have noticed masses in their inguinal regions, which can be a sequela of local inflammation and infection or evidence of lymph node metastases. Patients with advanced disease may complain of fatigue, weight loss, or bone pain.

There is often a delay in presentation with penile cancer, likely owing to the social stigma and denial. Between 15% and 50% of patients delayed seeking treatment for at least 1 year after first noticing symptoms.[15,28–32] For example, Narayana and colleagues[32] showed that of 176 patients with documentation of the interval between onset of symptoms and seeking medical attention, 85 (48.3%) sought treatment within 6 months, 37 (21.0%) waited between 6 and 12 months, and 54 (30.7%) waited for more than 1 year. Penile cancer is lethal once it has spread to regional lymph nodes and beyond, making any delay in diagnosis, whether because the patient delays seeking treatment or the physician delays a necessary diagnostic procedure, unacceptably perilous.

In addition to the generic histopathologic designation of squamous cell carcinoma there are 4 subtypes recognized by AJCC (verrucous, papillary squamous, warty, and basaloid); some investigators have also reported an adenosquamous subtype and a sarcomatoid variant.[33–35] A review of 61 cases in the United States by Cubilla and colleagues[34] found that 59% of patients had conventional squamous cell carcinoma, 15% papillary, 10% basaloid, 10% warty, 3% verrucous, and 3% sarcomatoid. A more recent study of 333 cases in Brazil by Guimarães and colleagues[35] showed a similar distribution: 65% of patients had conventional squamous cell carcinoma, 5% papillary, 4% basaloid, 7% warty, 7% verrucous, 1% sarcomatoid, 1% adenosquamous, and 10% mixed. In both studies, the basaloid and sarcomatoid variants carried the worst prognosis. Each subtype has a unique histopathologic appearance and natural history and may present in different ways.[35] For example, verrucous carcinomas, which rarely metastasize, are typically large, exophytic, fungating masses without other sites of involvement.[35–38] On the other hand, basaloid carcinomas often present at higher stages and have a higher likelihood of lymph node metastases than conventional squamous cell carcinomas.[32,35] Sarcomatoid carcinomas are also very aggressive. In a series of 15 cases, most tumors were large (2.5–7 cm) polypoid lesions, with surface ulceration affecting the glans in 93% cases and invading deeply into the corpora cavernosa in 80%.[39] Eight out of 9 patients who underwent lymphadenectomy had positive lymph nodes.

DIAGNOSIS

Clinicians must maintain a high index of suspicion for penile carcinoma in men with cutaneous lesions of the penis, particularly in men with risk factors for penile carcinoma. A careful history must be taken including the length of time the lesion has been present, the evolution of the lesion, and previous treatments for it. A complete review of systems is appropriate to identify symptoms of locally advanced disease (such as urinary obstruction), regional spread (such as lower extremity edema), and distant or advanced disease (such as constitutional symptoms).

The aims of the physical examination are to determine the need for biopsy, the local extent of disease, and the extent of spread. The physician should document the site of the lesion and describe its characteristics, including size, configuration (ulcerative, flat, warty, or exophytic), and a clinical assessment of the involvement of adjacent or deep structures (such as the scrotum, corporal bodies, urethra, pubic bone, and prostate).

A short trial of topical treatment for superficial, inflammatory-appearing lesions is acceptable, but prompt follow-up and further evaluation for incompletely treated lesions is imperative.

Ultimately, as stated in the European Association of Urology (EAU) guidelines, the AJCC, and the International Union Against Cancer (UICC), punch, excisional, or incisional biopsy is required to make a pathologic diagnosis.[4,33,40] Obtaining a deep biopsy specimen is essential for accurate staging, and thus superficial or shave biopsies are not appropriate.[41] Biopsy is followed by definitive local treatment, either after frozen-section diagnosis or as a separate procedure. In either case, the physician must obtain informed consent from the patient for the full extent of the expected procedure.

CLINICAL STAGING
Primary Tumor

Local extent of disease is determined clinically by physical examination. As described in the previous section, the aim is to document the location and estimate the extent and depth of local involvement. Specifically, the physician should determine whether there is involvement of the corporal bodies, urethra, scrotum, prostate, or pubic bone, because these factors impact the stage and, in turn, the likelihood of lymph node disease and prognosis.

There has been debate regarding the use of imaging for determining the clinical stage of the primary tumor.[42] This topic is covered in detail elsewhere in this issue by Inman. In brief, Lont and colleagues[42] compared physical examination with ultrasonography and magnetic resonance imaging (MRI) for clinical staging of penile cancer. Thirty-

three patients underwent physical examination and both imaging modalities before surgery. The investigators found that physical examination was highly accurate for detecting corpora cavernosa invasion, with a positive predictive value of 100%, sensitivity of 86%, and specificity of 100%. The respective figures were 75%, 100%, and 91% for MRI and a disappointing 67%, 57%, and 91% for ultrasonography. Other investigators have compared MRI with pharmacologically induced erection to physical examination and have found the imaging to add to clinical staging accuracy. For example, Petralia and colleagues[43] found that MRI and pharmacologically induced erection accurately staged 12 of 13 patients, whereas physical examination understaged 3 of 12 and overstaged 2 of 12 patients, for an overall accuracy of 8 of 13. Further studies are required to determine the best method for clinical staging of penile cancer.

Regional Lymph Nodes

Lymph node involvement is a critical component of treatment planning and prognosis. Up to 58% of patients have palpable inguinal lymph nodes at the time of presentation, whereas less than half of these patients have positive lymph nodes at final pathologic examination; other enlarged lymph nodes are caused by inflammatory conditions or infection at the primary site of disease.[9] On the other hand, 15% to 20% of patients with nonpalpable lymph nodes turn out to have disease. Status of the inguinal lymph nodes is ordinarily determined by physical examination augmented by computed tomography (CT) in obese patients or those with a previous inguinal surgery.

Because of the inadequacies of clinical staging of the inguinal lymph nodes, some clinicians have turned to the use of imaging and predictive models to guide management.[44] The roles of ultrasonography, CT, MRI (with and without nanoparticle enhancement), and positron emission tomography (PET) have been investigated.[44–47] Other researchers have investigated fine-needle aspiration (FNA),[48] but so far FNA has a limited role in evaluating lymphadenopathy in men with low-risk disease who otherwise lack indications for lymphadenectomy. Dynamic sentinel lymph node mapping[49] is another option for staging the lymph nodes that is taking hold in some centers of excellence. Each of these alternatives to traditional clinical staging is discussed by other investigators in this issue.

Many investigators have focused on identifying factors that predict positive lymph nodes in men with invasive squamous cell carcinoma of the penis. The aim of such efforts is to identify subclinical lymph node metastases and, perhaps, to avoid the morbidity of lymphadenectomy in men who are unlikely to harbor disease in the lymph nodes. For example, in 2006 Ficarra and colleagues[50] combined several of these factors into a nomogram designed to predict the presence of lymph node metastases based on clinical and tumor characteristics. The nomogram was based on 175 Italian men from 11 centers who underwent partial or total penectomy. Variables predictive of pathologically positive lymph nodes were tumor thickness greater than 5 mm, superficial growth pattern (compared with vertical), high-grade disease, lymphatic tumor embolization, corpora cavernosa invasion, corpus spongiosum invasion, urethral invasion, and clinically positive lymph nodes. The area under the receiver operating characteristic (ROC) curve was 0.876, suggesting excellent accuracy, but this result is yet to be validated in other cohorts. A more recently published nomogram, relying on age, clinical status of the lymph nodes, tumor stage, and grade has an area under the curve of 0.74.[51] Another model, based on 193 cases from Brazil and the United States, combines histologic grade, level of infiltration, and presence of perineural invasion to develop a prognostic index, which correlates with the likelihood of lymph node involvement.[52] Although this model is simpler in requiring fewer features to arrive at the risk group, the investigators did not rely on a standard staging system to categorize tumors with regard to depth of invasion. Furthermore, they assigned values to each feature (eg, 1 for lamina propria invasion, 2 for corpus spongiosum, urethra, or dartos, and 3 for corpus cavernosum or preputial skin) without the use of models to determine their relative contribution to the likelihood of lymph node metastases.

A slightly different approach was taken by Solsona and colleagues[53] in 2001, who developed a risk stratification system based on tumor stage and grade. These investigators used a retrospective series of 66 patients to develop the risk strata and a prospective series of 37 cases to test it. Patients were categorized as low risk (Tis or T1, G1), intermediate risk (T1 G2 or G3, or T2 G1), or high risk (T2 G2, or T2–3 G3). Including both the retrospective and prospective groups, positive lymph nodes were identified in 0 of 32 low-risk patients; 12 of 34 (35%) intermediate-risk patients; and 30 of 37 (81%) high-risk patients. The EAU guidelines adopted a similar risk stratification scheme but defined low risk as Tis, Ta G1–2 or T1 G1, intermediate risk as T1 G2, and high risk as pT2 or higher or G3 tumors.[4] The systems are similar with respect to the categorization of low-risk patients, but the approach adopted by Solsona and colleagues categorizes more patients as intermediate-risk and fewer as high-risk. These 2 systems were compared for their accuracy in predicting the presence of lymph node metastases in a large cohort of Italian patients with penile cancer.[54] The investigators found that each of the systems was an independent predictor of lymph node metastases when controlling for clinical stage of lymph nodes, tumor thickness, and lymphovascular invasion. However, the area under the ROC curve was only 0.632 (95% confidence interval [CI], 0.548–0.715) and 0.697 (95% CI 0.618–0.777) for the risk groups defined by the EAU guidelines and Solsona and colleagues, respectively, suggesting that both schemes are about equivalent but neither of them have high accuracy in predicting lymph node involvement.

In addition to grade and stage, individual factors that have been shown to be associated with the likelihood of lymph node involvement include lymphovascular invasion (embolization), perineural invasion, depth of tumor invasion, structures involved (ie, difference between urethral, corpus spongiosum, and corpora cavernosa invasion), size of the tumor, anatomic location, pattern of growth (superficial spreading vs vertical, and so forth), front of invasion (infiltrative vs pushing),

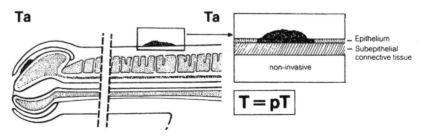

Fig. 1. Ta: noninvasive verrucous carcinoma. (*From* American Joint Committee on Cancer (AJCC). AJCC Cancer staging manual. 7th edition. Springer Science + Business Media LLC; 2010. Used with the permission of the American Joint Committee on Cancer (AJCC), Chicago, Illinois. The original source for this material is the AJCC Cancer Staging Manual, Seventh Edition (2010) published by Springer-Verlag New York, www.springer.com.)

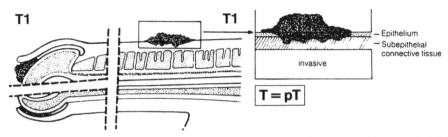

Fig. 2. T1: tumor invading subepithelial connective tissue; T1a: no vascular invasion and not poorly differentiated; T1b: high grade and/or poorly differentiated. (*From* American Joint Committee on Cancer (AJCC). AJCC Cancer staging manual. 7th edition. Springer Science + Business Media LLC; 2010. Used with the permission of the American Joint Committee on Cancer (AJCC), Chicago, Illinois. The original source for this material is the AJCC Cancer Staging Manual, Seventh Edition (2010) published by Springer-Verlag New York, www.springer.com.)

histologic subtype, percentage of poorly differentiated tumor, positive surgical margin, and palpable inguinal lymph nodes.[34,35,51,55–61] Genetic and molecular markers are also being investigated for this purpose.[62,63] Further studies are needed to determine the pathologic, genetic, and molecular markers that would be most valuable in predicting lymph node involvement. It should be emphasized that the use of predictive factors and prognostic models should be based on the final pathologic tumor specimen rather than on the result of a biopsy, because the biopsy can underestimate the depth of invasion and miss other key features of the tumor.[41]

Distant Metastases

Distant spread should be ruled out with chest radiograph and CT of the abdomen and pelvis in patients with pathologic risk factors for lymph node involvement or palpable lymph nodes. The EAU guidelines support the use of cross-sectional imaging only in patients with palpable lymph nodes.[4] However, cross-sectional imaging also has a role in patients in whom an inguinal examination is compromised (obese patients and those with previous inguinal surgery). It also may be important in patients with nonpalpable lymph nodes who have indications for lymphadenectomy. Although it could be argued that these patients would be staged surgically at the time of lymphadenectomy, preoperative evaluation of the pelvic lymph nodes with CT could guide the use of multimodal therapy, just as in patients with palpable lymph nodes. Staging should also include blood tests such as a complete blood count and comprehensive metabolic panel, and coagulation studies should be performed before any biopsy or intervention. Bone scan is performed in selected situations, such as bone pain, elevated alkaline phosphatase or serum calcium levels, or advanced disease.

STAGING SYSTEM

The aim of pathologic staging in penile carcinoma, or any cancer, is to provide standardized information to the patient, the clinician, and the researcher regarding the likelihood of disease recurrence, disease progression, and death from disease. As such, the staging system is designed to capture the best available prognostic information from the pathology report, and thus, staging systems evolve as new predictors of outcome are identified. In the newest AJCC staging manual, the

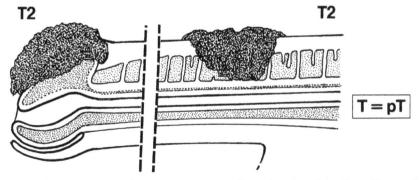

Fig. 3. T2: tumor invading corpus spongiosum or cavernosum. (*From* American Joint Committee on Cancer (AJCC). AJCC Cancer staging manual. 7th edition. Springer Science + Business Media LLC; 2010. Used with the permission of the American Joint Committee on Cancer (AJCC), Chicago, Illinois. The original source for this material is the AJCC Cancer Staging Manual, Seventh Edition (2010) published by Springer-Verlag New York, www.springer.com.)

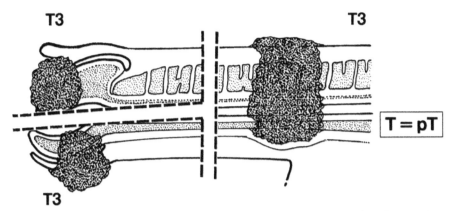

Fig. 4. T3: tumor invading urethra. (*From* American Joint Committee on Cancer (AJCC). AJCC Cancer staging manual. 7th edition. Springer Science + Business Media LLC; 2010. Used with the permission of the American Joint Committee on Cancer (AJCC), Chicago, Illinois. The original source for this material is the AJCC Cancer Staging Manual, Seventh Edition (2010) published by Springer-Verlag New York, www.springer.com.)

editors and investigators have made an effort to incorporate nonanatomic prognostic factors into the traditional TNM model.[33] A new edition of the UICC-TNM classification of malignant tumors has also been published recently and is virtually identical to the AJCC.[40]

The current staging system from AJCC is depicted in **Figs. 1–5** and **Tables 1** and **2**. The most notable change from the previous version is the substratification of T1 tumors into T1a and T1b, accounting for the influence of high-grade disease and lymphovascular invasion on outcome in patients with low-stage disease. With this change, T1b N0M0 is now included in stage II, along with T2–3 N0M0. In the previous (sixth) edition of the AJCC staging manual, both prostatic invasion and urethral invasion were considered T3, whereas in the current system only urethral invasion is considered T3, and prostatic invasion is

now considered T4 along with invasion of other adjacent structures. In addition, the AJCC now allows for separate designations for clinical and pathologic nodal staging. Finally, the AJCC has minimized the distinction between superficial and deep inguinal lymph nodes because there is no good evidence that these have different prognostic significance.

The AJCC did not separate corpus spongiosum invasion from corpora cavernosa invasion, as some have suggested, leaving both as T2 disease. Whereas most studies support grouping these 2 entities together,[64] others have found a higher rate of lymph node metastasis in corpus cavernosum invasion than in corpus spongiosum invasion (62% vs 36% in a recent series of 193 cases) and have suggested a new scheme for classifying the level of tumor invasion.[52,65] The AJCC seventh edition continued to define urethral invasion as

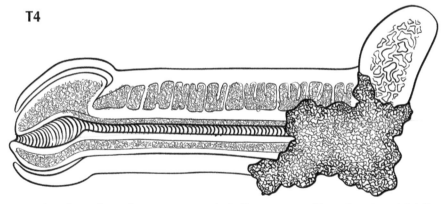

Fig. 5. T4: tumor invading other adjacent structures including prostate. (*From* American Joint Committee on Cancer (AJCC). AJCC Cancer staging manual. 7th edition. Springer Science + Business Media LLC; 2010. Used with the permission of the American Joint Committee on Cancer (AJCC), Chicago, Illinois. The original source for this material is the AJCC Cancer Staging Manual, Seventh Edition (2010) published by Springer-Verlag New York, www.springer.com.)

Table 1
Definitions of TNM

Primary Tumor (T)	
TX	Primary tumor cannot be assessed
T0	No evidence of primary tumor
Tis	Carcinoma in situ
Ta	Noninvasive verrucous carcinoma[a]
T1a	Tumor invades subepithelial connective tissue without LVI and is not poorly differentiated (ie, G3–4)
T1b	Tumor invades subepithelial connective tissue with LVI or is poorly differentiated
T2	Tumor invades corpus spongiosum or cavernosum
T3	Tumor invades urethra
T4	Tumor invades other adjacent structures

Regional Lymph Nodes (N)		
	Clinical Stage Definition	Pathologic Stage Definition
NX	Regional lymph nodes cannot be assessed	Regional lymph nodes cannot be assessed
N0	No palpable or visibly enlarged inguinal lymph nodes	No regional lymph node metastasis
N1	Palpable mobile unilateral inguinal lymph node	Metastasis in a single inguinal lymph node
N2	Palpable mobile multiple or bilateral inguinal lymph nodes	Metastasis in multiple or bilateral inguinal lymph nodes
N3	Palpable fixed inguinal nodal mass or pelvic lymphadenopathy unilateral or bilateral	Extranodal extension of lymph node metastasis or pelvic lymph node or lymph nodes unilateral or bilateral

Distant Metastasis (M)	
M0	No distant metastasis
M1	Distant metastasis[b]

Abbreviation: LVI, lymphovascular invasion.

[a] Broad pushing penetration (invasion) is permitted—destructive invasion is against this diagnosis. Clinical stage based on palpation and imaging; pathologic stage based on biopsy or surgical excision.

[b] Lymph node metastasis outside the true pelvis in addition to visceral or bone sites.

Table 2
Anatomic stage and prognostic groups

Stage	Group		
	T	N	M
Stage 0	Tis	N0	M0
	Ta	N0	M0
Stage I	T1a	N0	M0
Stage II	T1b	N0	M0
	T2	N0	M0
	T3	N0	M0
Stage IIIa	T1–3	N1	M0
Stage IIIb	T1–3	N2	M0
Stage IV	T4	Any N	M0
Any T	Any T	N3	M0
Any T	Any T	Any N	M1

T3 disease, despite the absence of a separate category in Cubilla's proposed system.[55]

The AJCC calls for a 4-tier grading system for tumors: G1, well differentiated; G2, moderately differentiated; G3, poorly differentiated; and G4, undifferentiated. The AJCC also recommends collection of additional prognostic factors that have been shown to be clinically significant and may affect outcome. These site-specific factors that are to be collected include: (1) the distinction between corpus spongiosum and corpus cavernosum involvement, (2) the percentage of tumor that is poorly differentiated, (3) the depth of invasion in verrucous carcinoma, (4) the size of the largest lymph node metastasis, and (5) HPV status. As mentioned in the previous section, there are other individual prognostic factors that are useful in predicting positive inguinal lymph nodes. Some of these also predict tumor recurrence and survival.

Table 3
Look-up table for individual prediction of 5-year CSM after surgical treatment of penile cancer according to stage and grade strata

Grade	Localized % 5-y CSM (95% CI)	Regional% 5-y CSM (95% CI)	Metastatic % 5-y CSM (95% CI)
1: well differentiated	6.5 (2.1–10.9)	22.2 (6.2–38.2)	–
2: moderately differentiated	19.4 (13.7–25.5)	54.6 (43.5–66.2)	–
3, 4: poorly differentiated or undifferentiated	34.4 (20.0–47.6)	54.7 (40.6–70.2)	67.8 (41.7–100)

Note: metastatic G1 and G2 5-year CSM could not be calculated because 1 patient and 8 patients were included in these 2 categories, respectively. The look-up table was developed within the cohort of 856 patients. The predictions of the look-up table were 73.8% accurate after internal validation. Point estimates are accompanied by their 95% confidence interval (CI).
Abbreviation: CSM, cancer-specific mortality.
Reprinted from Zini L, Cloutier V, Isbarn H, et al. A simple and accurate model for prediction of cancer-specific mortality in patients treated with surgery for primary penile squamous cell carcinoma. Clin Cancer Res 2009;15:1013; with permission.

Bilateral inguinal nodal metastasis, extranodal tumor extension, pelvic and iliac nodal involvement,[10,66] and lymph node density[67] are additional factors that are associated with outcome and are only ascertained in the final pathologic examination. In the United States, data describing these factors are recorded by the cancer registrars. For example, in a study of 49 patients with involvement of lymph node, Svatek and colleagues[67] found that the 5-year disease-specific survival was significantly higher in patients with lymph node density at or below the median (6.7%) than in patients with a lymph node density above the median (91.7% [95% CI, 53.9–98.8] vs 23.3% [95% CI, 7.0–45.1], $P<.001$).

Again, some researchers have used such individual prognostic factors in combination to develop predictive models or nomograms to predict disease recurrence after initial treatment and cause-specific survival.[8,68,69] For example, Kattan and colleagues[68] developed a nomogram based on 175 Italian patients who were treated for penile cancer. The nomogram created by Kattan and colleagues incorporates tumor thickness ($\leq$5 mm vs >5 mm), growth pattern (superficial vs vertical), grade, presence of lymphovascular invasion (embolization), presence of corpora cavernosa invasion, presence of corpus spongiosum invasion, and urethral invasion and nodal status to predict cancer-specific survival.[68] The area under the ROC curve was 0.747, indicating fair predictive value. This nomogram needs to be externally validated. Zini and colleagues[69] evaluated the surveillance epidemiology and end results (SEER) database, and found that categorizing patients with respect to pathologic grade and stage (local vs regional vs metastatic) predicted 5-year

cancer-specific mortality with approximately 74% accuracy in the internal validation cohort (**Table 3**).

SUMMARY

Invasive squamous cell carcinoma of the penis is an aggressive, lethal disease that often presents after substantial delay. All penile lesions must be evaluated promptly and thoroughly, and must be biopsied adequately if local treatment is not successful within a short period of time. Accurate staging with respect to local disease, regional lymph nodes, and metastatic disease is critical for risk stratification and treatment planning. Prognostic models can help the clinician predict the likelihood of lymph node metastases based on clinical factors, and predict the survival outcome from pathologic factors.

REFERENCES

1. Jemal A, Siegel R, Ward E, et al. Cancer statistics, 2009. CA Cancer J Clin 2009;59:225.
2. Hernandez BY, Barnholtz-Sloan J, German RR, et al. Burden of invasive squamous cell carcinoma of the penis in the United States, 1998–2003. Cancer 2008;113:2883.
3. Mobilio G, Ficarra V. Genital treatment of penile carcinoma. Curr Opin Urol 2001;11:299.
4. Solsona E, Algaba F, Horenblas S, et al. EAU guidelines on penile cancer. Eur Urol 2004;46:1.
5. Rippentrop JM, Joslyn SA, Konety B. Squamous cell carcinoma of the penis: evaluation of data from the surveillance, epidemiology, and end results program. Cancer 2004;101:1357.
6. Horenblas S. Lymphadenectomy for squamous cell carcinoma of the penis. Part 2: the role and

technique of lymph node dissection. BJU Int 2001; 88:473.

7. Lopes A, Bezerra AL, Serrano SV, et al. Iliac nodal metastases from carcinoma of the penis treated surgically. BJU Int 2000;86:690.

8. Novara G, Galfano A, De Marco V, et al. Prognostic factors in squamous cell carcinoma of the penis. Nat Clin Pract Urol 2007;4:140.

9. Ornellas AA, Seixas AL, Marota A, et al. Surgical treatment of invasive squamous cell carcinoma of the penis: retrospective analysis of 350 cases. J Urol 1994;151:1244.

10. Ravi R. Correlation between the extent of nodal involvement and survival following groin dissection for carcinoma of the penis. Br J Urol 1993;72:817.

11. Madsen B, Van Den Brule A, Jensen H, et al. Risk factors for squamous cell carcinoma of the penis—population-based case-control study in Denmark. Cancer Epidemiol Biomarkers Prev 2008;17:2683.

12. Maden C, Sherman KJ, Beckmann AM, et al. History of circumcision, medical conditions, and sexual activity and risk of penile cancer. J Natl Cancer Inst 1993;85:19.

13. Schoen EJ, Oehrli M, Colby C, et al. The highly protective effect of newborn circumcision against invasive penile cancer. Pediatrics 2000;105:E36.

14. Dillner J, von Krogh G, Horenblas S, et al. Etiology of squamous cell carcinoma of the penis. Scand J Urol Nephrol Suppl 2000;189.

15. Huben RP, Sufrin G. Benign and malignant lesions of the penis. In: Gillenwater JY, Grayhack JT, Howards SS, et al, editors. Adult and pediatric urology. 2nd edition. St. Louis (MO): Mosby; 1991. p. 1643.

16. Reddy CR, Devendranath V, Pratap S. Carcinoma of penis—role of phimosis. Urology 1984;24:85.

17. Miralles-Guri C, Bruni L, Cubilla AL, et al. Human papillomavirus prevalence and type distribution in penile carcinoma. J Clin Pathol 2009;62:870.

18. Boxer RJ, Skinner DG. Condylomata acuminata and squamous cell carcinoma. Urology 1977;9:72.

19. Smotkin D. Virology of human papillomavirus. Clin Obstet Gynecol 1989;32:117.

20. Wiener JS, Walther PJ. The association of oncogenic human papillomaviruses with urologic malignancy. The controversies and clinical implications. Surg Oncol Clin N Am 1995;4:257.

21. Engels EA, Pfeiffer RM, Goedert JJ, et al. Trends in cancer risk among people with AIDS in the United States 1980-2002. AIDS 2006;20:1645.

22. Daling JR, Madeleine MM, Johnson LG, et al. Penile cancer: importance of circumcision, human papillomavirus and smoking in in situ and invasive disease. Int J Cancer 2005;116:606.

23. Harish K, Ravi R. The role of tobacco in penile carcinoma. Br J Urol 1995;75:375.

24. Stern RS. Genital tumors among men with psoriasis exposed to psoralens and ultraviolet A radiation (PUVA) and ultraviolet B radiation. The photochemotherapy follow-up study. N Engl J Med 1990; 322:1093.

25. Depasquale I, Park AJ, Bracka A. The treatment of balanitis xerotica obliterans. BJU Int 2000;86:459.

26. Micali G, Nasca MR, Innocenzi D, et al. Penile cancer. J Am Acad Dermatol 2006;54:369.

27. Favorito LA, Nardi AC, Ronalsa M, et al. Epidemiologic study on penile cancer in Brazil. Int Braz J Urol 2008;34:587.

28. Burgers JK, Badalament RA, Drago JR. Penile cancer. Clinical presentation, diagnosis, and staging. Urol Clin North Am 1992;19:247.

29. Gursel EO, Georgountzos C, Uson AC, et al. Penile cancer. Urology 1973;1:569.

30. Hardner GJ, Bhanalaph T, Murphy GP, et al. Carcinoma of the penis: analysis of therapy in 100 consecutive cases. J Urol 1972;108:428.

31. Lynch HT, Krush AJ. Delay factors in detection of cancer of the penis. Nebr State Med J 1969;54:360.

32. Narayana AS, Olney LE, Loening SA, et al. Carcinoma of the penis: analysis of 219 cases. Cancer 1982;49:2185.

33. American Joint Committee on Cancer. Penis. In: Edge SB, Byrd DR, Compton CC, et al, editors. AJCC cancer staging manual. 7th edition. New York: Springer; 2010. p. 447.

34. Cubilla AL, Reuter V, Velazquez E, et al. Histologic classification of penile carcinoma and its relation to outcome in 61 patients with primary resection. Int J Surg Pathol 2001;9:111.

35. Guimarães GC, Cunha IW, Soares FA, et al. Penile squamous cell carcinoma clinicopathological features, nodal metastasis and outcome in 333 cases. J Urol 2009;182:528.

36. Masih AS, Stoler MH, Farrow GM, et al. Penile verrucous carcinoma: a clinicopathologic, human papillomavirus typing and flow cytometric analysis. Mod Pathol 1992;5:48.

37. McKee PH, Lowe D, Haigh RJ. Penile verrucous carcinoma. Histopathology 1983;7:897.

38. Seixas AL, Ornellas AA, Marota A, et al. Verrucous carcinoma of the penis: retrospective analysis of 32 cases. J Urol 1994;152:1476.

39. Velazquez EF, Melamed J, Barreto JE, et al. Sarcomatoid carcinoma of the penis: a clinicopathologic study of 15 cases. Am J Surg Pathol 2005; 29:1152.

40. International Union Against Cancer (UICC). Penis. In: Sobin LH, Gospodarowicz MK, Wittekind C, editors. TNM classification of malignant tumours. 7th edition. Chichester, West Sussex (UK): Wiley-Blackwell; 2009. p. 239.

41. Velazquez EF, Barreto JE, Rodriguez I, et al. Limitations in the interpretation of biopsies in patients with penile squamous cell carcinoma. Int J Surg Pathol 2004;12:139.

42. Lont AP, Besnard AP, Gallee MP, et al. A comparison of physical examination and imaging in determining the extent of primary penile carcinoma. BJU Int 2003;91:493.

43. Petralia G, Villa G, Scardino E, et al. Local staging of penile cancer using magnetic resonance imaging with pharmacologically induced penile erection. Radiol Med 2008;113:517.

44. Singh AK, Saokar A, Hahn PF, et al. Imaging of penile neoplasms. Radiographics 2005;25:1629.

45. Graafland NM, Leijte JA, Valdés Olmos RA, et al. Scanning with ^{18}F-FDG-PET/CT for detection of pelvic nodal involvement in inguinal node-positive penile carcinoma. Eur Urol 2009;56:339.

46. Kochhar R, Taylor B, Sangar V. Imaging in primary penile cancer: current status and future directions. Eur Radiol 2010;20:36.

47. Krishna RP, Sistla SC, Smile R, et al. Sonography: an underutilized diagnostic tool in the assessment of metastatic groin nodes. J Clin Ultrasound 2008; 36:212.

48. Saisorn I, Lawrentschuk N, Leewansangtong S, et al. Fine-needle aspiration cytology predicts inguinal lymph node metastasis without antibiotic pretreatment in penile carcinoma. BJU Int 2006;97:1225.

49. Spiess PE, Izawa JI, Bassett R, et al. Preoperative lymphoscintigraphy and dynamic sentinel node biopsy for staging penile cancer: results with pathological correlation. J Urol 2007;177:2157.

50. Ficarra V, Zattoni F, Artibani W, et al. Nomogram predictive of pathological inguinal lymph node involvement in patients with squamous cell carcinoma of the penis. J Urol 2006;175:1700.

51. Bhagat S, Gopalakrishnan G, Kekre N, et al. Factors predicting inguinal node metastasis in squamous cell cancer of penis. World J Urol 2010;28(1):93–8.

52. Chaux A, Caballero C, Soares F, et al. The prognostic index: a useful pathologic guide for prediction of nodal metastases and survival in penile squamous cell carcinoma. Am J Surg Pathol 2009;33(7):1049–57.

53. Solsona E, Iborra I, Rubio J, et al. Prospective validation of the association of local tumor stage and grade as a predictive factor for occult lymph node micrometastasis in patients with penile carcinoma and clinically negative inguinal lymph nodes. J Urol 2001;165:1506.

54. Novara G, Artibani W, Cunico SC, et al. How accurately do Solsona and European Association of Urology risk groups predict for risk of lymph node metastases in patients with squamous cell carcinoma of the penis? Urology 2008;71:328.

55. Cubilla AL. The role of pathologic prognostic factors in squamous cell carcinoma of the penis. World J Urol 2009;27:169.

56. Dai B, Ye DW, Kong YY, et al. Predicting regional lymph node metastasis in Chinese patients with penile squamous cell carcinoma: the role of histopathological classification, tumor stage and depth of invasion. J Urol 2006;176:1431.

57. Fraley EE, Zhang G, Manivel C, et al. The role of ilioinguinal lymphadenectomy and significance of histological differentiation in treatment of carcinoma of the penis. J Urol 1989;142:1478.

58. Lopes A, Hidalgo GS, Kowalski LP, et al. Prognostic factors in carcinoma of the penis: multivariate analysis of 145 patients treated with amputation and lymphadenectomy. J Urol 1996;156:1637.

59. McDougal WS. Carcinoma of the penis: improved survival by early regional lymphadenectomy based on the histological grade and depth of invasion of the primary lesion. J Urol 1995;154:1364.

60. Slaton JW, Morgenstern N, Levy DA, et al. Tumor stage, vascular invasion and the percentage of poorly differentiated cancer: independent prognosticators for inguinal lymph node metastasis in penile squamous cancer. J Urol 2001;165:1138.

61. Velazquez EF, Ayala G, Liu H, et al. Histologic grade and perineural invasion are more important than tumor thickness as predictor of nodal metastasis in penile squamous cell carcinoma invading 5 to 10 mm. Am J Surg Pathol 2008; 32:974.

62. Kayes O, Ahmed H, Arya M, et al. Molecular and genetic pathways in penile cancer. Lancet Oncol 2007;8:420.

63. Kroon BK, Leijte JA, van Boven H, et al. Microarray gene-expression profiling to predict lymph node metastasis in penile carcinoma. BJU Int 2008;102:510.

64. Ficarra V, Martignoni G, Maffei N, et al. Predictive pathological factors of lymph nodes involvement in the squamous cell carcinoma of the penis. Int Urol Nephrol 2002;34:245.

65. Cubilla AL, Piris A, Pfannl R, et al. Anatomic levels: important landmarks in penectomy specimens: a detailed anatomic and histologic study based on examination of 44 cases. Am J Surg Pathol 2001; 25:1091.

66. Srinivas V, Morse MJ, Herr HW, et al. Penile cancer: relation of extent of nodal metastasis to survival. J Urol 1987;137:880.

67. Svatek RS, Munsell M, Kincaid JM, et al. Association between lymph node density and disease specific survival in patients with penile cancer. J Urol 2009; 182:2721.

68. Kattan MW, Ficarra V, Artibani W, et al. Nomogram predictive of cancer specific survival in patients undergoing partial or total amputation for squamous cell carcinoma of the penis. J Urol 2006;175:2103.

69. Zini L, Cloutier V, Isbarn H, et al. A simple and accurate model for prediction of cancer-specific mortality in patients treated with surgery for primary penile squamous cell carcinoma. Clin Cancer Res 2009; 15:1013.

Imaging Tumors of the Penis and Urethra

Suzanne Biehn Stewart, MD[a], Richard A. Leder, MD[b],
Brant A. Inman, MD[c],*

KEYWORDS

- Penile cancer • Urethral cancer
- Imaging • Radiology • Staging

Although penile and urethral carcinomas represent less than 1% of all malignancies in North America,[1] imaging is of vital importance in their management, because therapeutic decisions depend on accurate determination of clinical stage.

PRESENT STAGING SYSTEMS

The 2010 TNM staging system proposed by the American Joint Committee on Cancer is the staging system of choice for penile and urethral cancers (**Table 1**).[2] For both sites, the T stage is defined by the depth of tumor invasion, the N stage by the number and/or size of cancer-affected lymph nodes, and the M stage by the presence of distant metastases. Unique to urethral cancer, a second substaging system exists for urothelial carcinoma (UC) of the prostatic urethra (see **Table 1**) because its histologic findings, prognosis, and management are distinct. Arriving at the correct clinical TNM stage involves integrating physical examination, imaging, and biopsy findings, a process that is not always obvious. For example, determining whether regional inguinal lymph nodes are enlarged and, if so, whether the cause is cancer or infection/inflammation can be difficult.[3]

IMAGING OF THE PRIMARY TUMOR
Retrograde Urethrography and Voiding Cystourethrography

Before computed tomography (CT) and magnetic resonance imaging (MRI), retrograde urethrography (RUG) and voiding cystourethrography (VCUG) were considered the cornerstones for defining and staging urethral tumors.[4] In men, RUG was commonly used for evaluation of the anterior urethra and VCUG was the preferred modality for the posterior aspect. In women, VCUG was the preferred modality.[5,6] Common signs of urethral cancer on RUG include narrowing of the urethral lumen, irregular margins with extravasation, filling defects, and obstructive changes.[6] Multiple small mucosal nodules seen after instrumentation or cystectomy may represent UC implants in the urethra.[7] Double-contrast RUG, a technique combining air and contrast dye, may improve the visualization of small distal urethral lesions.[4,8]

Although RUG and VCUG delineate intraluminal defects quite well, their capacity to stage tumors is limited because they are unable to determine the extent of local tissue invasion, such as tumor growth into the corpus spongiosum or cavernosum (**Fig. 1**A, B). If the

No financial disclosures.
[a] Division of Urology, Department of Surgery, Duke University Medical Center, Box 2922, Durham, NC 27710, USA
[b] Department of Radiology, Duke University Medical Center, Box 3808, Durham, NC 27710, USA
[c] Division of Urology, Department of Surgery, Duke University Medical Center, Box 2812, Durham, NC 27710, USA
* Corresponding author.
E-mail address: brant.inman@duke.edu

urologic.theclinics.com

Table 1
The 2010 TNM staging system for urethral and penile cancer

	Penile Cancer	Urethral Cancer	UC of the Prostate
T stage			
Tx	Tumor cannot be assessed	Tumor cannot be assessed	Tumor cannot be assessed
Tis	CIS	CIS	CIS of prostatic urethra; CIS of prostatic ducts
Ta	Noninvasive carcinoma	Noninvasive carcinoma	—
T1	Lamina propria invasion	Lamina propria invasion	Lamina propria invasion
T1a	Lamina propria invasion: low grade and no LVI	—	—
T1b	Lamina propria invasion: high grade or LVI present	—	—
T2	Invasion of corpus spongiosum or corpus cavernosum	Invasion of spongiosum, prostate, or periurethral muscle	Invasion of spongiosum, prostate, or periurethral muscle
T3	Invasion of urethra	Invasion of cavernosum, vagina, or bladder neck	Extraprostatic extension (cavernosum, bladder neck, prostate capsule)
T4	Invasion of adjacent structures	Invasion of adjacent structures	Invasion of adjacent structures (eg, bladder)
N stage			
N0	All regional nodes are negative	All regional nodes are negative	All regional nodes are negative
N1	Single positive inguinal node	Single positive node <2 cm	Single positive node <2 cm
N2	Multiple positive inguinal nodes	Single positive node >2 cm or multiple nodes	Single positive node >2 cm or multiple nodes
N3	Extranodal tumor extension or positive pelvic nodes	—	—
M stage			
M0	No metastases	No metastases	No metastases
M1	Distant metastases	Distant metastases	Distant metastases

Abbreviations: CIS, carcinoma in situ; LVI, lymphovascular invasion; UC, urothelial carcinoma.

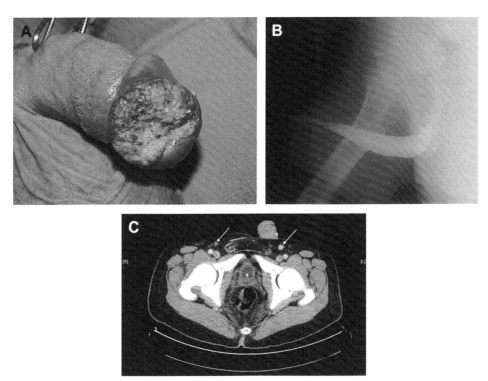

Fig. 1. Squamous cell carcinoma of the penis, stage pT3N0M0. (*A*) Clinical photograph. (*B*) RUG performed for obstructive urinary symptoms. A distal urethral stricture is identified and was biopsy proven to represent lichen sclerosis. Study did not aid in local staging. (*C*) Pelvic CT scan showing suspicious inguinal nodes identified by size criteria, which were negative by delayed inguinal lymph node dissection.

periurethral tissues cannot be imaged then a T stage cannot be determined. RUG and VCUG may also prove technically challenging if a high degree of urethral obstruction is present.[4,9,10] At present, cystourethroscopy has largely replaced RUG and VCUG in the evaluation of known urethral cancers because it allows for visualization and biopsy of lesions in 1 setting. However, RUG remains an important imaging modality for urethral stricture disease, and because roughly 50% of patients with urethral cancer have a history of urethral stricture, unusual findings on RUG obtained for urethral stricture should prompt evaluation for urethral cancer.[11]

Cavernosography

The injection of contrast media directly into the corpora cavernosa may show filling defects suggestive of tumoral invasion.[4,12] Raghavaiah[13] preformed preoperative cavernosography on 10 patients with penile cancer and found that it successfully staged patients when compared with pathologic examination. Cavernosography has also identified multifocal filling defects consistent with metastases.[14,15] At present,

cavernosography is not an imaging modality that is recommended for the evaluation of penile carcinoma because it is limited in its ability to evaluate tumor beyond the corporal bodies, and other imaging modalities that are more precise are available.

Ultrasonography

Although significant variation exists, squamous cell carcinoma of the penis most commonly presents as a heterogenous hypoechoic lesion on ultrasonography (US).[16–18] Agrawal and colleagues[16] found that of 59 patients with penile cancer, 36% had hyperechoic lesions, 47% had hypoechoic lesions, and 17% had lesions of mixed echogenicity. No association was found between echogenicity and tumor morphology or grade. A major benefit of US is that it can identify specific penile tissue planes, including the tunica albuginea, corpus cavernosum, corpus spongiosum, and urethra.[17,18] Delineation of tumor involvement with structures at the glans penis is more difficult. Horenblas and colleagues[18] found that US was not able to differentiate between subepithelial and spongiosal invasion at the glans. Despite this shortcoming, US was found to enhance the accuracy of clinical staging of local tumor extension (T). In the 2004 European Association of Urology (EAU) guidelines on penile cancer, penile US was deemed the initial diagnostic modality of choice to assist physical examination in determining the depth of tumor penetration, particularly if cavernosal invasion is suspected.[19]

Although US has not been evaluated as an imaging modality for urethral cancer, it has been used to evaluate urethral strictures. Some groups have found US superior to alternative imaging modalities for identifying the number, length, depth, and overall severity of strictures.[20,21] US can also demonstrate involvement of the corpus spongiosum, something that RUG cannot reliably identify.[4] Case reports also suggest that transvaginal US can be helpful in distinguishing urethral tumors from other urethral pathologic conditions such as urethral diverticulae.[22] The authors have found pelvic US to correctly identify a large urethral tumor in a woman complaining of pelvic pain (**Fig. 2**A). Similarly, transrectal US has been used to stage and biopsy UCs of the prostatic urethra. Invasion of the prostatic stroma, ejaculatory ducts, or periprostatic tissue by a hypoechoic tumor can be seen on transrectal US.[23,24]

Strengths of US include low cost, noninvasiveness, and the lack of ionizing radiation. Limitations include operator dependence, inability to assess tumor spread beyond the penis, and the inability to adequately stage lesions of the glans.[5,10,17]

CT and Positron Emission Tomography

With the advent of helical scanning and multiplanar reconstruction, multidimensional high-resolution CT is now possible. However, modern high-resolution CT still does not aid in adequate visualization of penile tissue planes and is therefore not considered an imaging modality of choice for evaluating the T stage of penile and urethral cancers (**Fig. 3**).[4,6,9,25] More recently, the fusion of CT and positron emission tomographic (PET) scanning has allowed functional and anatomic imaging to be combined in a single modality. At present, there are very little data published regarding PET combined with CT (PET/CT) in penile or urethral cancer. One small study of 13 patients with penile cancer found that PET/CT had a sensitivity and specificity of 75% for detecting primary penile tumors.[26] However, PET/CT remains no better than conventional CT in determining T stage because PET/CT continues to be similarly limited by poor soft tissue discrimination (**Fig. 4**A, B).

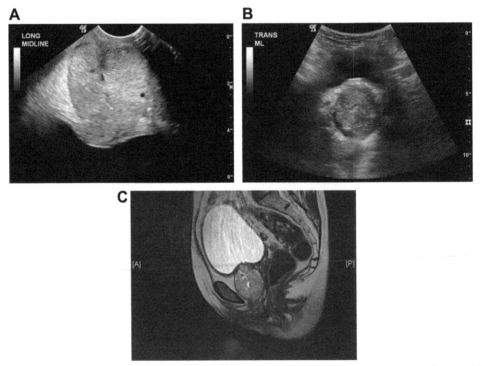

Fig. 2. UC of the female urethra, stage pT2N2M1. (*A*) Pelvic US showing large echogenic mass below the bladder. Extent of local tissue invasion or evidence of lymph node invasion was unable to be identified. (*B*) MRI scan, sagittal/coronal view.

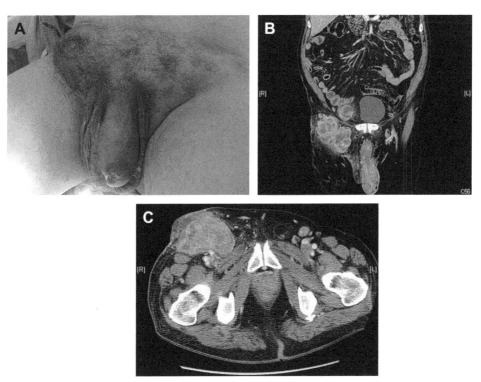

Fig. 3. Squamous cell carcinoma of the penis, stage pT3N3M0. (*A*) Clinical photograph. (*B*) CT scan, coronal view. Soft tissue mass involving distal tip of the penis causing severe distortion of normal penile anatomy. Pockets of gas within the mass, suggesting cutaneous extension. Large, heterogenous, enhancing, multilobulated, and septated mass in the right groin with cutaneous extension, suggesting necrotic right inguinal lymphadenopathy. (*C*) CT scan, axial view. Heterogenous enhancing mass in right hemipelvis abutting right external iliac vessels, suggesting pelvic lymphadenopathy.

Magnetic Resonance Imaging

MRI is the most sensitive imaging modality for the local staging of penile and urethral carcinomas. Advantages of MRI include superior soft tissue contrast, better spatial resolution, and lack of ionizing radiation. In addition, MRI provides better assessment of the penile fascial planes than physical examination.

Normal male anatomy

The penis is composed of 3 cylindrical bodies: 2 dorsal corpora cavernosa and a ventral corpus spongiosum. The corpora cavernosa and corpus spongiosum have a slightly higher signal intensity on T1-weighted images that is slightly higher than skeletal muscle. On T2-weighted images all 3 corporal bodies are hyperintense because of blood pooling. The penile bulb (dilated portion of corpus spongiosum where it attaches to the perineal membrane) has a higher T2 signal intensity than the corpora cavernosa because of differences in blood flow. The 3 corporal bodies enhance with gadolinium.[27,28] The corpus spongiosum completely encases the penile portion of the male urethra. On T2-weighted images, urethral smooth muscle appears less intense than the spongiosum.[28]

The corpora of the penis is surrounded by 3 fascial layers.[27–29] Each corpus cavernosum is contained within a layer of tunica albuginea. Buck fascia then wraps around the tunica albuginea and splits ventrally to cover the corpus spongiosum also. Therefore, Buck fascia is the layer that holds all 3 corporal bodies together. The tunica albuginea is not distinguishable from Buck fascia on MRI, and these 2 fascial layers appear jointly as a single low-intensity rim of tissue surrounding the corporal bodies on T1- and T2-weighted images. External to Buck fascia is the dartos fascia, which is also hypointense. A small quantity of fat lies between the Buck and the dartos fasciae and dorsally contains the deep dorsal vein of the penis and the dorsal penile arteries. This fat layer appears hyperintense on T2-weighted image. The cavernosal arteries of the penis are visible on T2-weighted axial images. They appear as 2 low-intensity foci within the dorsal medial third of the corpora cavernosa.

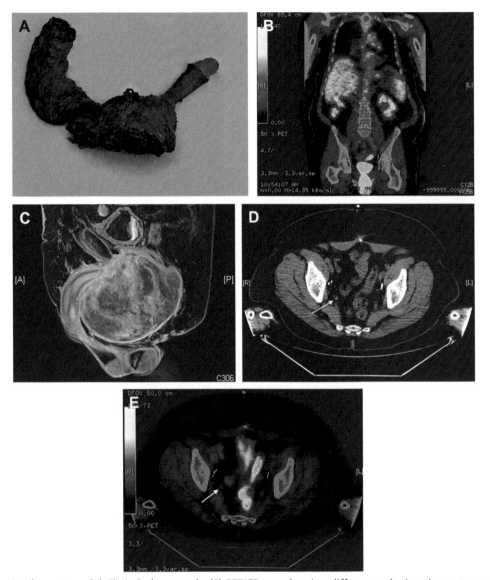

Fig. 4. Penile sarcoma. (*A*) Clinical photograph. (*B*) PET/CT scan showing diffuse uptake in primary tumor. Soft tissue planes to discriminate extent of invasion were unable to be identified. (*C*) MRI scan, sagittal view. Large, enhancing, heterogenous mass extending from the prostatic urethra to the penile urethra, where it infiltrates into the corpus spongiosum. The mass infiltrates the corpus cavernosa bilaterally, with greater involvement on the left side. (*D*) CT scan showing suspicious pelvic lymph node (*arrow*). (*E*) PET/CT scan showing no uptake in pelvic node, suggesting a benign morphology (*arrow*).

Normal female anatomy

The female urethra has a characteristic targetoid appearance on T2-weighted images because of concentric layers of different signal intensity.[30–32] The skeletal muscle of the rhabdosphincter appears as a low-intensity outer ring of tissue (**Fig. 5**). Moving inward, the next ring of tissue is the urethral smooth muscle, which has a higher signal intensity than the rhabdosphincter. The next inner layer represents the submucosa, which has a lower signal intensity. The innermost layer is the urethral mucosa, which is a bright hyperintense ring. The lumen of the urethra is demarcated as a small, dark, central focus.

Urethral tumors

Urethral tumors are typically best seen on sagittal images and present an obvious mass effect. Tumors tend to show a decreased signal intensity relative to that of the surrounding normal corporal tissue on T1- and T2-weighted images (**Fig. 6**).[7,33] In women, the characteristic targetoid appearance

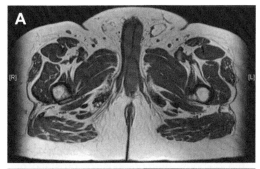

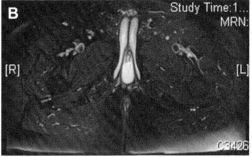

Fig. 5. Hypertrophic female rhabdosphincter mimicking urethral carcinoma. (*A*) MRI scan, axial view. (*B*) MRI scan, sagittal view. Prominent periurethral soft tissue representing the rhabdosphincter, which enhances after contrast administration. Prominent rhabdosphincter tissue indents the base of the bladder.

of the urethra often becomes disrupted (see **Fig. 2B**).[7,10,34] Malignant lesions usually enhance with gadolinium.[10] The accuracy of MRI for staging urethral cancer has been reported to be approximately 75%.[33,34] However, these studies reflect older technology, and newer applications have likely improved the accuracy of MRI. Still, MRI cannot reliably distinguish benign from malignant urethral tumors, and therefore, biopsy remains indicated for urethral masses.

Penile tumors

Penile tumors are best evaluated on T2-weighted images because of the superior contrast resolution between the hypointense fascial layers (Buck fascia and the tunica albuginea) and the adjacent hyperintense corporal bodies. Squamous cell carcinomas typically appear as hypointense lesions when compared with the adjacent corpora.[27–29,35] Although penile cancers enhance with gadolinium, the normal corporal bodies enhance even more, a property that makes contrast enhancement less useful for assessing the local tumor.[29,36]

On MRI, nonsquamous variants of penile cancer can appear different from squamous carcinomas (see **Fig. 4C**). For example, melanoma appears hyperintense on T1- and T2-weighted images and

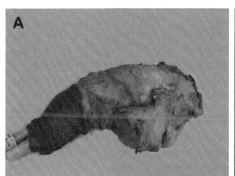

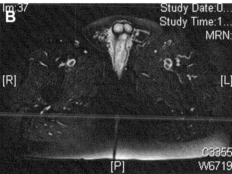

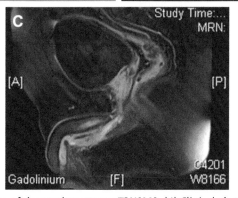

Fig. 6. Squamous cell carcinoma of the urethra, stage pT3N0M0. (*A*) Clinical photograph. (*B*) MRI scan, axial view. (*C*) MRI scan, sagittal view.

enhances much more avidly with gadolinium. Rhabdomyosarcoma of the penis, a tumor more common in pediatric populations, has an intermediate signal intensity on T1-weighted images and a heterogenous high signal intensity on T2-weighted images. This tumor shows heterogeneous enhancement after contrast administration.[28]

Intracavernosal alprostadil

Technical factors can affect the accuracy of MRI for penile and urethral tumors. For example, induction of an artificial erection with an intracavernosal injection of 10 μg of prostaglandin E_1 (alprostadil) may improve the ability of MRI to locally stage penile cancer.[36,37] In the flaccid penis, conventional MRI may have difficulty in distinguishing tumors that are confined to the tunica albuginea from those that invade into the corporal bodies (**Fig. 7**). The corporal bodies may have a low T2 signal intensity due to fibrosis or a transiently reduced blood flow when the penis is flaccid, which can cause the normally sharp interface between the corporal bodies and the tunica albuginea to degrade.[37] The erect penis is a larger imaging target, and its increased blood flow leads to a significantly stronger cavernosal signal intensity and thereby greater contrast from the tunica albuginea. Several reports have suggested better staging accuracy for penile cancer when MRI was combined with intracavernosal alprostadil.[36–38] Because of the potential for increased complications with intracavernosal alprostadil, some groups of investigators reserve its use for situations in which clinical uncertainty remains after imaging the flaccid penis.[27,28]

Endoluminal coils

Conventional MRI of penile and urethral cancers includes the use of a surface radiofrequency coil that is placed over the pelvis. Radiofrequency coils may be positioned in strategic configurations, which are closer to the anatomic location of imaging interest, to improve the signal-to-noise ratio of MRI and thereby produce sharper images.[39] With respect to perineal/pelvic MRI, coils have been developed for placement in the lumina of the rectum,[40,41] vagina,[41–43] and urethra.[44] The use of these endoluminal coils has been reported to improve the ability of MRI to diagnose urethral disease.[45] However, endoluminal coil technology is not standardized and is not available in most medical centers. In addition, endoluminal coil placement can be painful and may be not feasible in cases of large perineal masses.

IMAGING OF LYMPH NODES

One of the most important prognostic elements in staging penile and urethral cancers is the presence and degree of lymph node involvement.[2,46] Physical examination is the initial method used to screen for inguinal lymphadenopathy.[19] Generally, (although not absolutely) the lymphatic drainage from the female anterior urethra and the male penile urethra is to the inguinal lymph nodes, whereas tumors located in the bulbous, membranous, or prostatic male urethra or the female distal urethra tend to drain into the pelvic lymph nodes.[6,9] Whereas the lymphatic drainage from the penile skin and prepuce is to the inguinal nodes, the glans penis and corporal bodies tend to drain into the pelvic lymph nodes.[27,47] Cross-communication of the lymphatics commonly results in bilateral lymphadenopathy even in the presence of unilateral tumors.[19,35]

Approximately 25% of patients with urethral cancer have palpable inguinal lymphadenopathy at presentation and it almost always represents regional nodal metastases.[9,48,49] On the contrary, approximately 50% of patients with penile cancer have palpable inguinal lymphadenopathy at presentation but only half of these lymphadenopathies turn out to be nodal metastases.[19,50,51] An additional 25% of patients with penile cancer with nonpalpable inguinal lymph nodes actually have microscopic nodal metastases, a risk that depends on the stage and grade of the primary neoplasm.[19,52–54] To avoid operating on false-positive inguinal lymphadenopathy, the 2004 EAU consensus guidelines on penile cancer suggest that regional lymph nodes be evaluated several weeks after treatment of the primary lesion. The use of antibiotics for a 2- to 6-week period has been a common practice to help distinguish inflammatory nodal reaction from metastatic disease, although the evidence supporting this practice is sparse.[25,47] Lymph nodes that remain palpable after treatment of the primary penile lesion or after antibiotic therapy have a 90% likelihood of harboring a metastatic focus.[25] Lymphadenectomy is the most reliable method for staging inguinal lymph nodes and is also potentially curative if the nodes harbor cancer.[51,52,55] However, inguinal lymphadenectomy is associated with numerous complications and would ideally be reserved for patients with known nodal metastases.[19,51,55,56] The question therefore arises as to how to proceed in patients with nonpalpable inguinal lymph nodes and whether imaging can aid in ruling out occult nodal metastases and spare such patients the

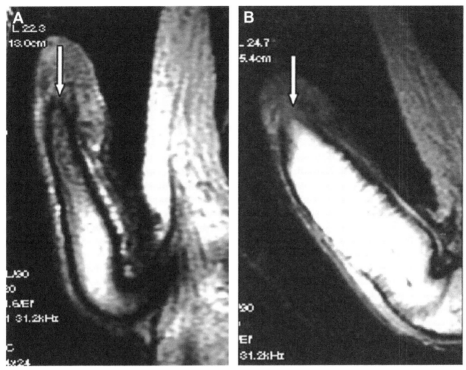

Fig. 7. Sagittal, T2-weighted MRI (*A*) before and (*B*) after penile erection. Tunica albuginea is evident as line of low-signal intensity relative to corpora cavernosa. (*A*) Arrow indicates very small interruption (lesion) of albuginea of corpora cavernosa. (*B*) Interruption is more evident and clearly indicates Stage T2 disease. (*From* Scardino E, Villa G, Bonomo G, et al. Magnetic resonance imaging combined with artificial erection for local staging of penile cancer. Urology 2004;63:1161; with permission.)

risk of inguinal lymphadenectomy. Historically, CT and lymphography were not found to improve clinical staging,[57] but with the advent of newer radiologic techniques the ability of imaging to aid in the clinical staging of penile and urethral cancers has matured.

Ultrasonography

US evaluates lymph nodes based on size, shape, outline, and echogenicity. An additional advantage of high-resolution US is that it is able to detect abnormalities in the architecture of the lymph node such as changes in the cortical contour, increasing thickness of the nodal cortex, and loss of hilar fat.[58,59] Color Doppler can be useful in evaluating changes in lymph node vascularity, with metastatic nodes showing peripheral vascularity and reactive nodes showing a hilar perfusion pattern.[60] A recent report of 64 patients with penile cancer with clinically negative nodes found US to have a sensitivity and specificity of approximately 75%, which is probably inadequate if used without ancillary studies such as fine-needle aspiration (FNA) cytology.[61]

FNA Cytology

FNA cytology is widely used in medicine and has shown excellent results.[62] For example, in patients with vulvar cancer (a tumor analogous to penile cancer), FNA has a sensitivity and specificity of 93% and 100%, respectively.[63] In penile cancer, the results have not been as good. In a study of 83 patients with penile cancer with nonpalpable inguinal nodes, the combination of FNA and US had a sensitivity of approximately 40% and a specificity of 100%.[64] It is likely that these results are because of the dependence of FNA on the identification of nodal structures that are sufficiently enlarged to permit aspiration.

Cross-sectional Imaging

CT and MRI are unable to visualize changes in internal lymph node architecture and are primarily reliant on changes in lymph node size to determine suspicion of metastasis. The use of size criteria to differentiate malignant change in lymph nodes is nonspecific, and, as mentioned earlier, inguinal lymph nodes frequently undergo a reactive inflammatory enlargement in patients with penile cancer (see **Fig. 1**C). As a result, cross-sectional imaging tends to have a high false-positive rate.[65] MRI does have the benefit of using differences in signal intensity to aid detection. Even without nodal enlargement, if the signal intensity is similar to the primary tumor then the lymph node should be considered suspicious for malignancy. In larger nodes, the presence of central necrosis increases the likelihood of metastatic disease (see **Fig. 3**).[35] One advantage of cross-sectional imaging over US is that CT and MRI help in the evaluation of the pelvic lymph nodes and distant sites of metastasis.

PET/CT

PET/CT allows for lymph nodes to be evaluated functionally and morphologically (see **Fig. 4**D, E). Graafland and colleagues[66] evaluated the ability of PET/CT to detect malignant pelvic lymph nodes in 18 patients with penile cancer with cytologically proven inguinal nodal metastases. PET/CT showed a sensitivity of approximately 90% and a specificity of 100%.[66] Although this imaging modality has revealed a high diagnostic accuracy in the setting of known positive inguinal nodes, its spatial resolution is restricted to structures that are larger than 2 mm in size, and this restriction can lead to an occasional false-negative examination.[66]

The diagnostic accuracy of PET/CT drops considerably for the evaluation of occult inguinal metastases in patients with penile cancer. It is in this patient population, with nonpalpable inguinal nodes, that accurate imaging is most needed. In a study of 24 patients, Leijte and colleagues[67] found that PET/CT correctly predicted only 1 out of 5 tumor-bearing groins, reflecting a sensitivity of approximately 20%. All false-negative findings occurred in lymph nodes that were less than 1 cm in size.[67] Although PET/CT was shown to have a specificity of 90%, this study revealed that in patients with nonpalpable inguinal nodes PET/CT does not enhance nodal staging accuracy.

Lymphotropic Nanoparticle-Enhanced MRI

Lymphotropic nanoparticle-enhanced MRI (LNMRI) is a promising noninvasive imaging modality recently introduced for lymph node staging.[68] Lymphotropic nanoparticle contrast agents are composed of ultrasmall particles of iron oxide that are coated with dextran to prevent their aggregation and rapid elimination from the circulation. The nanoparticles are so small that they move freely across the capillary endothelium and are picked up by local lymphatic channels, which then deliver them to the regional lymph nodes. Within normal lymph nodes the nanoparticles are phagocytosed by resident macrophages resulting in iron accumulation in the node. When seen on T2-weighted MRI, normal nodes containing the iron oxide nanoparticles show signal loss (**Fig. 8**). Because of the displacement of normal phagocytes by malignant cells, cancer-bearing nodes have relatively lower iron oxide uptake and as a result show either high or heterogenous signal intensity on T2-weighted images rather than the normal signal loss.[27,47,50]

Tabatabaei and colleagues[69] examined LNMRI in 7 patients with penile cancer, 2 of whom had palpable inguinal nodes. Imaging results were compared with the histologic findings of 113 nodes removed by inguinal lymphadenectomy, and LNMRI was found to have a sensitivity of 100% and a specificity of 97%. The high negative predictive value of LNMRI (100% in this small study) indicated a low likelihood of missing patients who had positive nodes and needed a therapeutic inguinal lymphadenectomy. If these results are confirmed in larger studies, unilateral lymphadenectomy could be possible when LNMRI detects the absence of metastases in the contralateral groin. A unique feature of LNMRI is that it is able to accurately diagnose nodal metastases in both patients with and without palpable inguinal nodes.[69] However, LNMRI is limited by the spatial resolution of the underlying MRI scanner and is also disadvantaged by the time required to interpret the images. LNMRI requires radiologists to make node-by-node pre- to postcontrast comparisons resulting in a very tedious and time-consuming process.

Diffusion-weighted MRI is another MRI technique that provides additional structural information about tissues.[70] Thoeny and colleagues[71] investigated the combination of diffusion-weighted MRI and nanoparticle enhancement in normal-sized pelvic lymph nodes of 21 patients with bladder and prostate cancers. Their technique of diffusion-weighted LNMRI correctly diagnosed 24 out of 26 positive nodes and had a significantly shorter interpretation time when compared with standard LNMRI (13 vs 80 minutes). At present, nanoparticle technology is not routinely available; however, for penile and urethral cancers the future of nanoparticle technology as a staging tool for lymph node disease is promising.

Dynamic Sentinel Lymph Node Biopsy

A sentinel node is theorized to be the first lymph node reached by metastasizing cancer cells from the primary tumor.[27,47] Dynamic sentinel lymph

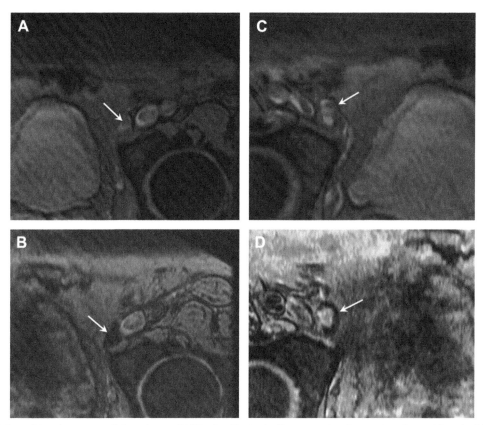

Fig. 8. Lymphtropic nanoparticle-enhanced MRI of pathologically proven benign and malignant inguinal lymph nodes in a patient with penile cancer. (*A*) Benign node: axial T2-weighted image shows hyperintense left inguinal lymph node (*arrow*). (*B*) Benign node: 24 hours after administration of ferumoxtran-10, the node shows homogeneous decrease in signal intensity indicating benign morphology. (*C*) Malignant node: axial precontrast T2-weighted image shows hyperintense right inguinal lymph node (*arrow*). (*D*) Malignant node: 24 hours after administration of ferumoxtran-10, there is no decrease in signal intensity indicating malignant infiltration. All findings were confirmed at surgery. (*From* Tabatabaei S, Harisinghani M, McDougal WS, et al. Regional lymph node staging using lymphotropic nanoparticle enhanced magnetic resonance imaging with ferumoxtran-10 in patients with penile cancer. J Urol 2005;174:925; with permission.)

node biopsy (DSNB) is a well-established modality for lymph node evaluation in patients with melanoma, and in this population, DSNB has a 95% sensitivity and a 10% complication rate.[72] DSNB involves injecting a technetium 99m–labeled nanocolloid intradermally into the peritumoral tissues and then performing lymphoscintigraphy. Hot spots (the sentinel nodes) are identified 1 to 2 hours after injection, and the skin is marked to indicate their anatomic location. The sentinel nodes can then be biopsied using US-guided FNA cytology or, more commonly, removed surgically with the aid of a second peritumoral injection of a patent blue dye (stains the sentinel nodes blue) and a handheld gamma probe (to locate the technetium 99m–containing nodes).

Early studies of DSNB in patients with penile cancer were plagued by high false-negative rates ranging from 22% to 75%.[73–75] The high false-negative rate was theorized to be due to suboptimal technique, and after a series of technical modifications the false-negative rate has dropped dramatically.[73,76–78] A recent prospective study of 64 patients with penile cancer and nonpalpable nodes revealed that the combination of DSNB and US-guided FNA had a negative predictive value of 100%, indicating that no patient with a negative result in DSNB developed a late inguinal node recurrence.[61] Leijte and colleagues[79] studied 323 patients with penile cancer and found DSNB to have a sentinel node identification rate of 97%, a false-negative rate of 7%, and an overall complication rate of 5%.

IMAGING OF DISTANT METASTASES

Distant metastases are found at the time of initial clinical presentation in about 5% of patients with penile cancer and 30% of those with urethral cancer. The most common distant organ sites of spread are nonregional nodes, lung, liver, and bone.[9,80] Patients at risk of metastases (positive nodes, high T stage, high grade, lymphovascular invasion) have historically been staged with a chest radiograph, a radionuclide bone scan, and a CT scan of the abdomen and pelvis.[4,9,25,27] There is little evidence supporting these 3 tests as the optimal modalities for staging.

PET and PET/CT

PET scanning can be done using several different radionucleotide-labeled biologically active molecules, although ^{18}F fluorodeoxyglucose (FDG) is by far the most common molecule in use at present. FDG is a glucose analogue that is actively taken up by metabolically active cells using glucose. However, once inside the cell, FDG cannot be metabolized because it lacks a $2'$-hydroxyl group that is required for further glycolysis and therefore, accumulates within the cell. Because cancer cells generally have a higher metabolic rate than normal cells, FDG tends to preferentially accumulate in malignant cells.[81] As FDG's radioactive ^{18}F label decays (half-life = 110 minutes), it emits positrons that can be detected by the PET scanner. Several other biologic molecules that are being used at present in PET scans include ^{11}C acetate, ^{11}C choline, ^{13}N ammonia, and ^{15}O water.[82] PET scans have been shown to be valuable in staging several malignancies.[81] Because of the infrequency of metastases in penile and urethral cancers, there are very little data regarding the ability of PET or PET/CT to diagnose metastases. One small study found that PET/CT detected distant metastases in 5 patients, 4 of whom were confirmed histologically to have distant metastases.[66]

SUMMARY

In penile and urethral cancers, imaging plays a crucial role in enhancing the precision of clinical staging and facilitating optimal surgical planning. Recently, great improvements have been made in imaging, affecting the ability to more precisely stage penile and urethral cancers. High-resolution MRI now represents the gold standard for evaluating the primary tumor and its local extension. LNMRI and DSNB combined with FNA seem to be superior modalities for imaging regional lymph nodes. PET/CT has shown great promise as a whole body screen for the detection of distant metastases. All these imaging modalities require further validation, but with the global burden of penile and urethral cancers located predominantly in the third world countries, it may be some time before knowing which imaging strategies are optimal.

REFERENCES

1. Fagan GE, Hertig AT. Carcinoma of the female urethra, review of the literature, report of eight cases. Obstet Gynecol 1955;6(1):1–11.
2. From the AJCC cancer staging manual. In: Edge SB, Byrd DR, Compton CC, et al, editors. Cancer staging handbook. 7th edition. New York: Springer; 2010. p. 515–84.
3. Leijte JA, Gallee M, Antonini N, et al. Evaluation of current TNM classification of penile carcinoma. J Urol 2008;180(3):933–8 [discussion: 938].
4. Vapnek JM, Hricak H, Carroll PR. Recent advances in imaging studies for staging of penile and urethral carcinoma. Urol Clin North Am 1992;19(2):257–66.
5. Kim B, Kawashima A, LeRoy AJ. Imaging of the male urethra. Semin Ultrasound CT MR 2007;28(4):258–73.
6. Wasserman NF. Urethral neoplasms. In: Pollack HM, McClennan BL, Dyer RB, et al, editors. Clinical urography. 2nd edition. Philadelphia: Saunders; 2000. p. 1699–715.
7. Kawashima A, Sandler CM, Wasserman NF, et al. Imaging of urethral disease: a pictorial review. Radiographics 2004;24(Suppl 1):S195–216.
8. Yokoyama M, Watanabe K, Iwata H, et al. Case profile: double-contrast urethrography for visualizing small lesions in distal urethra. Urology 1982;19(4):440.
9. Applewhite JC, Hall MC, McCullough DL. Urethral carcinoma. In: Gillenwater JY, Grayhack JT, Howards SS, et al, editors. 4th edition, In: Adult and pediatric urology, vol. 2. Philadelphia: Lippincott Williams and Wilkins; 2002. p. 1791–810.
10. Ryu J, Kim B. MR imaging of the male and female urethra. Radiographics 2001;21(5):1169–85.
11. Dalbagni G, Zhang ZF, Lacombe L, et al. Male urethral carcinoma: analysis of treatment outcome. Urology 1999;53(6):1126–32.
12. Sufrin G, Huben R. Benign and malignant lesions of the penis. In: Gillenwater JY, Grayhack JT, Howards SS, et al, editors. 2nd edition, In: Adult and pediatric urology, vol. 2. Philadelphia: Lippincott Williams and Wilkins; 2002. p. 1975–2009.
13. Raghavaiah NV. Corpus cavernosogram in the evaluation of carcinoma of the penis. J Urol 1978;120(4):423–4.
14. Escribano G, Allona A, Burgos FJ, et al. Cavernosography in diagnosis of metastatic tumors of the penis: 5 new cases and a review of the literature. J Urol 1987;138(5):1174–7.
15. Haddad FS, Kovac A, Kivirand A, et al. Cavernosography in diagnosis of penile metastases secondary to bladder cancer. Urology 1985;26(6):585–6.

16. Agrawal A, Pai D, Ananthakrishnan N, et al. Clinical and sonographic findings in carcinoma of the penis. J Clin Ultrasound 2000;28(8):399–406.

17. Bertolotto M, Serafini G, Dogliotti L, et al. Primary and secondary malignancies of the penis: ultrasound features. Abdom Imaging 2005;30(1):108–12.

18. Horenblas S, Kroger R, Gallee MP, et al. Ultrasound in squamous cell carcinoma of the penis; a useful addition to clinical staging? A comparison of ultrasound with histopathology. Urology 1994;43(5):702–7.

19. Solsona E, Algaba F, Horenblas S, et al. EAU guidelines on penile cancer. Eur Urol 2004;46(1):1–8.

20. Klosterman PW, Laing FC, McAninch JW. Sonourethrography in the evaluation of urethral stricture disease. Urol Clin North Am 1989;16(4):791–7.

21. McAninch JW, Laing FC, Jeffrey RB Jr. Sonourethrography in the evaluation of urethral strictures: a preliminary report. J Urol 1988;139(2):294–7.

22. Pavlica P, Bartolone A, Gaudiano C, et al. Female paraurethral leiomyoma: ultrasonographic and magnetic resonance imaging findings. Acta Radiol 2004;45(7):796–8.

23. Occhipinti K, Kutcher R, Gentile RL. Prolapsing inverted papilloma of the prostatic urethra: diagnosis by transrectal sonography. AJR Am J Roentgenol 1992;159(1):93–4.

24. Terris MK, Villers A, Freiha FS. Transrectal ultrasound appearance of transitional cell carcinoma involving the prostate. J Urol 1990;143(5):952–6.

25. Sufrin G, Huben R. Benign and malignant lesions of the penis. In: Gillenwate JY, editor. Adult and pediatric urology. 4th edition. Philadelphia (PA): Lippincott Williams and Wilkins; 2002. p. 1975–2009.

26. Scher B, Seitz M, Reiser M, et al. 18F-FDG PET/CT for staging of penile cancer. J Nucl Med 2005; 46(9):1460–5.

27. Kochhar R, Taylor B, Sangar V. Imaging in primary penile cancer: current status and future directions. Eur Radiol 2009;20(1):36–47.

28. Vossough A, Pretorius ES, Siegelman ES, et al. Magnetic resonance imaging of the penis. Abdom Imaging 2002;27(6):640–59.

29. Pretorius ES, Siegelman ES, Ramchandani P, et al. MR imaging of the penis. Radiographics 2001; 21(Spec No):S283–98 [discussion: S298–9].

30. Strohbehn K, Quint LE, Prince MR, et al. Magnetic resonance imaging anatomy of the female urethra: a direct histologic comparison. Obstet Gynecol 1996;88(5):750–6.

31. Suh DD, Yang CC, Cao Y, et al. Magnetic resonance imaging anatomy of the female genitalia in premenopausal and postmenopausal women. J Urol 2003; 170(1):138–44.

32. Prasad SR, Menias CO, Narra VR, et al. Cross-sectional imaging of the female urethra: technique and results. Radiographics 2005;25(3):749–61.

33. Hricak H, Marotti M, Gilbert TJ, et al. Normal penile anatomy and abnormal penile conditions: evaluation with MR imaging. Radiology 1988;169(3):683–90.

34. Hricak H, Secaf E, Buckley DW, et al. Female urethra: MR imaging. Radiology 1991;178(2):527–35.

35. Singh AK, Saokar A, Hahn PF, et al. Imaging of penile neoplasms. Radiographics 2005;25(6): 1629–38.

36. Scardino E, Villa G, Bonomo G, et al. Magnetic resonance imaging combined with artificial erection for local staging of penile cancer. Urology 2004;63(6): 1158–62.

37. Petralia G, Villa G, Scardino E, et al. Local staging of penile cancer using magnetic resonance imaging with pharmacologically induced penile erection. Radiol Med 2008;113(4):517–28.

38. Kayes O, Minhas S, Allen C, et al. The role of magnetic resonance imaging in the local staging of penile cancer. Eur Urol 2007;51(5):1313–8 [discussion: 1318–9].

39. Fujita H. New horizons in MR technology: RF coil designs and trends. Magn Reson Med Sci 2007; 6(1):29–42.

40. Lorenzo AJ, Zimmern P, Lemack GE, et al. Endorectal coil magnetic resonance imaging for diagnosis of urethral and periurethral pathologic findings in women. Urology 2003;61(6):1129–33 [discussion: 1133–4].

41. Blander DS, Rovner ES, Schnall MD, et al. Endoluminal magnetic resonance imaging in the evaluation of urethral diverticula in women. Urology 2001;57(4): 660–5.

42. Tan IL, Stoker J, Lameris JS. Magnetic resonance imaging of the female pelvic floor and urethra: body coil versus endovaginal coil. MAGMA 1997; 5(1):59–63.

43. Elsayes KM, Mukundan G, Narra VR, et al. Endovaginal magnetic resonance imaging of the female urethra. J Comput Assist Tomogr 2006;30(1):1–6.

44. Macura KJ, Genadry R, Borman TL, et al. Evaluation of the female urethra with intraurethral magnetic resonance imaging. J Magn Reson Imaging 2004; 20(1):153–9.

45. Chou CP, Levenson RB, Elsayes KM, et al. Imaging of female urethral diverticulum: an update. Radiographics 2008;28(7):1917–30.

46. Ficarra V, Zattoni F, Cunico SC, et al. Lymphatic and vascular embolizations are independent predictive variables of inguinal lymph node involvement in patients with squamous cell carcinoma of the penis: Gruppo Uro-Oncologico del Nord Est (Northeast Uro-Oncological Group) Penile Cancer data base data. Cancer 2005;103(12):2507–16.

47. Mueller-Lisse UG, Scher B, Scherr MK, et al. Functional imaging in penile cancer: PET/computed tomography, MRI, and sentinel lymph node biopsy. Curr Opin Urol 2008;18(1):105–10.

48. Ray B, Canto AR, Whitmore WF Jr. Experience with primary carcinoma of the male urethra. J Urol 1977;117(5):591–4.

49. Kaplan GW, Bulkey GJ, Grayhack JT. Carcinoma of the male urethra. J Urol 1967;98(3):365–71.

50. Hughes BE, Leijte JA, Kroon BK, et al. Lymph node metastasis in intermediate-risk penile squamous cell cancer: a two-centre experience. Eur Urol 2009; 57(4):688–92.

51. Horenblas S. Lymphadenectomy for squamous cell carcinoma of the penis. Part 1: diagnosis of lymph node metastasis. BJU Int 2001;88(5):467–72.

52. Hungerhuber E, Schlenker B, Karl A, et al. Risk stratification in penile carcinoma: 25-year experience with surgical inguinal lymph node staging. Urology 2006;68(3):621–5.

53. Kroon BK, Horenblas S, Lont AP, et al. Patients with penile carcinoma benefit from immediate resection of clinically occult lymph node metastases. J Urol 2005;173(3):816–9.

54. McDougal WS. Carcinoma of the penis: improved survival by early regional lymphadenectomy based on the histological grade and depth of invasion of the primary lesion. J Urol 1995;154(4):1364–6.

55. Horenblas S. Lymphadenectomy for squamous cell carcinoma of the penis. Part 2: the role and technique of lymph node dissection. BJU Int 2001; 88(5):473–83.

56. Bouchot O, Rigaud J, Maillet F, et al. Morbidity of inguinal lymphadenectomy for invasive penile carcinoma. Eur Urol 2004;45(6):761–5 [discussion: 765–6].

57. Horenblas S, Van Tinteren H, Delemarre JF, et al. Squamous cell carcinoma of the penis: accuracy of tumor, nodes and metastasis classification system, and role of lymphangiography, computerized tomography scan and fine needle aspiration cytology. J Urol 1991;146(5):1279–83.

58. Hughes B, Leijte J, Shabbir M, et al. Non-invasive and minimally invasive staging of regional lymph nodes in penile cancer. World J Urol 2009;27(2):197–203.

59. Esen G. Ultrasound of superficial lymph nodes. Eur J Radiol 2006;58(3):345–59.

60. Steinkamp HJ, Mueffelmann M, Bock JC, et al. Differential diagnosis of lymph node lesions: a semiquantitative approach with colour Doppler ultrasound. Br J Radiol 1998;71(848):828–33.

61. Crawshaw JW, Hadway P, Hoffland D, et al. Sentinel lymph node biopsy using dynamic lymphoscintigraphy combined with ultrasound-guided fine needle aspiration in penile carcinoma. Br J Radiol 2009; 82(973):41–8.

62. Kocjan G, Chandra A, Cross P, et al. BSCC code of practice–fine needle aspiration cytology. Cytopathology 2009;20(5):283–96.

63. Hall TB, Barton DP, Trott PA, et al. The role of ultrasound-guided cytology of groin lymph nodes in the management of squamous cell carcinoma of the vulva: 5-year experience in 44 patients. Clin Radiol 2003;58(5):367–71.

64. Kroon BK, Horenblas S, Deurloo EE, et al. Ultrasonography-guided fine-needle aspiration cytology before sentinel node biopsy in patients with penile carcinoma. BJU Int 2005;95(4):517–21.

65. Lont AP, Besnard AP, Gallee MP, et al. A comparison of physical examination and imaging in determining the extent of primary penile carcinoma. BJU Int 2003;91(6):493–5.

66. Graafland NM, Leijte JA, Valdes Olmos RA, et al. Scanning with 18F-FDG-PET/CT for detection of pelvic nodal involvement in inguinal node-positive penile carcinoma. Eur Urol 2009;56(2):339–45.

67. Leijte JA, Graafland NM, Valdes Olmos RA, et al. Prospective evaluation of hybrid 18F-fluorodeoxyglucose positron emission tomography/computed tomography in staging clinically node-negative patients with penile carcinoma. BJU Int 2009; 104(5):640–4.

68. Saksena MA, Saokar A, Harisinghani MG. Lymphotropic nanoparticle enhanced MR imaging (LNMRI) technique for lymph node imaging. Eur J Radiol 2006;58(3):367–74.

69. Tabatabaei S, Harisinghani M, McDougal WS. Regional lymph node staging using lymphotropic nanoparticle enhanced magnetic resonance imaging with ferumoxtran-10 in patients with penile cancer. J Urol 2005;174(3):923–7 [discussion: 927].

70. Koh DM, Collins DJ. Diffusion-weighted MRI in the body: applications and challenges in oncology. AJR Am J Roentgenol 2007;188(6):1622–35.

71. Thoeny HC, Triantafyllou M, Birkhaeuser FD, et al. Combined ultrasmall superparamagnetic particles of iron oxide-enhanced and diffusion-weighted magnetic resonance imaging reliably detect pelvic lymph node metastases in normal-sized nodes of bladder and prostate cancer patients. Eur Urol 2009;55(4):761–9.

72. Morton DL, Cochran AJ, Thompson JF, et al. Sentinel node biopsy for early-stage melanoma: accuracy and morbidity in MSLT-I, an international multicenter trial. Ann Surg 2005;242(3):302–11 [discussion: 311–3].

73. Gonzaga-Silva LF, Tavares JM, Freitas FC, et al. The isolated gamma probe technique for sentinel node penile carcinoma detection is unreliable. Int Braz J Urol 2007;33(1):58–63 [discussion: 64–7].

74. Spiess PE, Izawa JI, Bassett R, et al. Preoperative lymphoscintigraphy and dynamic sentinel node biopsy for staging penile cancer: results with pathological correlation. J Urol 2007;177(6):2157–61.

75. Tanis PJ, Lont AP, Meinhardt W, et al. Dynamic sentinel node biopsy for penile cancer: reliability of a staging technique. J Urol 2002;168(1):76–80.

76. Hegarty PK, Minhas S. Re: evaluation of dynamic lymphoscintigraphy and sentinel lymph-node biopsy for detecting occult metastases in patients with

penile squamous cell carcinoma. BJU Int 2008; 101(6):781 [author reply 781–2].

77. Horenblas S. Words of wisdom. Re: preoperative lymphoscintigraphy and dynamic sentinel node biopsy for staging penile cancer: results with pathological correlation. Eur Urol 2007; 52(4):1261.

78. Leijte JA, Kroon BK, Valdes Olmos RA, et al. Reliability and safety of current dynamic sentinel node biopsy for penile carcinoma. Eur Urol 2007;52(1): 170–7.

79. Leijte JA, Hughes B, Graafland NM, et al. Two-center evaluation of dynamic sentinel node biopsy for squamous cell carcinoma of the penis. J Clin Oncol 2009;27(20):3325–9.

80. Culkin DJ, Beer TM. Advanced penile carcinoma. J Urol 2003;170(2 Pt 1):359–65.

81. Poeppel TD, Krause BJ, Heusner TA, et al. PET/CT for the staging and follow-up of patients with malignancies. Eur J Radiol 2009;70(3):382–92.

82. Groves AM, Win T, Haim SB, et al. Non-[18F]FDG PET in clinical oncology. Lancet Oncol 2007;8(9):822–30.

Surgical Management of Carcinoma of the Penis

Richard E. Greenberg, MD

KEYWORDS

• Carcinoma • Penile cancer • Quality of life

Penile cancer is a rare malignancy primarily managed surgically since the end of the 19th century, as detailed in Young's Practice of Urology, published in 1926.[1,2] Pioneers in this field, include Thiersch (1875), MacCormack (1886), Curtis (1898), and Young (1907); the latter three surgeons actually espoused en-bloc surgical removal of the penis, partial or total, with bilateral inguinal lymph nodes. This procedure would be considered a formidable undertaking even now in the 21st century. However, Das[3] in 1992 actually credited Celsus in the 1st century AD with the description of the earliest definitive surgical excision of a penile lesion with a margin of healthy tissue. Methods have changed only minimally, although understanding of the nature of the pathology and its clinico–pathologic features has allowed urologists to better define appropriate and less aggressive methods of treatment for individual patients. Young in his 1926 text asserted that when lesions are confined to the prepuce it may be possible to radically excise by circumcision or by thorough cauterization, clearly not significantly different than today's approach, where surgery remains the cornerstone of the management of penile cancer.[2]

EPIDEMIOLOGY

The American Cancer Society estimated that in the United States about 1300 new cases of penile cancer would be diagnosed and an estimated 300 men would die of this cancer in 2009. The frequency of this rare cancer is about 1 in 100,00 men in the United States. The incidence in Europe is equally low, also accounting for less than 1% of male cancers. The prevalence of this malignancy is much greater in Asia, Africa, and South America, however, where it may account for up to 10% of cancers in men.[4] Almost all penile cancers arise from the normal skin cells of the penis. Approximately 95% of these tumors are squamous cell carcinomas (SCCa). These cancers may develop anywhere on the penis but have a predilection for the foreskin in uncircumcised males or the glans penis. In general, these cancers actually grow slowly and when found in the early stages are quite amenable to surgical cure using several modalities to be discussed later in this article. Unfortunately, little has changed since the turn of the 20th century when Young described the clinical presentation at that time. The patients continue to be asymptomatic and therefore the lesions frequently ignored. Rarely do they interfere with normal voiding, and pain or discharge frequently is a late manifestation of secondary infection or invasion.[2]

Verrucous carcinoma of the penis is an uncommon form of SCCa and usually felt to be of low malignant potential. Specifically, although they may grow quite large and they may invade the deep structures of the penis, they rarely metastasize. It is also referred to as a Buschke-Lowenstein tumor and may be mistaken for a large benign genital wart. Other cancers that may develop on the penis are also rare and represent less that 2% of penile malignancies. These include

> Melanomas, which usually are discovered late associated with systemic metastatic disease

Fox Chase Cancer Center, Department of Surgical Oncology, 333 Cottman Avenue, Philadelphia, PA 19111-2497, USA

E-mail address: richard.greenberg@fccc.edu

Urol Clin N Am 37 (2010) 369–378

doi:10.1016/j.ucl.2010.04.006

0094-0143/10/$ – see front matter © 2010 Elsevier Inc. All rights reserved.

Basal cell carcinoma, a slow-growing lesion unlikely to spread beyond the local disease

Adenocarcinoma, which arises from the sweat glands in the skin of the penis and is also called Paget disease of the penis

Rare sarcomas, which develop from blood vessels, muscle cells, and other connective tissues present in the penis.[5]

Carcinoma in situ (TIS) is the earliest stage of SCCa of the penis. It remains an intraepithelial process, and therefore preinvasive. When this lesion involves the glans penis, it is referred to as erythroplasia of Queyrat, first described in 1911.[6] Lesions on the shaft of the penis are called Bowen disease.[7] In this stage of penile cancer, the abnormal cells are confined to the upper layers of the skin and are amenable to local excision, yet have a potential to recur if the local therapy is inadequate. TIS when inadequately treated may indeed progress to invasive carcinoma, in approximately 10% of cases, although metastases rarely occur. Clearly, understanding the pathologic nature of the patient's cancer is essential to defining the appropriate initial management and establishment of his follow-up course of treatment or observation. Cancer eradication with attempts at organ preservation is the primary goal of this therapy.

The primary goal of the surgical management of penile cancer remains the complete eradication of the malignancy with minimal impact of function and cosmetic aspect of patient self-image, whenever possible. This aim should be readily achievable using modern methods of surgical intervention with stages TIS and T_1, noninvasive carcinoma, and limited early invasive disease. Stage T_1 is defined in the TNM classification of penile cancer as a lesion 2 cm or less in maximal dimension but strictly superficial in its invasiveness or primarily exophytic in character. T_2 disease is defined as larger tumors, between 2 and 5 cm, demonstrating minimal invasion. Invasive, stage T_3 SCCa represents larger tumors, which involve deep structures of the penis, including corpora and urethra. T_4 malignancies directly involve adjacent anatomic structures. Functional organ preservation recently has been shown feasible in selected cases of the more invasive lesions as well (T_1 and small anatomically suitable T_2 cancers). Standard therapy with necessary amputation of the penis in part or in total, however, still may be required, especially when there is delay in diagnosis and therefore extensive local disease or when local recurrence is documented following conservative primary treatments. A formal pathologic assessment via biopsy for histologic documentation and depth of invasion is the first necessary surgical step in diagnosis and staging required in order before consideration of the appropriate subsequent therapy. This may take the form of a punch biopsy, excisional biopsy of a relatively small tumor of the glans or foreskin, or an incisional biopsy of a larger lesion that cannot be excised completely. The biopsy always should include a portion of adjacent normal tissue with the specimen to allow optimal evaluation of the depth of invasion of the cancer. A dorsal slit may be required to gain adequate exposure of the preputial cavity. If a lesion involves the urethral meatus, urethroscopy is indicated to evaluate the urethra, and directed biopsies are performed if any suspicious areas are noted.[8] As with most cancers, prognosis depends upon both grade and stage, with higher-grade tumors and those tumors involving the corporal bodies or with lymph node involvement less likely to be cured regardless of treatment. Human papillomavirus (HPV) infection is an established causal agent for at least 40% of penile SCCa.[9]

ANATOMY

Intimate understanding of normal anatomy (**Fig. 1**) is a fundamental requirement for any surgical procedure, yet especially cogent when considering modifications of long-standing surgical approaches to maximize both oncologic outcome and quality of life. Functional and cosmetic results are paramount in modern penile cancer surgery. Fortunately, where surgical procedures and approaches have changed over the last several decades, penile anatomy has remained refreshingly unchanged, although vascular variations are noted.[10] The penis is comprised of three erectile bodies, the paired corporus cavernosum, and the corpus spongiosum. The corporus cavernosum is covered with a dense fibrous tunica albuginea and is incompletely separated by the septum penis. The erectile tissue is composed of endothelial-lined sinusoidal spaces, which are fed via multiple small helicine arteries, which with increase in blood flow flood these spaces and by virtue of compression of equally small emissary veins are responsible the maintenance of an erection. The corpus spongiosum surrounds the urethra and in its distal extent becomes the glans penis. There is a deep fascia (Bucks) and a superficial fascia (dartos). At the root of the penis, there is continuity between the deep penile fascia and the fascia of the external oblique muscles, which extends over the pubic symphysis. The crura are attached to the pubic arch, and two ligaments support the penis, the more superficial fundiform

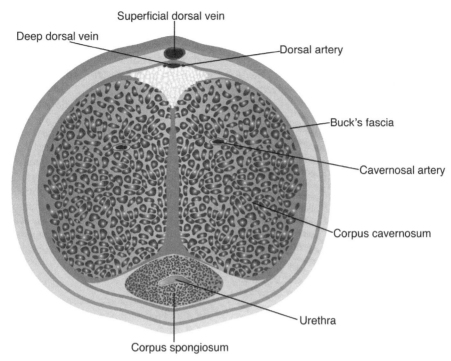

Fig. 1. Anatomy of the penis.

ligament and a deeper triangular suspensory liga-ment that apically attaches directly to the pubic symphysis. The main arterial blood supply of the penis is from the hypogastric artery, which continues as the internal pudendal artery and then as the penile artery. There are three terminal branches of the penile artery, the bulbomembra-nous artery, the cavernosal artery, and the dorsal penile artery. There is a superficial venous system of veins that drains to the saphenous system (primarily to the left saphenous vein when a single superficial dorsal vein is present), an intermediate drainage system comprised of the deep dorsal veins and circumflex veins, and the deep venous system of crural veins and the emissary veins from the proximal corporus cavernosum. There is both somatic and autonomic nerve innervation of the penis. The somatic innervation is supplied via the pudendal nerve (S2-S4), with a shared innerva-tion of the external sphincter (S2-S3). The para-sympathetic nerves arise from S2-S4 and the sympathetic of the pelvic plexus arises from T11-L2. Lymphatic drainage of the penis is also important, although not as it relates to surgical management of penile cancer, but rather as a source of predictable regional cancer spread. The skin of the penis and prepuce drain primarily to the superficial inguinal lymph nodes. The lymphatic drainage of the glans penis and corporal bodies are somewhat more unpredictable, with possible paths to superficial or deep inguinal no-des or even the external iliac lymph chain.[11]

LASER EXCISION OR ABLATION THERAPY

Penile laser surgery has been used clinically for treating selective penile cancers for 30 years. The lasers most commonly reported for this purpose are the carbon dioxide (CO_2), neodymiu-m:yttrium-aluminum-garnet (Nd:YAG), and less commonly, the potassium titanyl phosphate (KTP) lasers. The limitation of the CO_2 laser is its depth of penetration, which is only 0.1 mm and therefore thought only suitable for carcinoma in situ lesions. Recent data published by Bandiera-monte, however, demonstrate effective cancer control and 10-year recurrence-free survival of greater than 80% in patients with either in situ or T_1 cancers. The 10-year salvage amputation rate was 5.5%, and there was no significant difference between TIS and T_1 outcomes. Local recurrence was predictable using histologic parameters of margin status, depth of invasion, and tumor exten-sion.[12] This represents a significant improvement in long-term outcomes over earlier data reported by van Bezooijen in 2001, when local recurrence rates of up to 50% where documented.[13] Colec-chia recently reported using CO_2 laser surgery on 56 patients with T_1 SCCa. He noted that although 13 patients developed local recurrences, including

4 patients with multiple recurrences, that only 1 of the 13 patients required partial penectomy to control the local disease. With a median follow-up of 66 months, none of the patients died of penile SCCa, and the two patients found to have low-volume regional lymph node involvement were salvaged with lymphadenectomy.[14]

Localized surgical management with the Nd:YAG laser produces protein denaturation at a depth of 6 mm. This has led to a preferential use of the Nd:YAG laser in cases where there is concern regarding possibility of SCCa beyond CIS. In Sweden, Windahl reported on a prospective study where the primary treatment of localized SCCa was with the CO_2 laser, and the recurrences were then treated successfully with follow-up Nd:YAG laser therapy. The authors felt that the success of this combination local therapy was associated with highly satisfactory cosmetic results and function.[15] Organ-preserving Nd:YAG laser surgery for TIS, T1, and selected cases of T2 invasive cancers is a reasonable first approached to oncologic cure (control) of penile SCCa. Long-term follow-up studies clearly demonstrate a relatively high recurrence rate, yet oncologic outcome and ultimate disease-free survival do not appear to be compromised by local recurrence, when long-term (>4 years) follow-up is assured. Indeed, this may be the best initial treatment option for those patients with grade 2 stage T_1 tumors.[16,17] Meijer and colleagues[18] have suggested widening the field of initial laser excision as a means to successfully decrease the incidence of local recurrence, when laser therapy is used.

It is quite obvious that the cosmetic outcome of laser excision is superior to penile amputation. Laser treatment of localized penile carcinoma preserves satisfactory sexual function and self-image related to cosmesis allowing for improved quality-of-life assessment. Compared with other surgical options, men who undergo laser surgery are more likely to resume their normal sexual activities.[19,20]

CONSERVATIVE SURGERY

The standard therapies for invasive carcinoma of the penis include either amputative surgery or radical radiation therapy. Both of these options are associated with significant physical and psychosexual morbidity. Recent reports are compelling regarding equivalent oncologic outcomes with conservative organ-sparing techniques in selected patients with careful follow-up. Primary tumor stage clearly is the most important predictor of long-term outcome and potential cure. Compared with laser therapy, surgical

excision has the advantage of providing tissue for tumor grading and assessment of margins. Clinicopathologic features are necessary to design therapeutic strategies that will balance mortality risks with quality-of-life parameters. Mortality is highest within the fist 3 years of follow-up, whereas local recurrence depending on initial therapy may occur even after 11 years.[21] High-risk histology features, while rare, are important when considering attempts at conservative surgical treatments. Basaloid, sarcomatoid, and mixed SCCa-verrucous variants and invasion of the corpus cavernosum or preputial skin were noteworthy adverse prognostic characteristics of recurrent cancer. Local excisions with laser or scalpel as well as partial penectomy were usually inadequate treatments for sarcomatoid or basaloid penile carcinomas.[22–24]

Circumcision

The most common and direct management of SCCa of the penis is via circumcision. This is related to the fact that the most men with penile carcinoma are uncircumcised. The indication for circumcision as a potential curative intervention is with low-grade, small, low-stage tumors limited to the distal prepuce. It also may be indicated with acquired secondary phimosis often associated with preputial tumors and appropriate in patients undergoing radiation therapy. In these patients, circumcision allows improved narrow targeting, may prevent local toxicities related to the prepuce with radiation therapy and lastly, and most importantly, allows for improved local oncologic surveillance. In tumors that extend proximal to the coronal sulcus, the surgical margin must encompass that area of the penile shaft that will ensure an adequate negative tumor margin.[25]

Margins for Penile Cancer Surgery

A 2 cm surgical margin has been the standard of practice since the turn of the 20th century.[1] Whether this was a practice derived from surgical study and clinical observation or a practical consideration when attempting to perform conservative surgical intervention, this concept only recently has been challenged. In 2000, Hoffman and colleagues reported a small series of penile cancers treated with either partial or total penectomy where the average pathologic margin was 14.4 mm for these tumors, which were at minimum stage T_1. Three of the 10 patients undergoing partial penectomy actually had margins of less than 10 mm. None of this small cohort developed local or regional recurrence. In the seven patients

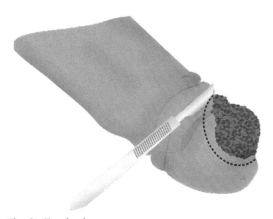

Fig. 2. Simple closure.

who required total penectomy, the average pathologic margin of resection was again less than the traditional 2 cm, at 14.8 mm. Four of these patients had margins less than 10 mm, all without local recurrence at time of follow-up (mean duration >2 years).[26]

Minhas reported a study of 51 patients selected for organ-sparing surgery in the United Kingdom between 2000 and 2004. Nine of these patients underwent local excision; 26 had glansectomy, and the remaining 9 patients had partial penectomy. Looking at both skin and deep margins, results demonstrated less than 10 mm in 48% and less than 20 mm in 90% of the cases. A positive surgical margin was noted

in three patients, and they subsequently had appropriate additional surgery to obtain a negative margin status. With follow-up, two patients did develop local recurrence in the nonpenectomy cohort and were salvaged satisfactorily with eventual partial penectomy.[27] A updated paper from the same institution illustrates a range of organ-preserving procedures that match the clinical spectrum of patients presenting with SCCa of the penis. These procedures provide excellent oncologic control while maximizing penile function and cosmetic form. This approach ameliorates some of the serious psychological and sexual morbidity historically linked with the diagnosis of cancer of the penis.[28]

Glansectomy

Because approximately 80% of penile carcinomas arise from the distal glans penis, many of these patients should be candidates for penile-preserving surgery. This type of extirpative surgery generally leaves a simple defect that may be closed either primarily with little cosmetic consequence (**Fig. 2**), closed using a lateral preputial skin flap (**Fig. 3**), or closed using split-thickness skin flap using a lateral thigh donor site.[22,29–32] This partial glansectomy should include frozen section diagnoses from the cavernosal bed and urethral stump if involved, to confirm negative

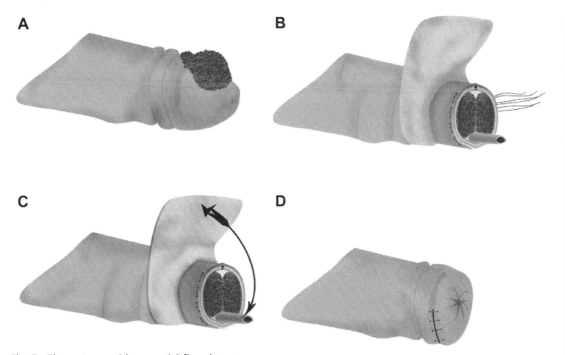

Fig. 3. Glansectomy with preputial flap closure.

margins and tumor clearance before reconstructive procedures. When grafting is required following glansectomy, a neoglans is created. Glansectomy when partial removes the portion of the glans affected by the tumor but does leave behind residual glandular epithelium, which may have malignant potential. This is essentially an excisional biopsy of a small distal cancer. A total glansectomy removes the entire glans, thus preventing any local recurrence from the glans tissue. When there is involvement of the underlying tunica albuginea of the corpora cavernosum, distal corporectomy should be included. The corporal defect can be directly closed. When a total glansectomy is oncologically necessary, split-thickness skin grafting and cavernosal tip reconstruction are used. Care must be maintained with glansectomy to avoid limiting oncologically essential surgical management when the primary lesion is within 5 mm or actually invading the urethral meatus. In these cases, excision including the urethral meatus with negative frozen sections directs the nature of the distal urethral reconstruction.[29] An additional issue associated with this type of conservative management remains penile sensitivity, which in turn affects ejaculation and orgasm as well as penile length and appearance.

An alternative approach to organ-preserving surgery for penile cancer recently has been developed. This is a modification of penile disassembly initially used in the surgical correction of congenital (hypospadias, extrophy–epispadias complex) and acquired deformities of the penis (penile curvature and Peyronie disease). This technique has been used principally in low-grade stage T_1 SCCa penile cancers to date with satisfactory early outcomes from both the oncologic and cosmetically acceptable and functional points of view. The technique involves urethral mobilization including Bucks fascia, after which the dorsal neurovascular bundle is dissected free. The glans with the urethra and the neurovascular bundle dorsally are completely separated from the corpus cavernosum. The neurovascular bundle is the divided 2 cm proximal to the glans cap, and the glans then is removed after incising the urethra. Mandatory frozen section biopsies are obtained to make certain than the procedure conforms to oncologic expectations. The urethra after mobilization then is spatulated and secured to the corpora with sutures. Then the spatulated distal urethra is used to reconstruct a neoglans.[33] While this approach appears to offer benefits beyond surgical amputation techniques, additional studies and longer follow-up are necessary before changing the management algorithm for this type of penile carcinoma, where total glansectomy and penile reconstruction replaces partial penectomy as the standard procedure offered to guarantee best possible survival.

Partial Penectomy

Partial penectomy (**Fig. 4**) remains the most common surgical procedure for treating the primary tumor in patients with invasive SCCa of the penis. The primary purpose of this procedure is to offer the patient excellent local control while

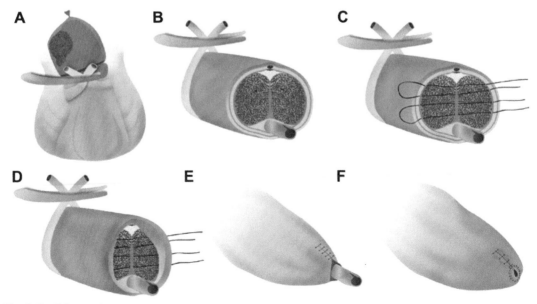

Fig. 4. Partial penectomy.

preserving the ability to void in a standing position and possibly to allow for adequate sexual function. It is interesting that the specifics of the surgical procedure have changed little since the earl 1900s. The major difference in the technique as described is in the available sutures.[1,8,34,35] Under tourniquet control to decrease blood loss and improve visualization (some authors are inclined to defer this part of the procedure), the distal tumor is covered with a surgical glove or impermeable

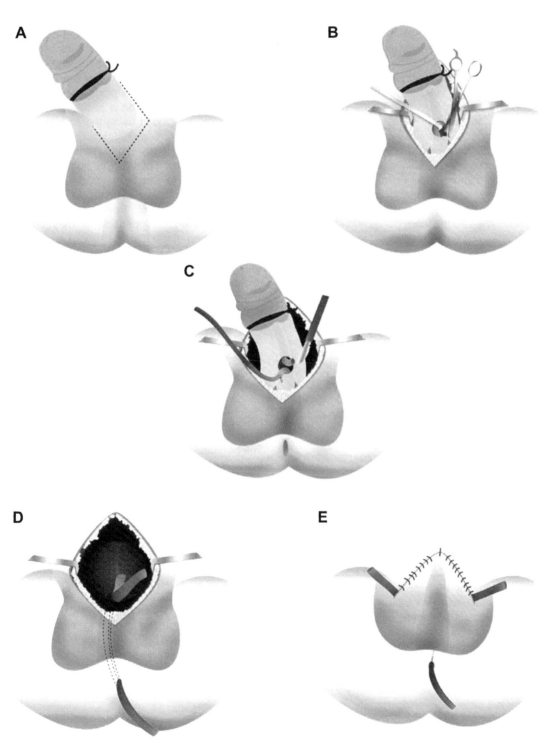

A

B

C

D

E

Fig. 5. Total penectomy.

dressing. This maneuver is designed to reduce the likelihood of wound seeding. A Foley catheter is placed to assist in the identification of the urethra. A circumferential skin incision is made 2 cm proximal to the proximal-most aspect of the distal penile cancer, through the skin and dartos fascia. At the level of Bucks fascia, the corpus cavernosum is incised laterally, allowing dissection and eventual ligation of the structures in the dorsal neurovascular bundle. The penile skin is retracted proximally to facilitate excision of approximately an additional 1 cm, thereby allowing for a tension-free skin closure over the ends of the closed corporal bodies. These corpora are closed using a horizontal mattress technique, using either a running or interrupted 3-0 suture method. The urethra, assuming it is uninvolved by the cancer, is left slightly more distal (1 to 1.5 cm) than the corpora cavernosal level before transection to facilitate posterior spatulation and Y-V plasty between the urethra and penile skin, using 4-0 chromic sutures. This helps to prevent the frequently noted complication of neo-meatal stenosis, reported in approximately 6% of patients. If additional stump length is needed to increase the probability of adequate voiding function, the suspensory ligament of the penis may be divided.[36]

Several series have been reported, citing excellent local control, low recurrence rate, and acceptable maintenance of urinary and sexual function using the partial penectomy approach. Many men after partial penectomy will sit to void secondary to spraying of their urinary stream, whereas 20% of these men report adequate sexual function postoperatively. Currently, partial penectomy must remain the gold standard for invasive distal penile malignancies not amenable to more conservative treatments options previously described, as well as for locally recurrent cancers after an attempt at penile-conserving surgical management.[37,38]

Total Penectomy

Total penectomy (**Fig. 5**) is indicated for penile tumors whose size or location would not allow excision with an adequate surgical margin and preservation of a remnant sufficient for upright voiding. This procedure requires additionally the supplemental creation of a perineal urethrostomy. This procedure should be distinguished from a radical penectomy, rarely necessary with penile cancer but often required for tumors that infiltrate the corporus cavernosum. These cases entail excision of the corporal bodies in their entirety. With total penectomy, other than positioning to allow access to the perineum, the process is essential identical to the partial penectomy as described in the previous section except the penis is amputated at or near the level of the suspensory ligament of the penis without removal of the corporus cavernosum more proximally. The patient should be placed in the lithotomy position, and a diamond-shaped skin incision is first created at the base of the penis. Dorsally, the dissection is carried down through subcutaneous fat and vessels, which are ligated when identified. The suspensory ligament of the penis then is divided. Proximal crural amputation is accomplished, and the corpora are closed using the standard horizontal mattress technique. Ventrally, near the penoscrotal junction, the urethra can be isolated and subsequently mobilized to obtain sufficient urethral length to reach the perineum without tension. Care must be taken to assure an adequate urethra margin free of cancer as large tumors requiring total penectomy may demonstrate invasion of the corpora spongiosum. Creation of the perineal urethrostomy is completed when the perineal skin flap is sutured to the full-thickness spatulated urethra with 3-0 sutures. The diamond-shaped skin defect then is closed transversely. Usually a small suction drain is placed and left in-situ for 24-48 hours. A Foley catheter is left for about 1 week. Long-term survival after penectomy depends upon tumor stage and specifically nodal involvement. Local recurrence remains less than 10%.[34]

SUMMARY

The potential devastating impact of curative traditional surgery on the anatomic, functional, and psychological aspects of the patient's quality of life should always be a consideration even as urologic oncologists attempt to cure this potentially life-threatening malignancy. The development of penile-preserving surgical techniques will reduce the negative impact of amputations on functional and cosmetic outcomes only if oncologists continue to place oncologic objectives first and foremost for patients. Clearly, there are highly selective cohorts of patients who will benefit from these new approaches, yet long-term data are necessary if indeed one is to place these phallus-preserving techniques above standard penile amputations.[39]

REFERENCES

1. Young HH, Davis DM. Operations on the penis. In: Young HH, Davis DM, editors. Young's practice of

urology, vol. 2. Philadelphia: WB Saunders; 1926. p. 648–54.

2. Young HH, Davis DM. Neoplasms of the urogenital tract. In: Young HH, Davis DM, editors. Young's practice of urology, vol. 1. Philadelphia: WB Saunders; 1926. p. 719–21.

3. Das S. Penile amputations for the management of primary carcinoma of the penis. Urol Clin North Am 1992;19(2):277–82.

4. American Cancer Society. Cancer Reference Information. Available at: http://www.cancer.org/docroot/CRI/content/CRI_2_4_1X_What_are_the_key_statistics_for_penile_cancer_35.asp?rnav=cri. Accessed October 7, 2009.

5. Grossman HB. Premalignant and early carcinomas of the penis and scrotum. Urol Clin North Am 1992;19(2):225.

6. Graham JH, Helwig EB. Erythroplasia of Queyrat: a clinicopathologic and histochemical study. Cancer 1973;32:1396–9.

7. Grossman HB. Premalignant and early carcinomas of the penis and scrotum. Urol Clin North Am 1992;19(2):22.

8. Mohler JL, Freeman JA. Penectomy for invasive squamous cell carcinoma of the penis. Glenn's urologic surgery. Philadelphia: Lippincott Williams & Wilkins; 1975. p. 553–57.

9. Hernadez BY, Barnholtz-Sloan J, Grman RR, et al. Burden of invasive squamous cell carcinoma of the penis in the United States, 1998–2003. Cancer 2008;113:2883–91.

10. Breza J, Aboseif S, Orvis B, et al. Detailed anatomy of penile neurovascular structures: surgical significance. J Urol 1989;141:347–51.

11. Devine Jr CJ, Angermeier KW. Anatomy of the penis and male perineum. AUA Update Series 1994;13: 10–23.

12. Bandieramonte G, Colecchia M, Mariani L, et al. Penoscopy controlled CO2 laser excision for conservative treatment of in situ and T1 penile carcinoma: report on 224 patients. Eur Urol 2008;54:875–82.

13. Van Bezooijen B, Horenblas S, Meinhardt W, et al. Laser therapy for carcinoma of the penis. J Urol 2001;166:1670–1.

14. Colecchia M, Nicolai N, Secchi P, et al. pT1 penile squamous cell carcinoma: a clinicopathologic study of 56 cases treated by CO2 laser therapy. Anal Quant Cytol Histol 2009;31:153–60.

15. Windahl T, Andersson SO. Combined laser treatment for penile carcinoma: results after long-term followup. J Urol 2003;169(6):2118–21.

16. Schlenker B, Tilki D, Gratzke C, et al. Intermediate-differentiated invasive (pT1 G2) penile cancer-oncological outcome and follow-up. Urol Oncol 2009. [Epub ahead of print].

17. Schlenker B, Tilki D, Seitz M, et al. Organ-preserving neodymium-yttrium-aluminium-garnet laser therapy

for penile carcinoma: a long-term follow-up. BJU Int 2010. [Epub ahead of print].

18. Meijer RP, Boon TA, van Venrooij GE, et al. Long-term follow-up after laser therapy for penile carcinoma. Urology 2007;69(4):759–62.

19. Windahl T, Skeppner E, Andersson SO, et al. Sexual function and satisfaction in men after laser treatment for penile carcinoma. J Urol 2004;172(2): 648–51.

20. Skeppner E, Windahl T, Andersson SO, et al. Treatment-seeking, aspects of sexual activity and life satisfaction in men with laser-treated penile carcinoma. Eur Urol 2008;54(3):631–9.

21. Adeyoju A, Thornhill J, Grainger R, et al. Prognostic factors in squamous cell carcinoma of the penis and implications for management. Br J Urol 1997;80: 937–9.

22. Pierrzak P, Corbishley C, Watkins N. Organ-sparing surgery for invasive penile cancer: early follow-up data. BJU Int 2004;94:1253–7.

23. Guimarães GC, Cunha IW, Soares FA, et al. Penile squamous cell carcinoma clinicopathological features, nodal metastasis and outcome in 333 cases. J Urol 2009;182(2):528–34.

24. Chaux A, Reuter V, Lezcano C, et al. Comparison of morphologic features and outcome of resected recurrent and nonrecurrent squamous cell carcinoma of the penis: a study of 81 cases. Am J Surg Pathol 2009;33(9):1299–306.

25. Bisssada N. Concervative extirpative treatment of cancer of the penis. Urol Clin North Am 1992; 19(2):283–90.

26. Hoffman M, Renshaw A, Joughlin K. Squamous cell carcinoma of the penis and microscopic pathologic margins. Cancer 2000;85:1565–8.

27. Minhas S, Kayes O, Hegarty P, et al. What surgical resection margins are required to achieve oncological control in men with primary penile cancer? BJU Int 2005;96(7):1040–3.

28. Hegarty P, Shabbir M, Hughes B, et al. Penile-preserving surgery and surgical strategies to maximize penile form and function in penile cancer; recommendations from the United Kingdom experience. World J Urol 2009;27:179–87.

29. Davis J, Shellhammer P, Schlossberg S. Conservative surgical therapy for penile and urethral carcinoma. Urology 1999;53:386–92.

30. Brown C, Minhas S, Ralph D. Conservative surgery for penile cancer: subtotal glans excision without grafting. BJU Int 2005;96:911–2.

31. Ubrig B, Waldner M, Fallahi M, et al. Preputial flap for primary closure after excision of tumors on the glans penis. Urology 2001;58:274–6.

32. Gulino G, Sasso F, Falabella R, et al. Distal urethral reconstruction of the glans for penile carcinoma; results of a novel technique at 1 year follow-up. J Urol 2007;178:941–4.

33. Ralph DJ, Garaffa G, García MA. Reconstructive surgery of the penis. Curr Opin Urol 2006;16(6): 396–400.

34. Horenblas S, van Tinteren H, Delemarre JF, et al. Squamous cell carcinoma of the penis. II. Treatment of the primary tumor. J Urol 1992;147(6):1533–8.

35. Rudy D, Borden T. Partial and total penile amputation. In: Crawford ED, Borden TA, editors. Genitourinary cancer. Philadelphia: Surgery Lea and Febiger; 1982. p. 313–5.

36. Parkash S, Ananthakrishnan N, Roy P. Refashioning the phallus stump and phalloplasty in the treatment of carcinoma of the penis. Br J Surg 1986;73:902–5.

37. Korets R, Koppie T, Snyder M, et al. Partial penectomy for patients with squamous cell carcinoma of the penis: the Memorial Sloan-Kettering experience. Ann Surg Oncol 2007;14:3614–9.

38. Opjordsmoen S, Fossa S. Quality of life in patients treated for penile cancer. A follow-up study. Br J Urol 1994;74:652–7.

39. Martins F, Rogrigues R, Lopes T. Organ-preserving surgery for penile carcinoma. Adv Urol 2008. [Epub ahead of print].

Reconstruction of the Penis After Surgery

Christopher J. Salgado, MD[a],*, Stan Monstrey, MD, PhD[b],
Piet Hoebeke, MD, PhD[c], Nicolaas Lumen, MD[d],
Moira Dwyer, MD[e], Samir Mardini, MD[f]

KEYWORDS

- Penis • Reconstruction • Cancer • Urethra
- Scrotum • Flap • Skin graft • Erectile

PATIENT CONSIDERATIONS IN RECONSTRUCTION

The primary goal of penile reconstruction following oncologic resection is to create a neophallus that enables the patient to void while standing and to achieve vaginal penetration, that has erogenous and tactile sensibility, and that is cosmetically acceptable in shape, size, and color. In addition, surgeons should aim to perform penile reconstruction in a single-stage procedure that is associated with low donor-site morbidity.[1–5] Success of such a complex endeavor depends on preoperative planning, which relies on a thorough evaluation of the patient that maximizes outcomes by guiding decisions regarding the method for reconstruction as well as elucidating possible challenges.

Because most recurrences and metastases following resection of penile carcinoma occur within 1 year of the initial resection, most surgeons await consideration of reconstruction until time has passed and the patient has been confirmed to be disease free.[6,7] Other elements of patient and procedure selection are the patient's baseline health status, social habits, and mental health status. The type of flap and the mechanism for providing rigidity should be determined with consideration of patient comorbidities[1] such as diabetes, steroid use,[3] obesity,[8] and connective tissue disorders, all of which can influence the predicted outcomes. Tobacco use should be assessed because smoking has been shown to produce a thrombogenic, peripherally ischemic state with impaired wound healing and poor surgical outcomes.[9] In particular, there is an increased risk of necrosing full-thickness skin grafts and local flaps in smokers.[10] The exact duration of time between cessation of smoking and surgery required to prevent wound healing complications is unknown although commonly it is preferred that patients cease smoking for 2 to 4 weeks before their reconstruction.[11] Summerton and colleagues[12] state the importance of seeking psychological counseling before the penectomy; however, office evaluation before reconstructive surgery should address the psychosexual elements of possible procedural results, which may also influence the type of procedure selected.[13] In addition, Khouri and colleagues[14] state that patients must be prepared to undergo up to 6 operations within the first 12 months after phalloplasty as a result of complications and revisions, a possibility that should be discussed in frank terms with the patient.

No author received financial support for any part of this manuscript.

[a] University of Miami Miller School of Medicine, Division of Plastic Surgery/Department of Surgery, 1611 NW 12th Avenue, ET 3019, Miami, FL 33136, USA
[b] Department of Plastic Surgery, Ghent University Hospital, De Pintelaan 185, 9000 Ghent, Belgium
[c] Diensthoofd Urologie, Kinderurologie & Urogenitale Reconstructie, Department of Urology, Ghent University Hospital, De Pintelaan 185, 9000 Ghent, Belgium
[d] Department of Urology, Ghent University Hospital, De Pintelaan 185, 9000 Ghent, Belgium
[e] Department of Urology, Mayo Clinic Rochester, Gonda Building 7 South, 200 1st Street SW, Rochester, MN 55905, USA
[f] Division of Plastic Surgery, Mayo Clinic Rochester, Gonda Building 7 South, 200 1st Street SW, Rochester, MN 55905, USA
* Corresponding author.
E-mail address: Salgado_plastics@hotmail.com

Urol Clin N Am 37 (2010) 379–401
doi:10.1016/j.ucl.2010.04.015

In selecting the type of penile reconstruction, additional variables exist such as donor-site hair distribution, scars, skin thickness, vascular supply, and vascular defects. Some surgeons use the Allen test, color duplex imaging, Doppler ultrasonography,[15–17] and even angiogram studies[18] for preoperative evaluation of pertinent vessels, given the vitality of understanding the vascular anatomy and viability of the vessels for successful outcomes. Some advocate application of antiscar ointment with associated massage beginning 3 months before the procedure to increase the dimension of the flap and facilitate closure of the defect.[17]

Selection of the appropriate surgery reduces long-term problems in cosmesis, sexual function, and psychology.[12] Although each reconstructive procedure has its unique benefits and drawbacks that should be tailored to the patient's particular anatomy and general health status, patient preferences and postoperative goals should be discussed, because these help to guide preoperative planning as related to penile reconstruction.

RECONSTRUCTION OF VARIED URETHRAL DEFECTS

Because the primary urethral tumor is a rare condition, no large-scale experience exists about this topic. If possible, urethral tumors may require resection of the affected part of the urethra with the corpus spongiosum (partial urethrectomy) to offer the patient a treatment with curative intent. After urethral resection, normal voiding can be made possible by several reconstructive techniques replacing the resected urethra. These reconstructive techniques are based on the principles of urethroplasty for urethral stricture disease, but in urethral replacement, a whole new urethral tube must be created. To bridge the urethral gap, several techniques can be used:

1. Anastomotic repair (AR)
2. Augmented AR
3. One-stage substitution urethroplasty
   Free graft urethroplasty
   Pedicled flap urethroplasty
4. Two-stage urethroplasty.

General Principles of Urethroplasty

Preoperative preparation
The presence of urinary infection is one of the major causes of failure of urethral reconstruction, and for this reason it is advocated that the urine is sterile during reconstruction. It is advised to perform a urine culture the week before operation and to start with the appropriate antibiotics in case of infection 24 hours before operation.

Patient positioning
For tumors at the penile urethra, a common supine position is advised. When the tumor is situated deeper than the penile urethra, it is necessary to place the patient in the high lithotomy position. If there is any doubt about the extent of the urethral tumor, the patient should also be placed in the lithotomy position, which guarantees access to the penile and bulbar urethra.

Access to the urethra
Penile urethra A circumferential incision about 0.5 cm below the glans is the best access to the penile urethra. This access provides an excellent and well-vascularized coverage of all sutures, grafts, or flaps at the end of the operation. Fistulation is uncommon with this incision. The tissue is incised and dissected perpendicular to Buck's fascia, which can be easily identified because of its white aspect. The surgical plane following Buck's fascia is virtually avascular and can be easily followed to the base of the penis without jeopardizing the vascularization of the penile skin.

Bulbar urethra For exposure of the bulbar (and posterior) urethra, a perineal incision is necessary. Although an inverted-U or -λ incision has been described, a midline incision provides good access even to the posterior urethra and has the advantage of less postoperative pain. The subcutaneous tissue is incised until the level of the musculus bulbospongiosus. The bulbospongiosus is then incised at the midline and separated from the corpus spongiosum. The muscle can be fixated with 4 sutures at the perineal skin to provide good exposure.

Urinary diversion After every reconstructive procedure of the urethra, a urinary diversion is mandatory. Leakage and extravasation of urine in a recently reconstructed urethra can cause significant complications. For one-stage urethroplasty and in the second stage of a 2-stage urethroplasty, the urinary diversion is important. In most cases, diversion can be assured by a 16- to 20-Fr urethral catheter or a suprapubic catheter. After 10 to 14 days (depending on the type of urethroplasty) a cystourethrogram is performed. In no or only minimal urinary extravasation, the urinary diversion can be removed. In significant urinary extravasation, the diversion is maintained and the examination is repeated after 1 week.

SURGICAL TECHNIQUES OF URETHRAL RECONSTRUCTION
AR

This type of urethral reconstruction is the best technique because the diseased urethra is resected and replaced by its own healthy tissue without the interposition of foreign material. The good results are maintained in the long-term.[19–22] The anastomosis must be made with 2 well-vascularized urethral ends without any tension. When these 2 basic principles are neglected, failure can occur. To assure a broad anastomosis, both healthy urethral ends are spatulated for about 1 cm. With this technique, the intrinsic elasticity of the urethra is used to bridge the gap: the urethra can be elongated about 20% of its original length. The urethra must therefore be mobilized by dissecting it away from the corpora cavernosa. To avoid chordee and shortening of the penis, this mobilization should not go beyond the penoscrotal angle distally. In an already impotent patient, this is of no importance and the urethra can be mobilized up to the glans. Proximally, the urethra can be mobilized up to the urogenital diaphragm. To free the bulbous urethra the centrum tendineum must be sectioned. Additional length can be gained by separating the corpora cavernosa and placing the mobilized urethra between them. In the absence of any residual tension, the anastomosis is started at the dorsal side of the urethra using 4 or 5 interrupted resorbable 4.0 sutures. Thereafter a 16-Fr urethral catheter is introduced to avoid adhesions at the level of the anastomosis. The anastomosis is further completed ventrally with another 4 or 5 interrupted resorbable 4.0 sutures. If the patient already has a suprapubic catheter, the urethral catheter can be removed after 5 days. If not, the urethral catheter is maintained for 10 days. Postoperative antibiotics are not necessary unless there is urinary infection.

In general, only 2 to 3 cm can be bridged with these maneuvers and only at the proximal bulbar urethra. Because surgical resection of the tumor requires a sufficient tumor-free margin and AR requires spatulation of the healthy urethral ends, AR is in most cases impossible. The only exception is leiomyoma of the male urethra, which most often occurs at the bulbar urethra. These tumors do not recur or metastasize. If the affected segment is short, resection and primary AR are sufficient to treat this condition.[23–25]

Augmented AR

If an AR is attempted, but during the operation a tension-free anastomosis cannot be provided, a graft can be used to bridge the defect. This technique was initially described by Guralnick and Webster,[26] whereby the urethral ends are spatulated at the dorsal side and the ends are sutured to each other. A graft is then fixed at the corpora cavernosa at the place of the defect and the urethral edges are sutured against this graft using a running suture on both sides. It is essential that the graft is placed against a well-vascularized graft bed.

One-stage Substitution Urethroplasty

This type of urethroplasty obtains the reconstruction of a new urethra within the same time as the urethral resection. Two major different types of substitution urethroplasty are described:

1. Free graft urethroplasty:

To survive, the graft must be sutured against a well-vascularized graft bed. This is a problem in urethral replacement, because the corpus spongiosum is resected as well. Dorsally, the graft can be sutured against the corpora cavernosa but laterally and ventrally, a well-vascularized graft bed is lacking when creating a tube of a free graft. It has been shown that creating a tube of a free graft has disappointing results. For this reason, this type of urethroplasty is not indicated for urethral replacement.

2. Pedicled flap urethroplasty:

This is a one-stage urethroplasty in which a (pedicled) flap is used as a tube to reconstruct the urethra. A flap remains connected to the donor area with a vascular pedicle that provides vascularity to the flap. Flaps are thus not dependent on the vascularization of the surrounding tissues to survive and to defend themselves against infection. Harvested at the prepuce, the penile shaft or the scrotum, they can be used along the whole length of the urethra (**Fig. 1**).

Penile skin flaps

During dissection of penile skin flaps, it is essential not to damage the vascular pedicle. It is essential to follow the avascular surgical plane along Buck's fascia, which lies on the corpora cavernosa and spongiosum, to preserve all vessels of the subcutaneous tissue of the penis. The dissection must be performed far enough to allow mobilization of the flap without any traction. After harvesting the flap, a tube is made around an 18- to 20-Fr catheter using a resorbable running suture 4.0. It is important that the skin of the flap is healthy, without scar tissue, and that the vascularization is intact and not altered. This situation is not guaranteed if there have been previous interventions or lichen sclerosus.

Penile skin flaps can be harvested by several techniques:

Transverse island flap

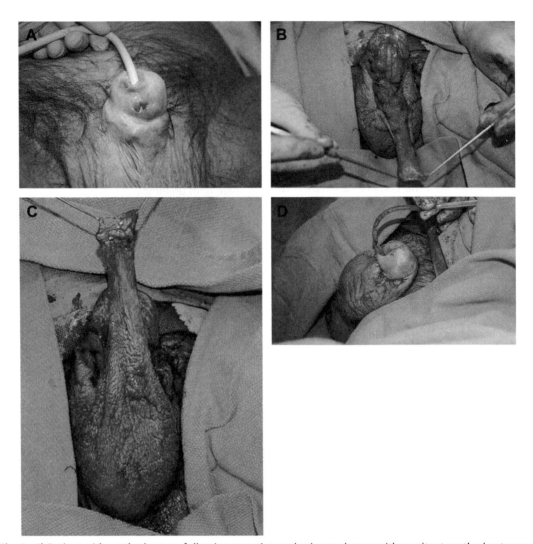

Fig. 1. A) Patient with urethral cancer following resection and primary closure with resultant urethral-cutaneous fistula. (B) Penile urethra is exposed (marked arrows) and scrotal flap is raised as a random pattern flap. (C) The distal half of the scrotal flap is de-epithelialized and turned over to become the penile urethra and the proximal half of the flap advanced for closure. (D) Immediate postoperative view of scrotal flap for urethra reconstruction.

The most distal part of the penile skin is used in a circular fashion. This technique was developed by Duckett[27] in the treatment of hypospadias. In a noncircumcised man, the flap is taken at the inner surface of the prepuce. The dimensions of a transverse island flap are limited by the circumference of the penis and seldom exceed 10 to 12 cm (**Fig. 2**).

Procedures for the person with hypospadias who has undergone numerous prior repairs and remains with residual strictures, fistulas, and chordee, in addition to those patients who have undergone prior radiation therapy with injured genitalia and impaired wound healing, represent a subset of complex problems that require transfer of extragenital tissues for successful resolution. Muscle-assisted full-thickness skin and buccal graft urethroplasty using gracilis, rectus abdominis, gluteus maximus, and free latissimus dorsi muscle transfers used for urethral and genital reconstruction has been successful in the past.[28] These muscle flaps may be prelaminated with skin for the urethral component with muscle transfer 2 to 4 weeks later using the muscle to obliterate the dead space and aid in microbial clearance. Skin may also be placed for the urethral component at the time of inset. The gracilis muscle remains the workhorse of perineal reconstruction as it is the most readily available for transfer to the urethra and other perineal conditions.

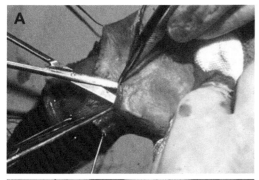

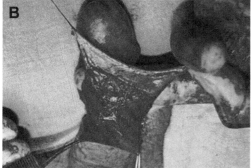

Fig. 2. (*A*) Transverse island flap using the inner surface of prepuce. Pre-elevation. (*B*) Elevated transverse island flap.

RECONSTRUCTION OF SCROTAL AND TESTICULAR DEFECTS

Cancer of the penis that extends into the scrotum and bulky penile tumors may require the resection of scrotal skin.[29] The resilient and vascular nature of the scrotum allows for primary closure of the scrotum even with skin losses of up to 50%,[30] a figure that can be improved to 67% with tissue expansion of the remnant scrotum.[31] Even so, reconstruction of the scrotum using grafts and flaps remains associated with the surgical treatment of advanced penile carcinomas. Given that tissue loss of the scrotum is frequently associated with Fournier gangrene (**Fig. 3**), much of the literature surrounding scrotal reconstruction is based on experiences with this disease; however, techniques and lessons learned are directly applicable to urologic oncology patients who have undergone surgical resection or complete removal of the scrotum.

The primary concerns in repairing scrotal defects are to protect the testes and to obtain a closed wound. These objectives have been achieved with split-thickness skin grafts, subcutaneous thigh pockets, and various myocutaneous and fasciocutaneous flaps. Definitive reconstruction of the scrotum can be delayed for several weeks from the time the testicles are denuded.

During this time, each testis is treated either with repeated wet dressing changes, thereby protecting the tissues from the increased systemic temperatures that can impair spermatogenesis, or with burial in an ipsilateral, medial, subcutaneous thigh pouch (**Fig. 4**). Relocation of the testicles to a more anatomic position is supported by concerns about pain, adverse psychological outcomes, and thermoregulation.[32] Wang and colleagues[33] reported that spermatogenesis, which requires a temperature $2°$ to $8°$ lower than the abdominal environment, is significantly abnormal after 2 years of follow-up in cases of thick skin flaps and buried testicles. Consequently, these methods are not recommended for patients who desire to maintain fertility. In patients in whom the creation of a flap is deferred from the time of cancer resection, perioperative considerations should include minimizing the infection rate, with complete shaving of the remaining scrotum within the operating room[34] as well as administration of a first-generation cephalosporin just before surgery.[35] In addition, the spermatic cord or testicles are typically sutured together before reconstruction to minimize the surface area, facilitate closure, and prevent a bifid neoscrotum.[5,36] Following the procedure, the scrotum should be elevated, and all patients should be advised that the neoscrotum may seem tight for 6 to 12 months until the testicles have expanded it fully.[2]

Although the denuded testicles are more commonly covered with meshed split-thickness skin grafts[5] that are aesthetically satisfactory, conform well to irregular defects, and enable the drainage of exudate, thus improving the success of the graft take to nearly 100%,[4] with 95% skin survival in extended defects,[37] these grafts cannot be used if the tunica vaginalis is affected or if there is no granulation tissue. Furthermore, grafts have the disadvantages of being insensate, demanding a long and time-consuming period of wound care,[38] and potentially adhering to the testes to cause contractures that hinder the cremasteric reflex.[10] In addition, the incidence of testicular torsion and vascular compromise in healed grafts is not uncommon and patients need to be aware of these occurrences. Skin grafts are not recommended in defects so large as to expose the spermatic cords because a greater amount of procedural difficulty is associated with the increasing size of the defect.[39] Because local flaps are the preferred option for providing testicular coverage when the remnant scrotum is insufficient, alternatives have been extensively developed over the years; options for testicular coverage use pedicled flaps, which can be completed safely in single-stage repairs.[40] These

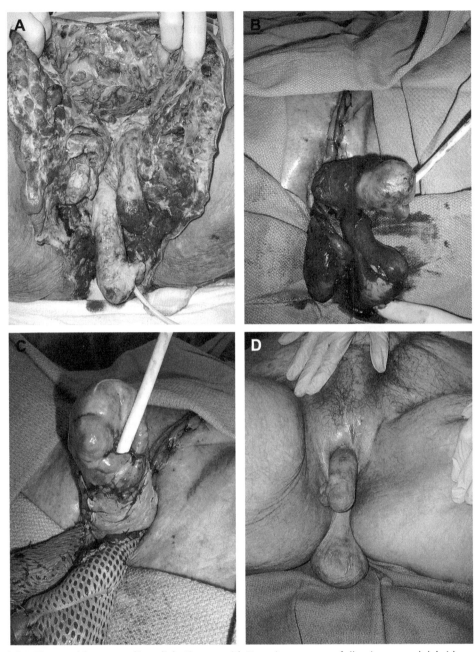

Fig. 3. (*A*) A 59-year-old noncompliant diabetic man with Fournier gangrene following several debridements and ongoing necrosis. The right testicle has been buried in subcutaneous tissues of the right thigh. (*B*) Following multiple debridements and at the time of skin graft reconstruction. (*C*) A meshed partial-thickness skin graft is used for coverage of the testicles and a pie-crusted skin graft used for the penile shaft. (*D*) Final postoperative view at 6 months after right orchiectomy for a necrotic testicle after torsion and ischemia which occurred 1 month following skin graft procedure (one of the complications of skin graft reconstruction of the testicle).

flaps tend to avoid the complications of skin grafting such as skin maceration and breakdown secondary to fecal and urinary contamination. In addition, the complicated postoperative care and the duration of anesthesia that are required for free-flap repairs are obviated with the use of a pedicled flap for scrotal reconstruction.

Reconstruction of the scrotum and perineum may be accomplished with vertical rectus abdominis myocutaneous flaps and is the flap of choice

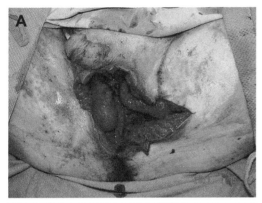

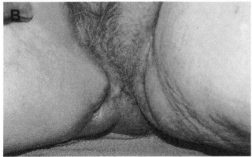

Fig. 4. (*A*) A 58-year-old man following debridement of the scrotum for Fournier gangrene. (*B*) Testicles are buried under medial thigh skin and flaps advanced for closure.

of the authors for perineal defects (**Fig. 5**). Many flaps, however, are based on tissue from the perineum, groin, or lower extremities as opposed to the abdomen, and Hallock[41] describes a medial circumflex femoral artery perforator flap that is based on the musculocutaneous perforators of the gracilis muscle. This technique is suggested as an improvement on the medial thigh fasciocutaneous flap and is regarded as superior to the sensory anterolateral thigh (ALT) flap, which is typically based on discrete perforators and requires a more extensive dissection.[4] Hallock's technique uses a nonhirsute donor site and spares one lower extremity from violation; however, it results in an insensate neoscrotum that may be attached to the medial thigh, thereby begging a second-stage procedure. Hsu and colleagues[42] illustrate the use of the well-established gracilis myofasciocutaneous advancement flap for cases of scrotal and perineal skin loss. This graft is elevated with a robust portion of the perigracilis fascia, and the associated skin incision is simply repaired with a V-to-Y primary closure. Kayik-çioğlu[43] advocates a short gracilis flap with a more proximal skin island to minimize problems caused by the traditional pedicle base location, which is 8 to 10 cm from the pubic tubercle, and

the bulky nature of the original flap. In the short gracilis flap procedure, the main pedicle, derived from branches of the medial femoral circumflex artery and vein, is ligated and the motor nerve transected with the aim of inducing muscle atrophy. Despite these maneuvers, the flap is left as a peninsula or an island. A disadvantage of such myofasciocutaneous flaps is the sacrifice of normally functioning muscle tissue in a setting in which bulk is an unnecessary flap feature. Thus, attention has been directed to developing thinner fasciocutaneous flaps. One such flap is the neurovascular pedicled pudendal thigh flap that Karacal and colleagues[44] described for use in scrotal reconstruction. With this technique, the superficial perineal artery supplies a posterior flap from the level of the scrotoperineal junction. The flap, used for defects with a mean area of 300 cm^2, includes the deep fascia of the thigh and the fibrous tissue covering the adductor muscles, leaving a donor defect that can be closed primarily. The superficial perineal nerve is incorporated into the flap, eliminating numbness in spite of the associated denervation of the genitofemoral and ilioinguinal nerves.[11] In cases of pelvic radiation, however, this flap is not always reliable. A novel technique published by Payne and colleagues[45] is the use of local perforator lotus petal flaps that are based on the internal pudendal arteries. In this method, the skin flaps are raised from the gluteal folds and rotated 90° to create a neoscrotum. Maharaj and colleagues[46] have used the Singapore flap, which was originally used in vaginal reconstruction, as a testicular sling, dissecting from the posterior perineum along the groin crease to the medial thigh as deep as the subfascial layer. The flap is elevated and then tunneled under the remaining bridge of skin between the groin crease and the scrotum. The donor site is closed primarily after the flap is secured to the edges of the defect. In search of a functionally and aesthetically ideal outcome for reconstructing a wide scrotal defect, Atik and colleagues used a skin expander for 3 weeks at a location 5 cm inferolateral to the anterior superior iliac spine. The area of expansion extended toward the lateral aspect of the groin where the subcutaneous fat tissue is notably less than in the peri-inguinal region. The flap, based on the superior circumflex iliac artery with nerve input from the lateral cutaneous femoral nerve, was dissected subfascially, tunneled subcutaneously to the scrotum, and sutured to the defect. The donor site was closed primarily and the capsule that had formed around the expander prevented any adhesion of the testes to the flap. The result of this procedure was a superthin neoscrotum with

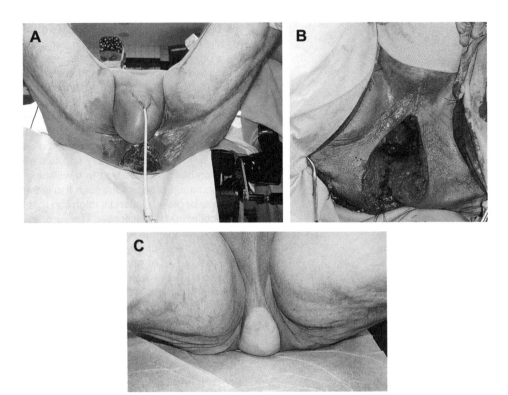

Fig. 5. (*A*) A 62-year-old man with recurrent colorectal cancer involving the perineum and posterior scrotum. (*B*) Following oncologic resection and awaiting immediate reconstruction. (*C*) Six months following vertical rectus abdominis myocutaneous flap for perineum and posterior scrotum reconstruction.

an average, uncomplicated hospital stay of 33 days.[10] Various other flaps that use similar principles to these procedures have been described, with a more recent emergence of technical modifications that are based on advancements in technology and engineering. For instance, fibrin sealant intended to prevent fluid accumulation in reconstruction with split-thickness skin grafts and flaps has had success as a tissue glue for genital skin reconstruction.[47] New tools to aid the surgeon in scrotal reconstruction will be developed as science and technology continue to advance.

The need for testicular reconstruction associated with penile cancer is rare. The testicles have an independent blood supply compared with the surrounding tissue, and thus, even with extensive debridement, they can be completely exposed and remain viable. Nonetheless, for damage to the testicle that requires repair, free grafts of tunica vaginalis are superior to synthetic grafts, which have a high infection rate, often requiring orchiectomy. Serial Doppler ultrasonography can be used to assess the testicles following repair, and testicular volume can be monitored.[48]

Many options exist for scrotal reconstruction following resection or complete excision of the scrotum in association with surgical procedures aimed at eradicating local penile carcinoma. With the application of basic principles and the individualization of therapy based on the size of the defect and patient desires such as continued spermatogenesis and cosmesis, an appropriate technique can be selected and used in a single-stage procedure.

RECONSTRUCTION OF THE PENILE SHAFT
Patient Evaluation

History
The evaluation of the patient requiring penile reconstruction begins at the time the surgeon greets the patient. Typically the patient who has suffered from the loss of any portion of his penis finds himself in a desperate frame of mind and at times does not fully understand your reconstructive plan. It is therefore imperative to obtain informed consent of your proposed procedures and to enquire about previous psychiatric history because often these patients have some form of depression. A significant percentage of patients may even have attempted to injure themselves because of the loss of their penis. This situation should not exclude them from being a surgical

candidate; this deformity has caused some patients to commit suicide.

A questionnaire may be given to the patient before the consultation to include a more detailed sexual history and desired goals. These goals are then reviewed by the surgeon and a picture of the patient's expectations may be evaluated to determine if they are realistic or not. If a questionnaire is used then directed questions need to be made to elicit your defects and to formulate the operative plan. Ask if the patient is able to urinate voluntarily or not and whether it is via a perineal or penile urethrostomy. Is the patient able to have an orgasm currently and in what manner (eg, by penetration, masturbation)? Is the tactile sensation necessary for the patient to obtain an orgasm and are nerves such as the pudendal, ilioinguinal, and iliohypogastric sensate or not? When was the last time the patient was able to obtain an orgasm and has he been able to obtain one following the extirpation procedure? These are all important questions and the surgeon must feel comfortable asking them, because often the questionnaire may not elicit the answers.

The patient needs to be aware that you will do whatever you can within your surgical capabilities to perform a successful reconstruction, accomplishing as many of the desired goals as possible. Commonly more than one operation is necessary to accomplish your reconstructive goals and the patient needs to be as committed as you are to the process. A patient who desires only one quick operation is often not a good surgical candidate, because revision surgery is often required to accomplish all goals. In addition realistic expectations should be sought. A patient who states that his erect penis was 25 cm long preoperatively and desires this result postoperatively should be referred to the Kinsey Institute study and one in the *Journal of Urology* showing that the top 1% of patients have penises at most 22.5 cm in length when erect, with the top 10% measuring just more than 15.5 cm in length. The average penile length is 15 cm when erect.[49]

Patient-controlled factors such as smoking and diabetes need to be addressed and a commitment from the patient to cease smoking or control his blood sugars if he is diabetic is vital. Hemoglobin A_{1C} should be evaluated and an endocrinologist should be consulted to ensure there is hypoglycemic control. Urine nicotine levels should be measured to ensure that the patient (if a smoker) has ceased smoking. Although smoking is considered by some surgeons to be a contraindication for surgery, if the patient abstains for a minimum of 3 weeks then surgery may be entertained. The patient should be aware of the increased risks of surgery if he has a previous smoking history. Surgical scars and prior history of trauma should be addressed because this dictates the use of flap tissue for the reconstruction. A detailed medical and surgical history should be taken so that any complicating factors to the proposed reconstruction may be addressed before surgery.

Physical examination

The patient should be in a gown for easier access for examination of the genital and perineal region. A lithotomy position is beneficial, particularly for the patient with a perineal urethrostomy, so that the abdominal and perineal regions are visualized together. The patient is often best evaluated in the surgical position in which he will be placed during surgery. Patient hygiene should be observed. The importance of good hygiene for any patient undergoing genitoperineal surgery cannot be overemphasized. If a partial penectomy has been performed and a remnant portion of penile shaft exists then measurement should be made with tape from the pubic symphysis to the distalmost aspect of the glans penis. This measurement should be recorded in the flaccid and erectile state if the patient is potent. Circumference in the midshaft axis should also be measured and recorded. Tactile sensation is evaluated at the distalmost aspect of the penis, midshaft, and at the pubic base. This sensation is evaluated in the perineum as well because this is particularly important in the patient with a perineal urethrostomy.

Suprapubic fat excess is recorded because a simpler buried penis operation may correct the patient deformity and achieve the patient's goals. Previous infections and associated microbes are recorded so that they may be treated with perioperative antibiotics. Surgical scars are also noted and appropriate preoperative studies obtained to ensure adequate arterial inflow and venous outflow of the surrounding vasculature. One must ensure that the recipient vessels are suitable for free tissue transfer and that any local flap option maintains flap vessel patency if it is an axial pattern flap.

Goals in penile reconstruction:

- Allow patient to void through reconstructed penile urethra conduit
- Allow patient to have intercourse with new penis
- Allow patient (if possible) to have orgasm during sexual intercourse
- Allow patient to have sensitivity to distal shaft/glans
- Create an aesthetically pleasing phallus
- Avoid infection and other complications if possible.

TIMING OF RECONSTRUCTION
When is Reconstruction Necessary?

The penis is an exceptionally composite organ with several and complex roles (transport of urine through a flaccid organ, transport of semen through an erected organ, allowing intercourse, essentiality for sexual function); it thus has a psychosexual effect on the man. When the penis is absent or inadequate, surgery is unable to replace it totally, recreating an anatomically and functionally normal organ with adequate sensation, erection, and capability to convey sperm and urine. Recently, there has been increasing interest in phallic substitution in adults and some fascinating procedures have been introduced that may partially reproduce an efficient penis. Many of these procedures were introduced in the treatment of female-to-male gender dysphoria as the main indication for phalloplasty. These technical proposals give new perspectives in male reconstructive surgery in infants, children, and adolescents affected by congenital penile malformations or early acquired serious penile deficiencies. Severe penile insufficiency or absence of a penis is a devastating condition for men, with significant psychological and physical effects. Although uncommon, they are challenging lesions to treat. As well as congenital conditions in which the penis has failed to develop, traumatic events, medically necessary penile amputations, and failed reconstructions of congenital anomalies are the main reasons for penile insufficiency (**Box 1**).

Possible treatment options are tailoring of the penile stump, phallic reconstruction (phalloplasty), and more recently penile transplantation. Tailoring of the penile stump by means of penile degloving, division of the suspensory ligament, and rotational skin flaps has been reported.[50,51] However, this procedure can be applied only to moderate penile defects with a reasonable penile stump. Men with defects with a remnant penile length of 2 to 3 cm are capable of urination in a standing position and often do not require aggressive reconstruction, depending on patient comorbidities and age.

LOCAL PEDICLED FLAPS IN PENILE RECONSTRUCTION

The use of pedicled flaps for phalloplasty has fallen out of favor as new techniques have been developed that compensate for the shortcomings of local flaps in the creation of a neopenis. Although pedicled flaps such as the extended groin skin flap, the rectus abdominis myocutaneous flap, the superficial inferior epigastric skin flap, and the tensor fascia lata myocutaneous flap have been

---

> **Box 1**
> **Conditions leading to severe penile insufficiency**
>
> Congenital conditions (disorders of sexual development)
>
> - Aphallia or penile agenesis
> - Ideopathic micropenis
> - 46,XY disorder of sexual development
> - Exstrophy
> - Cloacal exstrophy
>
> Genital trauma
>
> - Injuries
> - Surgery
>
> Penile amputation
>
> Female-to-male gender dysphoria

---

used recently for total penile reconstruction, the resultant neophalluses can have poor to no sensation, which precludes the use of stiffeners or inflatable prostheses, and can be aesthetically inferior to the alternatives. By comparison, microsurgical free-flap techniques can have significantly improved functional and aesthetic outcomes in respect to the neophallus and, consequently, the urologic and plastic surgery communities have begun to embrace these methods for total penile reconstruction. Whereas pedicled flaps have a diminishing role in the primary creation of the neophallus, peninsular and island flaps continue to have a predominant role in genitourinary reconstructive surgical procedures.

Although microsurgical free-flap phalloplasty tends to be the favored method of penile reconstruction given advancements in free tissue transfer and microsurgical techniques, the use of pedicled flaps continues to provide a method of total penile reconstruction that has a decreased risk of total failure, a decrease in visible donor-site morbidity, and a decrease in the operative time that microsurgical techniques necessitate.[4,5,52] Much of the literature regarding total penile reconstruction reports on transsexual and trauma patients; however, principles and lessons from these populations easily translate to guide total penile reconstruction after surgical amputation for penile carcinoma. Uniformly, the ideal flap for phalloplasty is one that is safe, sensate, hairless, and based on a long pedicle. Operative goals include providing an aesthetically satisfactory neophallus, tactile and erogenous sensation of the neophallus, the ability to urinate while standing, the ability to achieve vaginal penetration, and minimal scarring at the donor site. It is generally understood, in addition, that it is most desirable to perform the reconstruction in a single-stage procedure as well as to create a stricture-free, fistula-free urethra with its meatus located at the tip of the neoglans.[2,53] These objectives have been met to varying degrees throughout the history of peninsular and island flaps in phalloplasty, which began in 1936 when Bogaraz[54] reported a multistage reconstruction with an abdominal tubularized skin flap. A wide array of pedicled flaps have been attempted since then and, although no standard procedure has been established for pedicled flap phalloplasty, the more recent techniques have had the greatest advantages and relevance to contemporary practice.

One method for neophallic reconstruction is the use of a pedicled island ALT flap, the center of which can be identified by the location of the most distal perforating artery detected by Doppler ultrasonography. In 2009, Rubino and colleagues[52] described the creation of a neophallus for a female-to-male transsexual patient in a procedure that combined this type of flap with the creation of a neotunica albuginea intended to provide a protective barrier against infection, extrusion, and trauma for the malleable prosthesis that was inserted at that same time. The material for the neotunica was harvested during the flap elevation as a 3-cm-wide strip of vascularized fascia lata, which was then wrapped around the prosthesis. To render the neophallus sensate, the lateral cutaneous femoral nerve, which distributes to the ALT flap, was isolated at this time, with special care taken to protect this nerve during the proximal dissection of the pedicle. The nerve stump was then coapted with the dorsal clitoris branch of the pudendal nerve in hopes of providing erogenous sensibility. Hage and colleagues[53] also reported in 2009 on the pedicled island ALT flap after 3 patients with aphallia had been reconstructed with this flap. In their series, the investigators passed the flap, after it was tubularized, through a tunnel directed toward the pubis and located deep to the sartorius and rectus abdominis muscles. Once centrally located, a circular skin excision allowed for the neophallus to be sutured into place in a tension-free manner. Full-thickness grafts were harvested from the groin and applied to the ALT fascia in anticipation of neourethral construction as a second-stage procedure. Although Rubino and colleagues had reserved urethral reconstruction for the future, no preparatory actions were taken with their patient. As a result, the success of the procedure was measured in terms of satisfactory aesthetic results and sexual activity, both of which were present 6 months following surgery. An obvious disadvantage to the use of the pedicled island ALT flap is that the width of the donor site may be so extensive as to require split-thickness skin grafting, which, although easily concealed with trunk-length undergarments, can lead to an unpleasant cosmetic result.

In 2006, Mutaf[5] described a technique that combined an ALT flap, which was used to create the shaft and neoglans, with a sartorius perforator flap, from which the neourethra was created, allowing for a single-stage phalloplasty. The modification was inspired by the desire for a nonhirsute neourethra and the procedure used the tube-within-a-tube technique to unite the 2 flaps. These flaps were then passed through a subcutaneous tunnel for appropriate positioning. Similarly to Rubino and colleagues, these investigators created a neotunica albuginea from vascularized fascia lata to protect a prosthesis that was placed at the time of the procedure. For reconstruction using an alloplastic prosthesis, which, because of disappointing late-term results with autogenic materials, is the current trend, the investigators recommended the creation of such a neotunica albuginea. With this advancement, this patient had no mechanical or wound complications 2 years following the procedure. Erogenous sensibility, reported at 1 year, was facilitated by the coaptation of the lateral femoral cutaneous nerve to the paired pudendal nerves. This procedure was felt to be reliable, meeting the goals of total penile reconstruction in one stage without the use of microsurgery.[2]

Akoz and Kargi[55] felt that the use of vascularized autogenic material would provide the rigidity necessary for sexual penetration in a more durable fashion and, in 2001, described a double-pedicle procedure in a transsexual that sought to use this principle. The first stage of the procedure entailed defining the superficial iliac circumflex artery and deep iliac circumflex artery by Doppler ultrasound before parallel incisions were made down to the iliac crest. This procedure allowed for excision of a 14- $\times$ 3-cm piece of bone, which was left attached to the deep iliac circumflex artery. While still connected superiorly and inferiorly, the skin of this flap was then tubularized. A full-thickness skin graft from the opposite side of the body was tubularized in an inverted fashion around a silicone rod and then inserted into the flap to become the neourethra, because it was believed that this prefabrication would be beneficial for healing of the skin graft. The initial incisions made around the flap were closed together beneath the now tubularized tissue. After 2 weeks, the flap was raised on the inferior pedicle, which included the aforementioned arteries, and passed through a tunnel to be delivered to the pubic region. The neourethra was anastomosed and urine was diverted for 1 week via a suprapubic tube. The patient required repair of an anastomotic fistula, and an asymmetry was noted at follow-up, because the neopenis seemed directed toward the donor side. Nonetheless, this procedure allowed for limited donor-site morbidity in an easily concealed location.

Sun and Huang[56] described a lateral groin skin flap based on the superficial circumflex iliac artery that also incorporated the iliac crest as rigid supporting tissue. In such a procedure, the distance between the pubic symphysis and the femoral origin of the superficial circumflex iliac artery should be exceeded by the length of the flap pedicle. The bone is harvested beginning at the posterosuperior iliac spine and moving toward the base, and its attachments to the skin flap are maintained. To be soft and hairless, the neourethra is made from a separate scrotal septal skin flap, a technique preferable because of the rich blood supply of the scrotum; otherwise, a superficial inferior epigastric vessel island skin flap or a free skin graft, which has a lower survival rate, can be used. The principal flap is transferred to the midline via a subcutaneous tunnel and the iliac crest bone is then sutured to the corpus cavernosum. The neourethra is tubularized and placed into the composite flap, where the proximal end is anastomosed to the remnant urethra. The distal end is then anastomosed to the composite flap before tubularization of the neophallus. This technique takes advantage of the thin and hairless skin of the lateral groin flap, the donor site of which is easily closed and well concealed, as well as its good blood supply and the easy transfer of the flap within a one-stage procedure. There is little sensation in the neophallus. Despite the poor sensibility, Koshima and colleagues[57] have more recently described the use of bilateral superficial circumflex iliac artery perforator flaps for penile and urethral reconstruction, citing minimal donor-site morbidity and ability for single-stage reconstruction as advantages.

Perovic[17] described a modified version of the phalloplasty described by He and colleagues[58] and Lai and colleagues[59] in which he created an extended pedicle island groin flap based on the superficial circumflex iliac and epigastric vessels. The base of the flap is located below the inguinal ligament and extends cranially and laterally. This groin flap consists of a 2-cm lateral nonhirsute strip for the neourethra, which is first tubularized itself before being rolled within the shaft of the neophallus. The flap pedicle is lengthened with 4 to 5 cm of de-epithelialization on which the flap is rotated 90° to 180° as it is tunneled toward the recipient site. The donor defect is closed primarily

and anastomosis of urethra to neourethra can be performed primarily or in a secondary procedure at the time of sculpting of the neoglans or implantation of penile stiffeners. Sensibility was found to be slight to moderate in follow-up of this cohort of children and adolescents.

Hage and colleagues[60] evaluated 31 phalloplasties of different types in the Amsterdam experience and, although they favored microsurgical methods, they concluded that the rectus abdominis myocutaneous pedicled flap is a reliable technique. Similarly, Santi and colleagues[61] acknowledge the superiority of microsurgical techniques or even multistage procedures for enhanced aesthetic and functional results; however, they advocate the inferiorly based rectus abdominis myocutaneous flap in cases in which the psychological needs of the patient may make penile reconstruction at the time of penectomy most beneficial. The skin island portion of this flap, which is based on the deep inferior epigastric artery, becomes the ventral surface of the penis after the flap is passed through a subcutaneous tunnel; however, the dorsal surface of the reconstructed penis must be covered with a split-thickness skin grafts after tubularization. Vicryl mesh or other biologic implants may be used to reinforce the anterior rectus fascia, which, like the abdominal skin at the donor site, is closed primarily. Concerns for risk of abdominal hernia were addressed by the investigators, who state that muscular function and abdominal competence should not be significantly affected. Their patient returned at 12 months with no evidence of abdominal weakness, in part because of the small amount of muscular tissue that was included in the flap. These investigators propose that fibrosis of this muscle may allow for sufficient rigidity for sexual penetration; however, sensitivity is not provided with this procedure. Hanash and Tur[7] performed a unilateral myocutaneous gracilis flap on a 36-year-old man who had a total penectomy for carcinoma and, on the contrary, reported preservation of deep penile sensation and successful intercourse.

Penile skin itself is an apt medium to use as a flap for the urethral component of penile reconstruction, because its vascular supply is collateralized from the left and right superficial external pudendal vessels, which complements the superlative thinness and mobility of this tissue. Elevation of the fascia to create a subcutaneous pedicle allows for the transfer of a penile skin flap to almost any segment of the neourethra.[62] These same favorable characteristics of penile skin apply to preputial skin, which can be used as a local flap in patients with glanular disease. When primary closure becomes an impossibility secondary to the need for an acceptable negative surgical margin, the preputial skin flap serves as an alternative to full-thickness penile skin grafts or extragenital split-thickness skin grafts as a means to cover the resultant, wide defect of the glans.[63] Because these last 2 options are such excellent sources of resilient and compliant tissue, local flaps are seldom necessary for repair of lesions limited to the penile skin.[35] Integra, which is bovine collagen with silicone outlayer (Integra Life Sciences Corp, Plainsboro, NJ, USA) has also been shown to be useful for penile skin coverage as a dermal substitute to be followed by skin grafting after removal of the silicone sheeting 1 month later.

The scrotum is an ideal substrate for providing skin coverage because it stretches easily and is pliable, making it useful for penile shaft coverage. In patients in whom there is excess mons pubis fat a buried penis corrective technique may be used with fat excision with or without penopubic suspensory ligament transaction (**Fig. 6**). In addition, the scrotum has a dual blood supply and scrotal flap necrosis is rare. Even if a main vessel is transected, the scrotal skin flap can survive on its fascial vessel network.[64] These features lend themselves to reconstructive procedures. Emsen[65] took advantage of such valuable characteristics in his use of a bilateral vascularized scrotal pedicle flap to cover a defect at the penoscrotal junction in a patient who, after refusing total penectomy, had undergone wide surgical excision of a squamous cell carcinoma with resection down to the capsule of the cavernosum. Emsen remarks that, unlike reconstructive efforts that use the expanded scrotal musculocutaneous flap, the superiorly based flap allowed for reconstruction in a single procedure. In addition, this procedure overcame the poor cosmetic results of a split-thickness skin graft and avoided the multiple incisions associated with a rotary multiflap. Zhao and colleagues[20] also used the advantages of scrotal skin for reconstruction in addressing a partial surgical amputation with penile lengthening and coronoplasty that involved scrotal flaps. No significant breakdown was noted and recovery of deep and superficial sensation was observed, with 15 of 18 patients reporting satisfied sexual intercourse during the 0.5- to 5-year follow-up. Perhaps even more exemplary of the plasticity of the scrotal skin is the 2-stage pedicled flap, which can be considered in select patients as a means of reconstructing the glans after partial penectomy. In this technique, which Mazza and Cheliz[66] described in 34 patients, the distal end of a scrotal flap is initially sutured to the penile stump after a buttonhole has been created for the urethra, which is also sutured into place. The pedicle of the flap is resected secondarily about 4 to 6 weeks after the initial procedure. Follow-up revealed that 17.6% of patients required definitive depilation of the neoglans and that 20.5% of patients had preservation of sexual potency by self-report. Although scrotal skin is hirsute, this technique does allow for preservation of the penile skin, which is not usually redundant. It avoids retraction seen with the use of penile skin as well as the risks of skin grafting onto the poorly vascularized albuginea, and it uses tissue with pigmentation similar to the natural glans. Based on experience with hypospadias and penoscrotal transposition, Liu and colleagues[67] observe the success with which scrotal skin flaps with arterial supply from the lateral braches of the posterior scrotal arteries can resurface ventral wounds of the penis. Scrotal flaps have also been used in combination with suprapubic flaps to reconstruct the phallus after partial penectomy, restoring directional voiding with adequate cosmesis. Greenberger and Lowe[68] describe a patient with retained cutaneous sensation and orgasmic response following bilateral, anterolateral-based, full-thickness, rotational scrotal myocutaneous flaps, with complete wound healing at 2 weeks.

The strategic uses of local flaps in reconstruction apart from the creation of a strict neophallus represent the variety and versatility of the pedicled flap, which can offer a wide array of advantages. The deep inferior epigastric perforator flap is used for the reconstruction of lower abdominal, inguinal, and genital defects, with the benefits of minimal donor-site morbidity, a wide arch of rotation, and a versatile flap design.[69] Zeng and colleagues[70] describe the use of this flap for penoscrotal resurfacing after resection of Paget disease and also for groin defects following the resection of inguinal lymph nodes containing metastatic penile carcinoma. With application of the techniques described, the patient may benefit from ambulation on the first postoperative day, a primary closure of the donor site, excellent cosmesis, and a low complication rate because of the exceptional blood supply of these flaps. The deep inferior epigastric perforator flap was also used by Demirtas and colleagues[71] in the reconstruction of a glans after the flap was tunneled subcutaneously. Similarly, Shaeer and El-Sebaie[72] describe the construction of a neoglans using a rectus abdominis myofascial flap as a component of total phalloplasty or as a solitary procedure, referencing the superiority of the consistency of the muscle for its semblance to the consistency of the natural glans plus its ability to tolerate the effect of a prosthesis. The associated tunneled flap procedure is combined with

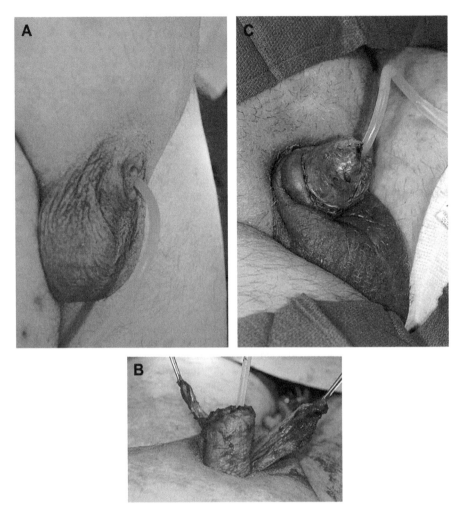

Fig. 6. (*A*) A 76-year-old following near total penectomy with excess suprapubic fat. Desires to "pee standing up." (*B*) Patient treated with mons lipectomy, transection of penopubic ligaments, scrotal flaps for base of penis coverage, and skin grafting of distal penile shaft. (*C*) 3 weeks following reconstruction.

urethral lengthening using penile skin and allows for sculpting of the neoglans before anastomosis to fashion a corona. Subsequently, the neoglans is covered by a split-thickness graft that, over the muscle layer, mimics the typical pigmentation of the glans. Jordan and Schlossberg[17] adopted the practice of covering the neourethral-urethral anastomosis with a gracilis muscular flap, which resulted in a decreased occurrence of anastomotic fistulae and stricture formation in their series of patients undergoing penile reconstruction, an improvement believed to be secondary to increased vascularity. In addition, the gracilis muscle has been shown to be advantageous when combined with a bipedicled flap from the base of the penile shaft to cover the junction of the flap and the base of the neoscrotum. Such a bipedicled flap could provide stability to the neophallus as well, and this principle has been used

in transsexual patients, in whom the flap was transposed to the undersurface of the neopenis after it had been implanted onto the area from which the flap had been elevated.[17] Kayes and colleagues[8] have described the use of the vertical rectus abdominis flap in patients with advanced penile cancer following radical resection of extensive cutaneous metastatic disease. The potential of this flap, which has excellent blood supply through segmental perforators, in the setting of large, soft-tissue defects, shows the broad usefulness of local pedicled flaps in reconstruction for patients with penile cancer, as well as the use of such pedicled flaps for scrotal reconstruction, as described earlier.

Although local flaps have proved to be a versatile and useful component of reconstruction after surgery for penile carcinoma, total penile reconstruction or phalloplasty is often unsatisfactory when dependent on regional flaps alone, because these can result in an insensate neopenis and a technical inability to place an inflatable penile prosthesis.[18] Nonetheless, pedicled flaps remain a favorable option when compared with the use of skin grafts and cultured grafts for tissue coverage in the genital, perineal, inguinal, and lower abdominal regions during reconstruction.

DISTANT FREE-TISSUE TRANSFER IN PENILE RECONSTRUCTION
Soft-tissue Flaps and Prosthetic Implantation

Varied flaps available
Performing a penile reconstruction is a challenging procedure. In the ideal situation, the surgeon should reconstruct an aesthetically appealing phallus, with erogenous and tactile sensation, which enables the patient to void while standing and to have sexual intercourse. Moreover, this should best be achieved in a single-stage operative procedure that is predictably reproducible and that leaves the patient without functional loss in the donor area and with only minimal scarring or disfigurement.[2,3] These ideal phalloplasty requirements have not been met yet.

Looking back on the history of this kind of surgery, Bogoras[73] was the first to report on the reconstruction of the entire penis by using a single abdominal tube, a technique later applied by many others. Subsequently the term phalloplasty was used to describe penile reconstruction. Following World War II, some leading plastic surgeons showed an interest in the penile reconstructive procedure. A neourethra could be reconstructed with inlay skin grafts and Gillies and Millard[74] popularized the technique when they added a costal cartilage graft as a rigidity prosthesis. Different attempts evolved[75–77] to further refine this complex procedure and reduce the number of stages previously necessary for phalloplasty.

However, after McGregor[78] introduced the groin flap in 1972, Hoopes[79] commented that "the groin flap may prove the method of choice for phallus reconstruction." On the other hand, the Norfolk team used a (multistaged) unilateral gracilis myocutaneous flap for phalloplasty and claimed it produced cosmetically and functionally superior results.[80] Other surgeons advocated a combination of flaps to further increase the functional and aesthetic outcome.[81]

More recently, however, microsurgical free flaps have been considered state-of-the-art in penile reconstruction[82] because they allow for the selection of distant flaps with the transfer of free vascularized tissue and the co-optation of nerves from the donor flap to recipient nerves in the perineum.

The most frequently used free flap is the radial forearm flap, or Chinese flap, which was originally described by Song.[83] Various other free flaps have been described, including the dorsalis pedis flap,[1] the deltoid flap,[84] the lateral arm flap,[3] the fibular flap,[85] the tensor fasciae latae flap,[86] and the ALT flap.[87]

The existence of so many techniques for penile reconstruction is evidence that none is considered ideal.

Flap of Choice?

Despite the multitude of free flaps that have been used and described (often as case reports), the radial forearm is the most frequently used technique (>90% of reported cases) and is the most accepted form of penile reconstruction.[2,3,88–90]

To achieve a functional and aesthetic phallic reconstruction, it is essential to perform a procedure that can be replicated with minimal complications. The main advantages of the radial forearm flap include the thinness and pliability of the flap, allowing the reconstruction of a well-vascularized and skin-lined urethra with the so-called tube- (the urethra) within-a-tube (the penis) technique. Moreover, the flap is easy to dissect, has a long vascular pedicle, and is predictably well vascularized, with the greatest sensitivity of all flaps used for penile reconstruction because of its multiple and easily identifiable sensory nerves, which play an important role in the extent of the recovery of tactile and erogenous sensation in the reconstructed penis.[2]

Radial Forearm Flap

Monstrey and colleagues[91] in a recent article described the largest series to date, of 287 radial forearm phalloplasties performed by the same surgical team. Many different outcome parameters had been described separately in previously published articles but the main purpose of this review was to critically evaluate to what degree this supposed gold-standard technique had been able to meet the ideal goals of penile reconstruction. These investigators' results showed that radial forearm phalloplasty is a reliable technique for the creation, mostly in 2 stages, of a normal-looking penis, which allows the patient to void while standing and also to experience sexual satisfaction. The unique feature of this series was that all patients were ultimately able to urinate through the newly reconstructed penis and all patients who were sexually active were able to reach an orgasm. These investigators admit that the cosmetic outcome of a phalloplasty procedure with a radial forearm flap is subjective; the ability of most patients undergoing phalloplasty to shower with other men or to go to a sauna was considered an acceptable cosmetic barometer. Features that seem important for increasing the aesthetic aspect of the reconstructed penis are preoperative depilation of the forearm, reconstruction of the corona and glans of the penis, and tattooing of the glans.

The relative disadvantages of this technique were the high number of initial fistulas (the majority closed spontaneously), the residual scar on the forearm, and the potential long-term urologic complications (including those that are prosthesis related). None of the patients in this large series showed any long-term donor-site problem (such as functional limitation, chronic pain, cold intolerance, or evidence of vascular compromise) after harvesting from the large radial forearm. With regard to the aesthetic outcome of the donor site, the patients were accepting of the donor-site scar, viewing it as a worthwhile trade-off for the creation of a phallus (**Fig. 7**).

Although when comparing these investigators' (radial forearm) results with the rest of the literature, one might think that for most patients who need a phalloplasty, the alternatives are rarely considered as a better option, it is still up to the individual surgeon to judge which technique for penile reconstruction should be chosen for each individual patient. Surgeons performing phalloplasty operations mainly stick to one preferred technique, because they are convinced this gives the best results and also because they have the most experience with this technique. The most valuable alternative techniques or new developments for penile reconstruction include the fibular free flap and the use of perforator flaps.

Radial Forearm Osteocutaneous Flap

Before each radial forearm procedure, an Allen test should be performed and a total and permanent depilation of the entire nondominant forearm preoperatively if prelamination is not planned. In a typical phalloplasty operation 2 surgical teams operate at the same time: in the perineal area, the urologist performs the oncologic resection (eventually with lymphadenectomy) and they also prepare the urethral stump, which will be connected with the neourethral tube of the flap (in complete or near-complete penile reconstruction). In a perineal urethrostomy versus a penile urethra a longer neourethral conduit is required for adequate penile length. In addition, the dissection of the perineal urethrostomy allows for a more facile dissection of pudendal recipient nerves.

At the same time the plastic surgeon dissects the free vascularized flap on the nondominant forearm. If prelamination is not performed, the ulnar aspect of the flap is often more hairless and, therefore, is usually preferred as lining for the urethra and dissected 2 cm more proximally. The medial and lateral antebrachial nerves are easily identified at the beginning of the flap elevation, and dissected an additional 5 cm proximal to the skin paddle to facilitate the anastomosis to the nerves in the groin area. The forearm flap itself is dissected in a suprafascial plane and the creation of a phallus as a tube-in-a-tube technique is performed with the flap still attached to the forearm by its vascular pedicle in nonprelaminated cases. A small skin flap and a skin graft are used to create a corona and simulate the (circumcised) glans of the penis. Once the urethral stump is prepared and the vessels are dissected in the groin area (through a lower abdominal incision), the free flap is transferred to the pubic area. First the urethral anastomosis is performed, after which the radial artery is microsurgically connected to the common femoral artery or a branch of this vessel in an end-to-side fashion, if necessary with an interpositional vein graft. Alternatively the inferior epigastric vessels may be used as recipient vessels. Careful dissection distally at the level of the umbilicus is necessary for adequate vessel length and a Pfannenstiel approach may be used. The venous anastomosis is performed between the cephalic vein and the greater saphenous vein or inferior epigastric venae comitantes. One forearm nerve is connected to the ipsilateral ilioinguinal nerve for protective sensation and the other nerve of the arm is anastomosed to one of the dorsal penile nerves or pudendal nerves for erogenous sensation.

When a radial forearm osteocutaneous flap is harvested, iliac crest bone graft may be used and screw fixated to the radius defect with a titanium plate along the ulnar aspect of the radius to prevent potential late fracture of the radius (**Fig. 8**).

The defect on the forearm can be covered with full-thickness skin grafts taken from the groin area or with split-thickness skin grafts harvested from the thigh (sometimes in combination with a dermal substitute). A better aesthetic aspect of the grafted donor site on the forearm might be obtained by a suprafascial dissection of the flap, sparing the paratenon, as well as by advancing the skin edges after harvesting of the flap and by paying extra attention to obtaining a flat contour of the underlying muscle surface, with careful graft placement to avoid additional wrinkling and scarring. All patients receive a suprapubic urinary diversion postoperatively.

Like in any free-flap procedure, the vascularization of the penile flap is monitored postoperatively

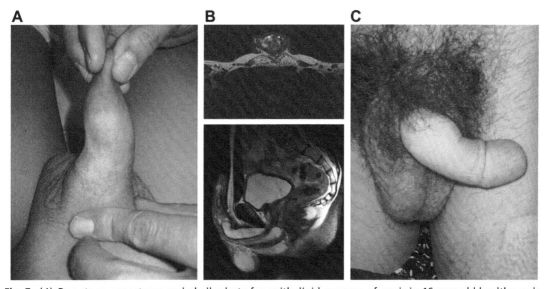

Fig. 7. (*A*) One-stage penectomy and phalloplasty for epithelioid sarcoma of penis in 16-year-old healthy male, who was referred for curvature of the penis based on a clinical diagnosis of Peyronie disease. He recalled having a lump at the base of the penis for more than a year. Furthermore he complained of urinary frequency. Three months previously he was treated for cystitis, which was not further investigated. On clinical examination an atypical lump was felt at the base of the penis. A hard 1-cm lesion involving the total circumference of the penile body was palpated. On uroflowmetry an obstructive flow pattern was seen. Retrograde urethrography showed a compressing lesion of the urethra, narrowing the lumen. (*B*) Magnetic resonance imaging revealed a 3-cm irregular rounded mass at the base of the penis. It was contained within both cavernous corpora, compressing the urethra and corpus spongiosum, but without evidence of direct invasion of the latter. Distal to the mass, the penile body enhanced poorly, suggesting severely disturbed blood flow. Cystoscopy showed a white tumorlike structure in the urethra, filling more than 80% of the lumen. An excisional biopsy was performed through a penile skin incision and pathologic examination revealed epithelioid sarcoma. Metastatic evaluation, including physical examination and computerized tomography of the pelvis, abdomen, and chest, was negative. After multidisciplinary discussions with pediatric and adult oncology and radiotherapy consultants it was recommended to perform surgery at once without any neoadjuvant therapy. It was decided that penectomy was needed. (*C*) A penectomy and reconstruction in one stage were planned. A total penectomy was performed. As the lesion was at the base of the penis, we needed to remove the whole penile body to remove the tumor. The neurovascular bundle was identified and 3 dorsal nerves could be identified. The cavernous bodies were transected just below the pubic bone and ligated. The urethra was transected and the spongeous tissue was oversewn. At the same time, the team of plastic surgeons prepared the radial forearm flap and reconstructed a phallus in a tube fashion. At the forearm level, 3 nerves could be identified to connect with the dorsal nerves. The vascular connection was made with the femoral artery and vein. Microscopic examination of the penectomy specimen showed a tumor with a nodular growth pattern, composed of a mixed proliferation of eosinophilic, epithelioid, and spindle cells. Focal necrosis was present. Diagnosis of epithelioid sarcoma was made. Perineural invasion was present; there was no evidence of lymphovascular invasion. Surgical margins were negative. Recovery after surgery was uneventful. Next to surgical follow-up, the patient was also seen by a psychologist. The phallus healed and voiding was started after 12 days. Voiding was normal on uroflowmetry and no fistulae occurred. The patient was discharged from hospital after 16 days. The final result is aesthetically good and patient satisfaction is high. On follow-up we decided that he would be seen every 6 weeks for clinical evaluation during the first year with computed tomography of the pelvis, abdomen, and chest every 3 months. He was also seen by his psychologist. After 1 year an erectile device was implanted.

and revision of the vascular anastomosis is performed if necessary.[92]

Fibular Osteocutaneous Flap

The advantage of the fibular flap is that it makes sexual intercourse possible without a penile prosthesis. The disadvantages are less sensation, more urethral complications (despite prelamination techniques), a pointed deformity to the distal part of the penis (where the extra skin can glide around the end of fibular bone), and a permanently erected phallus may be considered to be impractical. Some investigators specifically advocate the fibular osteocutaneous flap for penile reconstruction in a biologic male patient.[93] A case

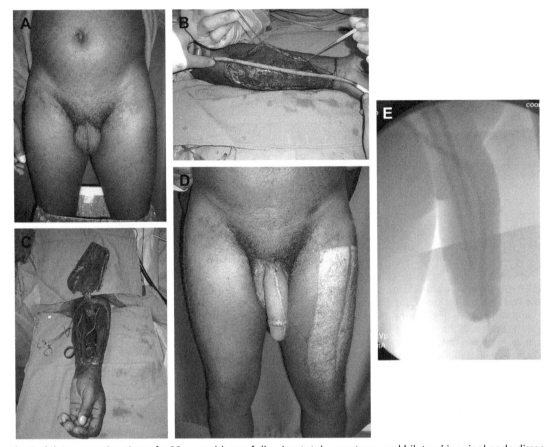

Fig. 8. (*A*) Preoperative view of a 38-year-old man following total penectomy and bilateral inguinal node dissection for invasive squamous cell cancer 8 months previously. The patient has perineal urethra. (*B*) Left radial forearm osteocutaneous flap prelamination of neourethra. (*C*) Radial forearm osteocutaneous flap shown following flap harvest before pedicle division and transfer. (*D*) The patient at 4 months following total phalloplasty with radial forearm osteocutaneous flap and adjunctive palmaris longus tendon graft for coronoplasty. (*E*) Retrograde cystourethrogram obtained before suprapubic tube removal showing patent urethra at 4 weeks.

example is shown in **Fig. 9**. An example of management of a postoperative urethral-cutaneous fistula is also given.

Alternative Flaps

Another alternative is reconstruction with a perforator flap, which is now considered as the ultimate form of tissue transfer. Donor-site morbidity is minimized, and the usually large vascular pedicles provide an additional range of motion or an easier vascular anastomosis. The most promising perforator flap for penile reconstruction is the ALT flap, which has been used as a free flap[87] and as a pedicled flap (S. Suominen, personal communication, 1994),[94] thus avoiding the problems related to microsurgical free-flap transfer. However, there is still a higher number of urinary problems following this ALT flap related to the more difficult reconstruction

of a well-vascularized urethra and to the thickness of the flap. However, this flap may become an interesting alternative to the radial forearm flap, particularly as a pedicled flap. The donor site is less conspicuous, and secondary corrections at that site are easier to make. In certain centers a pedicled ALT flap has become the first choice for phallic reconstruction if no urinary reconstruction is required, such as in patients with bladder extrophy.

VARIED FORMS OF PROSTHESES

A drawback of the radial forearm soft-tissue flap is the need for a rigidity prosthesis and its associated risks of placement. A prosthesis is therefore required to engage in sexual intercourse postoperatively. Implantation of a penile erection prosthesis is commonly performed 6 to 12 months after the phalloplasty procedure because it usually takes

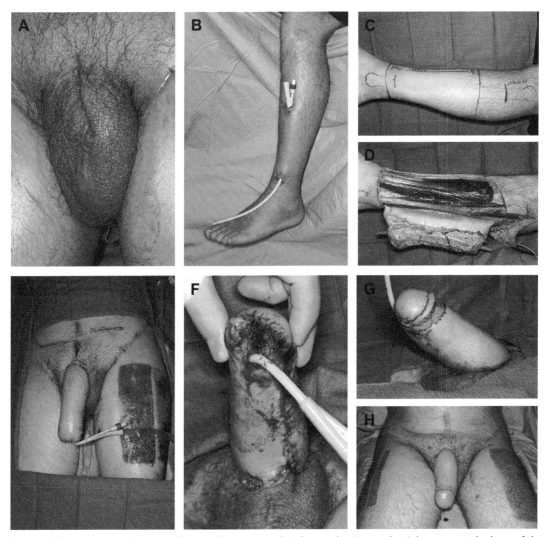

Fig. 9. (*A*) The patient is a 43-year-old man who presented with an enlarging and painless mass at the base of the penis and a malignant-appearing mass at the right distal shaft. The mass measured 3 cm by 2 cm and was present at the right distal penile shaft. Biopsy and final staging showed grade 3 squamous cell carcinoma. The patient underwent radical penectomy, scrotal urethrostomy, bilateral deep and superficial inguinal lymph node dissections, and bilateral extensive pelvic lymph node dissection. (*B*) At 8 months he was tumor free and he underwent prelamination of a urethra in the left leg using a thinned full-thickness skin graft from the left groin. (*C*) After skin graft maturation in the lateral leg, the patient underwent total phalloplasty using the prelaminated fibula osteocutaneous flap. A large skin island was designed to wrap around the fibula bone. (*D, E*) Creation and inset of the flap. The flap was harvested based on the peroneal artery and vein, and including branches of the lateral sural cutaneous nerve, a branch off the common peroneal nerve. The lateral leg skin was wrapped around the fibula bone, and the periosteum of the fibula proximally was sutured to the periosteum of the pubic bone. A primary urethra neourethrostomy was performed and a Foley catheter was kept in place for 6 weeks. The deep inferior epigastric artery and veins were harvested through an incision in the anterior rectus sheath. Dissection was carried cephalad to allow for the vessels to be turned down to reach the pubic region for convenient anastomosis with the peroneal vessels. The peroneal artery was anastomosed to the deep inferior epigastric artery and the venae comitantes of the peroneal artery were anastomosed to the venae comitantes of the deep inferior epigastric artery. The lesser saphenous vein was included in the flap given the large size of the skin island and was anastomosed to the great saphenous vein (this vein was dissected distally in the thigh, ligated, and turned up; it reached the medial groin region). The patient was noted to have superficial epidermolysis on the ventral side of the neophallus and a dehiscence of the inferior portion of the abdominal wound. He was taken to the operating room, where he underwent debridement and closure of the abdominal wound and debridement of the ventral penis wound, which healed by secondary intention. (*F, G*) Three weeks postoperatively he developed a urethrocutaneous fistula on the right side. Two months after the initial surgery he underwent closure of the fistula with a scrotal flap, and a coronoplasty and skin grafting. (*H*) The patient is able to use the penis for intercourse, and is able to urinate spontaneously. He has had to undergo one procedure for urethral dilation.

at least 1 year before sensation has returned to the distal end of the penis.

Hoebeke and colleagues[95] reported on the largest series to date on penile implants after a radial forearm reconstruction for female-to-male transsexualism. In their opinion, the rigid and semirigid prostheses seem to have a high perforation rate and therefore are no longer used in their patients. Instead they prefer the hydraulic systems available for impotent men, and these erection prostheses have been implanted in more than 129 patients. Initially, a one-piece hydraulic prosthesis was used (Dynaflex American Medical Systems, Minnetonka, MN, USA), usually in combination with 2 testicular prostheses. When this implant became unavailable, they switched to the 3-piece AMS CX prosthesis. In this device, the pump replaced one testicular prosthesis. Good results were reported with the 3-piece prosthesis, but these investigators recently encountered an increase in technical failure because of leakage, probably because there was no limit to the amount of fluid that can be pumped into the cylinders because the cylinders are not placed in cavernous bodies; overpumping seemed to be the basis of the problem. More recently, these investigators shifted to the 2-piece device (Ambicor, American Medical Systems, Minnetonka, MN, USA), a system that limits the amount of fluid available. A long-term follow-up study indicated that in about one in 4 patients, a reintervention was required because of malpositioning, technical failure, or infection. A more recent long-term follow-up study showed an explantation rate of 48% in 129 patients, although more than 80% of the patients were able to have normal sexual intercourse with penetration.[96] Another study reported that patients with an erection prosthesis were more able to attain their sexual expectations than those without prostheses, although the group with prostheses more often reported pain during intercourse.[97] A major concern regarding erectile prostheses is long-term follow-up. These devices were developed for impotent men who are older and have a shorter life expectancy and a lower sexual drive than the younger patients after oncologic resection (or female-to-male transsexual patients who are receiving these devices).

MANAGEMENT OF COMPLICATIONS FOLLOWING PENILE RECONSTRUCTION

Complications:

- Flap loss (total or partial): wound closure with local flap or second free flap

- Urethral fistula, stenosis, obstruction: suprapubic cystostomy, closure with tissue plug, obstruction alleviation: full-thickness skin graft, buccal mucosa
- Implant infection: implant removal and either reinsertion or bone graft after 6 months.

Sequelae:

- Dyspareunia in sexual partner (possible): fascial interposition with bone osteotomies[98]
- Embarrassment from constantly erect penis: place to side, wear briefs underwear
- Immediate or gradual loss of corona of glans penis: palmaris longus graft, fat, fascia graft.[99]

POSTOPERATIVE CARE IN PENILE RECONSTRUCTION PATIENT

The patients remain in bed during a 1-week postoperative period, after which the transurethral catheter may be removed. At that time, the suprapubic catheter is clamped, and voiding is begun. Effective voiding may not be observed for several days. Before removal of the suprapubic catheter, a cystography with voiding urethrography is performed followed by bladder training. The average hospital stay for the phalloplasty procedure is 2.5 weeks.

Postoperative complications can include fistula and/or stenosis: smaller fistulas usually close by themselves, whereas most strictures can be resolved by simple dilatation and/or incision. Only a few patients require a second surgical procedure (usually urethroplasty). As mentioned earlier, from a urological point of view and even independent of the oncologic aspect, lifelong follow-up is required. Tattooing of the glans can be performed after 2 to 3 months, before sensation returns to the penis, and is preferred by most patients.

PENILE TRANSPLANTATION

Recently, one case report has been published on penile transplantation.[100] Penile transplantation is possible because of microsurgical techniques (including anastomosis of neurovascular structures, corporal bodies, and urethra) and because of knowledge of immunosuppressive medication from other transplant surgery. The transplanted penis was cut off 14 days postoperatively as a result of psychological problems of the patient and his partner. This technique is still experimental and is not a current treatment option. Future options like tissue engineering for penile reconstruction are to date not science fact but rather science fiction.

REFERENCES

1. Cheng K, Hwang W, Eid AE, et al. Analysis of 136 cases of reconstructed penis using various methods. Plast Reconstr Surg 1995;95(6):1070–80.
2. Gilbert DA, Horton CE, Terzis JK, et al. New concept in phallic reconstruction. Ann Plast Surg 1987;18(2):128–36.
3. Hage JJ, de Graaf FH. Addressing the ideal requirements by free flap phalloplasty: some reflections on refinements of technique. Microsurgery 1993;14:592–8.
4. Descamps MJL, Hayes PM, Hudson DA. Phalloplasty in complete aphallia: pedicled anterolateral thigh flap. J Plast Reconstr Aesthet Surg 2009; 62(3):51–4.
5. Mutaf M, Isik D, Bulut O, et al. A true one-stage nonmicrosurgical technique for total phallic reconstruction. Ann Plast Surg 2006;57(1):100–6.
6. Hage JJ. Simple, safe, and satisfactory secondary penile enhancement after near-total oncologic amputation. Ann Plast Surg 2009;62(6):685–9.
7. Hanash KA, Tur JJ. One-stage plastic reconstruction of a totally amputated cancerous penis using a unilateral myocutaneous gracilis flap. J Surg Oncol 1986;33(4):250–3.
8. Kayes OJ, Durrant CA, Ralph D, et al. Vertical rectus abdominis flap reconstruction in patients with advanced penile squamous cell carcinoma. BJU Int 2007;99(1):37–40.
9. Payne CE, Southern SJ. Urinary point-of-care test for smoking in the pre-operative assessment of patients undergoing elective plastic surgery. J Plast Reconstr Aesthet Surg 2006;59:1156–61.
10. Atik B, Tan O, Ceylan K, et al. Reconstruction of wide scrotal defect using superthin groin flap. Urology 2006;68(2):419–22.
11. Rohrich RJ, Coberly CM, Krueger JK, et al. Planning elective operations on patients who smoke: survey of North American plastic surgeons. Plast Reconstr Surg 2002;191(1):350–5.
12. Summerton DJ, Campbell A, Minhas S, et al. Reconstructive surgery in penile trauma and cancer. Nat Clin Pract Urol 2005;2(8):391–7.
13. Hoebeke PB, Rottey S, Van Heddeghem N, et al. One-stage penectomy and phalloplasty for epithelioid sarcoma of the penis in an adolescent: part 2. Eur Urol 2007;51(6):1744–7.
14. Khouri RK, Young VL, Casoli VM. Long-term results of total penile reconstruction with a prefabricated lateral arm free flap. J Urol 1998;160(2):383–8.
15. Garaffa G, Raheem AA, Christopher NA, et al. Total phallic reconstruction after penile amputation for carcinoma. BJU Int 2009;104:852–6.
16. Hallock GG. Doppler sonography and color duplex imaging for planning a perforator flap. Clin Plast Surg 2003;30(3):347–57.
17. Perovic S. Phalloplasty in children and adolescents using the extended pedicle island groin flap. J Urol 1995;154:848.
18. Taylor GI, Corlett R, Boyd JB. The extended deep inferior epigastric flap: a clinical technique. Plast Reconstr Surg 1983;72(6):751–65.
19. Andrich DE, Dunglison N, Greenwell TJ, et al. The long-term results of urethroplasty. J Urol 2003; 170:90.
20. Zhao YQ, Zhang J, Yu MS, et al. Functional restoration of penis with partial defect by scrotal skin flap. J Urol 2009;182(5):2358–61.
21. Santucci RA, Mario LA, McAninch JW. Anastomotic urethroplasty for bulbar urethral stricture: analysis of 168 patients. J Urol 2002;167:1715.
22. Micheli E, Ranieri A, Peracchia G, et al. End-to-end urethroplasty: long-term results. BJU Int 2002;90:68.
23. Mira JL, Fan G. Leiomyoma of the male urethra: a case report and review of the literature. Arch Pathol Lab Med 2000;124:302.
24. Jalon Monzon A, Garcia Rodriguez J, Sanchez Trilla A, et al. [Obstructive urethral angioleiomyoma]. Arch Esp Urol 2004;57:1128 [in Spanish].
25. Saad AG, Kaouk JH, Kaspar HG, et al. Leiomyoma of the urethra: report of 3 cases of a rare entity. Int J Surg Pathol 2003;11:123.
26. Guralnick ML, Webster GD. The augmented anastomotic urethroplasty: indications and outcome in 29 patients. J Urol 2001;165:1496.
27. Duckett JW Jr. Transverse preputial island flap technique for repair of severe hypospadias. Urol Clin North Am 1980;7:423.
28. Zinman L. Muscular, myocutaneous, and fasciocutaneous flaps in complex urethral reconstruction. Urol Clin North Am 2002;29:443.
29. Sharp DS, Angermeier KW. Surgery of penile and urethral carcinoma. In: Wein AJ, Kavoussi LR, Novick AC, et al, editors. Campbell-Walsh urology. Philadelphia: Saunders Elsevier; 2007. p. 993–1022.
30. Morey AF, Rozansky TA. Genital and lower urinary tract trauma. In: Wein AJ, Kavoussi LR, Novick AC, et al, editors. Campbell-Walsh urology. Philadelphia: Saunders Elsevier; 2007. p. 2649–62.
31. Por YC, Tan BK, Hong SW, et al. Use of the scrotal remnant as a tissue-expanding musculocutaneous flap for scrotal reconstruction in Paget's disease. Ann Plast Surg 2003;51(2):155–60.
32. Yu P, Sanger JR, Matloub HS, et al. Anterolateral thigh fasciocutaneous island flaps in perineoscrotal reconstruction. Plast Reconstr Surg 2002; 109(2):610–6.
33. Wang D, Zheng H, Deng F. Spermatogenesis after scrotal reconstruction. Br J Plast Surg 2003;56(5): 484–8.
34. Alexander JW, Fischer JE, Boyajian M, et al. The influence of hair-removal methods on wound infections. Arch Surg 1983;118:347–52.

35. Friedman JD. Reconstruction of the perineum. In: Thorne CH, Beasley RW, Aston SJ, et al, editors. Grabb and Smith's plastic surgery. Philadelphia: Lippincott Williams & Wilkins; 2007. p. 708–16.

36. Sandlow JI, Winfield HN, Goldstein M. Surgery of the scrotum and seminal vesicles. In: Wein AJ, Kavoussi LR, Novick AC, et al, editors. Campbell-Walsh urology. Philadelphia: Saunders Elsevier; 2007. p. 1098–128.

37. Ying J, Yao DH, Cheng KX, et al. [Reconstruction of extended skin defect after the radical resection procedure for penile scrotum skin cancer]. Zhonghua Wai Ke Za Zhi 2007;45(18):1257–9 [in Chinese].

38. Karacal N, Livaoglu M, Kutlu N, et al. Scrotum reconstruction with neurovascular pedicled pudendal thigh flaps. Urology 2007;70(1):170–2.

39. Altchek ED, Hoffman S. Scrotal reconstruction in Fournier's syndrome. Ann Plast Surg 1979;3: 523–8.

40. Perovic SV, Djinovic RP, Bumbasirevic MZ, et al. Severe penile injuries: a problem of severity and reconstruction. BJU Int 2009;104:676–87.

41. Hallock GG. Scrotal reconstruction following Fournier gangrene using the medial circumflex femoral artery perforator flap. Ann Plast Surg 2006;57(3):333–5.

42. Hsu H, Lin CM, Sun TB, et al. Unilateral gracilis myofasciocutaneous advancement flap for single stage reconstruction of scrotal and perineal defects. J Plast Reconstr Aesthet Surg 2007; 60(9):1055–9.

43. Kayikçioğlu A. A new technique in scrotal reconstruction: short gracilis flap. Urology 2003;61:1254–6.

44. Karaçal N, Livaoglu M, Kutlu N, et al. Scrotum reconstruction with neurovascular pedicled pudendal thigh flaps. Urology 2007;70(1):170–2.

45. Payne CE, Williams AM, Hart NB. Lotus petal flaps for scrotal reconstruction combined with Integra resurfacing of the penis and anterior abdominal wall following necrotising fasciitis. J Plast Reconstr Aesthet Surg 2009;62(3):393–7.

46. Maharaj D, Naraynsingh V, Perry A, et al. The scrotal reconstruction using the "Singapore Sling". Plast Reconstr Surg 2002;110(1):203–5.

47. Morris MS, Morey AF, Stackhouse DA, et al. Fibrin sealant as tissue glue: preliminary experience in complex genital reconstructive surgery. Urology 2006;67(4):688–91.

48. Ferguson GG, Brandes SB. Gunshot wound injury of the testis: the use of tunica vaginalis and polytetrafluoroethylene grafts for reconstruction. J Urol 2007;178(6):2462–5.

49. Schonfeld W, Beebe GW. Normal growth and variation in the male genitalia from birth to maturity. J Urol 1942;48:759.

50. Ochoa B. Trauma of the external genitalia in children: amputation of the penis and emasculation. J Urol 1998;160(3 Pt 2):1116–9 [discussion: 1137].

51. Amukele SA, Lee GW, Stock JA, et al. 20-year experience with iatrogenic penile injury. J Urol 2003;170(4 Pt 2):1691–4.

52. Rubino C, Figus A, Dessy LA, et al. Innervated island pedicled anterolateral thigh flap for neo-phallic reconstruction in female-to-male transsexuals. J Plast Reconstr Aesthet Surg 2009;62(3):45–9.

53. Hage JJ, Bloem JJ, Suliman HM. Review of the literature on techniques for phalloplasty with emphasis on the applicability in female-to-male transsexuals. J Urol 1993;150(4):1093–8.

54. Bogaraz N. Plastic restoration of the penis. Sovet Khir 1936;8:303.

55. Akoz T, Kargi E. Phalloplasty in a female-to-male transsexual using a double-pedicle composite groin flap. Ann Plast Surg 2002;48:423–7.

56. Sun GC, Huang JJ. One-stage reconstruction of the penis with composite iliac crest and lateral groin skin flap. Ann Plast Surg 1985;15:519.

57. Koshima I, Nanba Y, Nagai A. Penile reconstruction with bilateral superficial circumflex iliac artery perforator (SCIP) flaps. J Reconstr Microsurg 2006;22(3):137–42.

58. He QL, Lin ZH, Liu Q, et al. One-stage penis reconstruction with the abdominal fasciocutaneous flap based on the double arteries. Report of 16 cases. Chin Med J 1987;100:255.

59. Lai CS, Chou CK, Yang CC, et al. Immediate reconstruction of the penis with an iliac flap. Br J Plast Surg 1990;43:621.

60. Hage JJ, Bouman FG, de Graaf FH, et al. Construction of the neophallus in female-to-male transsexuals: the Amsterdam experience. J Urol 1993;149:1463–8.

61. Santi P, Berrino P, Canavese G, et al. Immediate reconstruction of the penis using an inferiorly based rectus abdominis myocutaneous flap. Plast Reconstr Surg 1988;8:961–4.

62. Jordan GH, Schlossberg SM. Surgery of the penis and urethra. In: Wein AJ, Kavoussi LR, Novick AC, et al, editors. Campbell-Walsh urology. Philadelphia: Saunders Elsevier; 2007. p. 1023–97.

63. Ubrig B, Waldner M, Fallahi M, et al. Preputial flap for primary closure after excision of tumors on the glans penis. Urology 2001;58:274–6.

64. Zhao YQ, Zhang J, Yu MS, et al. Functional restoration of penis with partial defect by scrotal skin flap. J Urol 2009;182(5):2358–61.

65. Emsen IM. A different application of the unilobed flap: bilateral vascularized scrotal pedicle flap for reconstruction on the scrotal and peno-scrotal defects. Dermatol Surg 2009;35(4):714–6.

66. Mazza ON, Cheliz GM. Glanuloplasty with scrotal flap for partial penectomy. J Urol 2001;166:887–9.

67. Liu Y, Li S, Li Y, et al. Clinical applications of the scrotal skin flaps pedicled on lateral branches of the posterior scrotal arteries. Zhonghua Zheng Xing Wai Ke Za Zhi 2002;18(6):367–8.

68. Greenberger ML, Lowe BA. Penile stump advancement as an alternative to perineal urethrostomy after penile amputation. J Urol 1999;161:893.

69. Seyhan T, Borman H. Pedicled deep inferior epigastric perforator flap for lower abdominal defects and genital reconstructive surgery. J Reconstr Microsurg 2008;24(6):405–12.

70. Zeng A, Xu J, Xiaoqing Y, et al. Pedicled deep inferior epigastric perforator flap: an alternative method to repair groin and scrotal defects. Ann Plast Surg 2006;57(3):285–8.

71. Demirtas Y, Ozturk N, Kelahmetoglu O, et al. Glans penis reconstruction with the pedicled deep inferior epigastric artery perforator flap. J Reconstr Microsurg 2008;24(5):323–6.

72. Shaeer O, El-Sebaie A. Construction of neoglans penis: a new sculpturing technique from rectus abdominis myofascial flap. J Sex Med 2005; 2(2):259–65.

73. Bogoras N. Über die volle plastische Wiederherstellung eines zum Koitus fähigen penis (Peniplastica totalis). Zentralbl Chir 1936;22:1271–6 [in Danish].

74. Gillies H, Millard DR Jr. The principles and art of plastic surgery, vol. 2. London: Butterworth; 1957. p. 368–84.

75. Snyder CC. Intersex problems and hermaphroditism. In: Converse JM, editor. Reconstructive plastic surgery. Philadelphia: Saunders; 1964. p. 2078–105.

76. Biber SH. A method for constructing the penis and scrotum. Presented at the VIth international symposium on gender dysphoria. San Diego (CA); 1979.

77. Hester TR Jr, Nahain F, Beeglen PE, et al. Blood supply of the abdomen revisited, with emphasis on the superficial inferior epigastric artery. Plast Reconstr Surg 1984;74(5):657–66.

78. McGregor IA, Jackson IT. The groin flap. Br J Plast Surg 1972;25:3–16.

79. Hoopes JE. Surgical construction of the male external genitalia. Clin Plast Surg 1974;1(2):325–34.

80. Horton CE, McCraw JB, Devine CJ Jr, et al. Secondary reconstruction of the genital area. Urol Clin North Am 1977;4:133–41.

81. Exner K. Penile reconstruction in female to male transsexualism: a new method of phalloplasty. Xth International Congress on plastic and reconstructive surgery. Madrid; 1992.

82. Hage JJ, Winters HA, Van Lieshout J. Fibula free flap phalloplasty: modifications and recommendations. Microsurgery 1996;17:358–65.

83. Song R, Gao Y, Song Y, et al. The forearm flap. Clin Plast Surg 1982;9(1):21–6.

84. Harashima T, Ionque T, Tanaka I, et al. Reconstruction of penis with free deltoid flap. Br J Plast Surg 1990;43:217–22.

85. Sadove RC, Sengezer M, McRobert JW, et al. One-stage total penile reconstruction with a free sensate osteocutaneous fibula flap. Plast Reconstr Surg 1993;92(7):1314–25.

86. Santanelli F, Scuderi N. Neophalloplasty in female-to-male transsexuals with the island tensor fascia lata flap. Plast Reconstr Surg 2000;105(6): 1990–6.

87. Felici N, Felici A. A new phalloplasty technique: the free anterolateral thigh flap phalloplasty. J Plast Reconstr Aesthet Surg 2006;59:153–7.

88. Chang TS, Hwang WY. Forearm flap in one stage reconstruction of the penis. Plast Reconstr Surg 1984;74(2):251–8.

89. Fang RH, Kao YS, Ma S, et al. Phalloplasty in female-to-male transsexuals using free radial osteocutaneous flap: a series of 22 cases. Br J Plast Surg 1999;52(3):217–22.

90. Monstrey S, Hoebeke P, Dhont M, et al. Surgical therapy in transsexual patients: a multi-disciplinary approach. Acta Chir Belg 2001;101:200–9.

91. Monstrey S, Hoebeke P, Selvaggi G, et al. Penile reconstruction: is the radial forearm flap really the standard technique. Plast Reconstr Surg 2009;124:510–8.

92. Salgado CJ, Moran SL, Mardini S. Flap monitoring and patient management [review]. Plast Reconstr Surg 2009;124(Suppl 6):e295–302.

93. Sengezer M, Ozturk S, Deveci M, et al. Long term follow-up of total penile reconstruction with sensate osteocutaneous free fibula flap in 18 biological male patients. Plast Reconstr Surg 2004;114(2):439–50.

94. Ceulemans P. The pedicled antero-lateral thigh (ALT) perforator flap: a new technique for phallic reconstruction. XIX Biennial Symposium of the Harry Benjamin International Gender Dysphoria (HBIGDA) Association. Bologna (Italy), April 2005.

95. Hoebeke P, de Cuypere G, Ceulemans P, et al. Obtaining rigidity in total phalloplasty: experience with 35 patients. J Urol 2003;169(1):221–3.

96. Hoebeke P, De Cuypere G, Ceulemans P, et al. Obtaining rigidity in total phalloplasty: experience with 35 patients. J Urol 2003;169:221–3.

97. De Cuypere G, T'Sjoen G, Beerten R, et al. Sexual and physical health after sex reassignment surgery. Arch Sex Behav 2005;36(6):679–90.

98. Salgado CJ, Rampazzo A, Xu E, et al. Treatment of dyspareunia by creation of a pseudojoint in rigid bone following total penile reconstruction with fibular osteocutaneous flap. J Sex Med 2008; 5(12):2947–50.

99. Salgado CJ, Licata L, Fuller DA, et al. Glans penis coronaplasty with palmaris longus tendon following total penile reconstruction. Ann Plast Surg 2009; 62(6):690–2.

100. Hu W, Lu J, Zhang L, et al. A preliminary report of penile transplantation. Eur Urol 2006;50(4):851–3.

Mohs Micrographic Surgery for Penoscrotal Malignancy

Michael J. Wells, MD[a],*, R. Stan Taylor, MD[b]

KEYWORDS

- Male genitalia • Penis • Scrotum • Mohs
- Carcinoma • Extramammary Paget disease

The inability to adequately assess margins of tumor excision specimens hampers the surgeon's ability to obtain cure. False-negative histologic findings can result in leaving tumor behind and highlights the importance of careful and complete microscopic visualization of excision margins. Vertical sections through the center of an excision specimen (eg, bread loafing) are adequate for diagnostic purposes but often fall short of providing sufficient visualization of the margins of the excision specimen. It has been calculated that 0.1% or less of the margins is assessed using this approach (Ronald P. Rapini, MD, 2009, personal communication).[1,2] Other methods of evaluating the surgical margins have been developed, but when applying the concept of surgical margin control to lesions of the skin and mucous membranes, perhaps the most effective is the Mohs surgery technique.[1–5] Most commonly used for removal of skin cancers of the head and neck region, Mohs surgery also can be used in the eradication of skin cancers of the external genitalia. This article highlights the documented uses of Mohs surgery for treating malignancies of the genitalia and perigenital regions.

MOHS MICROGRAPHIC SURGERY

While using zinc chloride paste as a medical student involved in research at the University of Wisconsin in the 1930s, Frederic E. Mohs developed the technique that now bears his name. Mohs applied the paste directly to the surface of skin cancers and left it in place for 24 hours. While on the patient's lesion, the paste acted as a fixative that preserved the histologic features of the cells and tissue architecture. When fixation was complete, he would dissect the fixed tissue sample off the patient and, using a microtome, slice thin sections from the undersurface of the fixed specimen. If tumor was found in these sections, then the process was repeated with application of more paste for another 24-hour fixation period. These horizontal sections cut from the undersurface of the fixed tissue and examination microscopically by the surgeon became the distinguishing features of the Mohs technique. They are the hallmark features of what is now referred to as Mohs micrographic surgery (MMS).

The original zinc chloride paste used by Mohs included 40 g of black granular antimony (stibnite), 10 g of Sanguinaria canadensis (blood root), and 34.5 mL of saturated zinc chloride solution. When compounded, it had a tarlike consistency and color (**Fig. 1**). Tissue debulking with curettage or a saturated solution of dichloroacetic acid often was performed before applying the zinc chloride paste to aid paste penetration into the skin. The paste caused an intense localized inflammatory reaction where it was applied; therefore "chemosurgery,"

[a] Department of Dermatology, Texas Tech University Health Sciences Center, 3401 West 4th Street, MS 9400, Lubbock, TX 79407, USA
[b] Department of Dermatology, University of Texas Southwestern, 5323 Harry Hines Boulevard, Room DF03.432, Dallas, TX 75390-7208, USA
* Corresponding author.
E-mail address: mjwells@pol.net

Urol Clin N Am 37 (2010) 403–409
doi:10.1016/j.ucl.2010.04.012

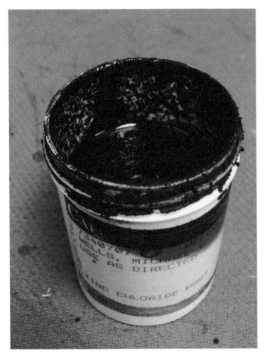

Fig. 1. Zinc chloride (Mohs) paste for chemosurgery.

as it was called, had significant morbidity associated with it. Drawbacks included severe discomfort for the patient and the fact that it often took several days to clear the tumor. In addition, patients had to wait several more days once the tumor margins were clear to allow the wound to mature before a repair of the defect could be considered.

In 1953, Mohs experimented with the use of fresh-frozen specimens to speed up the process for an educational film he was making on the removal of skin cancers of the eyelids.[3] He noted that microscopic detail was preserved with this approach, and he continued to use this thereafter for removal of tumors in the periorbital area. In 1969, he reported on a series of tumors of the eyelid removed in this manner and noted a 5-year cure rate of 100%.[3] In 1974 and later in 1976, Stegman and Tromovitch published a series of skin cancer removals from head and neck sites in which they used the fresh-frozen method to process tissue margins.[3–5] The speed at which tissue could be processed allowed the surgeon to perform multiple stages in a matter of hours instead of days, and resultant defects could be repaired immediately following tumor clearance. Consequently, today it is rare to see the chemosurgery approach used by Mohs surgeons.

MMS is most successful when tumors grow in a contiguous fashion. For most mucocutaneous malignancies treated with MMS, visible and palpable tumor is debulked using a curette or scalpel. Then a 2 to 3 mm margin of tissue is excised from around and underneath the debulk defect. The excision most commonly is performed by beveling the incisions toward the center of the debulk defect during removal (**Fig. 2**). These beveled incisions follow the contour of the debulk defect and usually approach 45°. Margin removal can be accomplished in a more completely horizontal fashion when removing from convex sites. Incisions that parallel the contour of the debulk defect usually result in a bowl- or pancake-shaped excision specimen that can facilitate manipulation of the entire surgical margin into a flat plane for laboratory processing. On occasion, a beveled incision is not possible when harvesting an MMS surgical margin. In these situations, one must provide relaxation cuts on the debulked side of the specimen to facilitate the flattening of the specimen.

Orientation of the excised margin specimen relative to where it was removed is maintained by marking the margin specimen edge at two or more spots. These marked spots correspond to marks on the patient at the edge of the defect resulting from removal of the margin specimen. Also referred to as hash marks, these marks routinely are made at the 12, 3, 6 and 9 o'clock positions on both the margin specimen and the patient's defect. The marks on the margin of the specimen are made as short shallow nicks using the scalpel. The patient is marked either with corresponding surgical nicks or an ink mark. The ink used on the margin specimen is applied in a unique fashion that is recorded on a map showing the margin specimen and its relation to the location

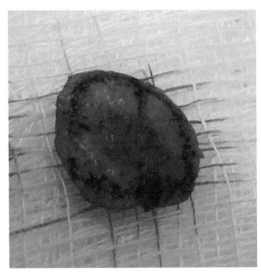

Fig. 2. Tissue excised in beveled fashion.

of removal from the patient (**Figs. 3–5**). Ink applied to the margin of the specimen can be visualized under microscopic examination, so that when residual tumor is visualized in microscopic sections from the margin specimen, its location is correlated relative to the inked hash marks and then documented on the map. The surgeon then returns to the patient and removes the involved areas with another 2 to 3 mm margin of tissue around and underneath the sites of tumor as noted on the map.

Hematoxylin and eosin or Toluene blue stains are used routinely for all frozen tissue Mohs specimens. Occasionally immunohistochemical stains are used to highlight tumor cells not easily seen on routine stains.[3–5]

Standard excision for malignancy involving the male genitalia often involves extensive surgical margins resulting in defects that range from extensive loss of skin to total penectomy. Due to the tissue sparing capabilities of MMS many have attempted to apply the use of the technique to treat cutaneous malignancies of the male genitalia and perigenital regions.

TREATMENT OF PENILE SQUAMOUS CELL CARCINOMA

Mohs and colleagues reported data on 35 patients with invasive squamous cell carcinoma (SCC) who were treated using the fixed-tissue (chemosurgery) technique over a 50-year period.[6,7] Five-

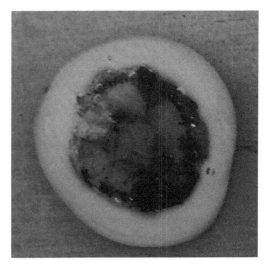

Fig. 4. Tissue covered with freezing media.

year follow-up data were available on 31 patients, which revealed a recurrence rate of 26%. Two of the 8 patients with recurrence had local recurrence due to extensive urethral involvement. The remaining six were reported to have occult lymph node metastasis at the time of MMS and died of SCC. In the first case series of MMS using the fixed-tissue technique for invasive penile SCC, Mohs and colleagues reported 0% recurrence in 5 years if the tumor size was less than 1 cm, 17% with tumors 1 to 2 cm, 25% if tumor size was between 2 and 3 cm, and 50% if tumor size was greater than 3 cm.[7,8]

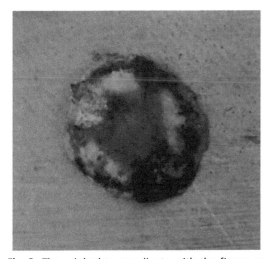

Fig. 3. Tissue inked to coordinate with the figure on the Mohs micrographic surgery map. This margin specimen is processed by pressing the edges of the specimen, which corresponds to the peripheral margins, into the same plane as the deep margin. This allows for histologic analysis of both the peripheral and deep excision margins in the same tissue section.

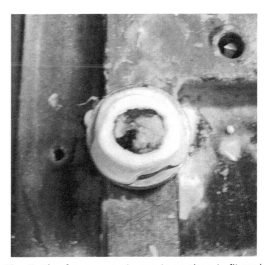

Fig. 5. The frozen margin specimen then is flipped over so that the excised margin is exposed and mounted to a cryostat chuck. Thin sections are cut from the exposed excision margin, placed on glass slides, stained ,and then evaluated under the microscope by the Mohs surgeon.

Brown and colleagues[9] studied 20 patients with penile malignancies treated with Mohs surgery. Eleven patients had invasive SCC; seven had SCC in situ. One had verrucous carcinoma, and one had leiomyosarcoma. They reported a 29% recurrence rate over a mean follow-up period of 3 years. One of the 17 patients had only local recurrence, and four patients developed lymph node involvement, with one patient dying of metastatic disease.

Shindel and colleagues[7] reported on 41 penile cancers in 33 patients treated with MMS. Twenty-five patients were identified, with overall average follow-up data of 58 months. Eight patients developed recurrence (32%), of whom seven were retreated with MMS. The eighth patient had a T3 SCC of the glans and was reported to be tumor-free for 4 years. Initially he was treated with a partial penectomy for recurrent distal T3 disease. Another recurrence 1 year later resulted in the patient receiving a total penectomy. One patient developed inguinal lymph node involvement, and one patient died of metastatic disease. Of the original 41 cases, 10 were invasive SCC; 25 were squamous cell carcinoma in situ. Four cases were verrucous carcinoma; one was epidermoid carcinoma, and one was basal cell carcinoma. The authors concluded their discussion by pointing out that despite a higher recurrence rate in their patients treated with MMS as compared with those receiving traditional surgery, recurrence was managed effectively in most by retreatment with MMS and did not have an adverse effect on overall survival rate or tumor progression. Their patients reported that they were satisfied with the resulting sexual and urinary function following MMS compared with the option of penectomy. The authors report they terminated five MMS procedures due to urethral involvement or size of defect during MMS with continued positive margins. They suggested that very large tumors may not be best treated by MMS, especially if they deeply involve the corpora, urethra, or urethral meatus.[7,10]

MMS may be most helpful in SCC in situ (SCCIS) of the penis (**Figs. 6–10**). SCCIS of the penile shaft can be removed easily using MMS with the resultant defect allowed to heal by second intention for smaller defects or with primary closure or local skin flaps. SSCIS of the glans is more difficult because of the possibility of urethral involvement. Therefore for lesions located on the distal glans it is imperative that a careful cystoscopic examination be performed before formulation of the treatment plan. Rare reports of good outcomes using MMS for urethral SCCIS with or without distal urethrectomy have been described. Especially when used alone, MMS is not considered as effective

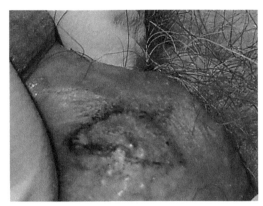

Fig. 6. Squamous cell carcinoma in situ persistent after treatment with topical 5-fluorouracil.

when urethral involvement is present and should be discouraged.[7,11,12]

TREATMENT OF PENILE BASAL CELL CARCINOMA

Basal cell carcinoma (BCC) rarely involves the penis. BCC of the penis accounts for less than 1% of all BCCs. Gibson and Ahmed report that they were only able to identify fewer than 200 cases involving the perineum or genitalia.[13] Recurrence is rare even with wide local excision.[13] On the other hand, MMS has been shown to be superior to standard excision of aggressive histologic presentations of BCC such as those that exhibit sclerosis or the morpheaform or micronodular growth patterns. Nguyen and colleagues were only able to find two cases (0.03%) of penile BCC in 6688 male cases of BCC referred for MMS over a 25-year period.[14] Their review of the literature only yielded one other case reported.

TREATMENT OF EXTRAMAMMARY PAGET DISEASE

Extramammary Paget disease (EMPD) is known for its clinically unapparent margins and the development of satellite lesions, making it difficult to surgically excise. Consequently, patients with this malignancy experience recurrence rates up to 44% when treated with wide local excision.[15–17] Still for EMPD of the penis and scrotum, surgical excision is considered the standard. Zhu and colleagues[18] were able to show a reduced recurrence rate of 16% (6 of 38 cases) for primary penoscrotal EMPD treated with wide local excision (2 cm) and intraoperative frozen-section margin control. Mean follow-up was 33.5 months. O'Connor and colleagues[17] reported on 95 patients with

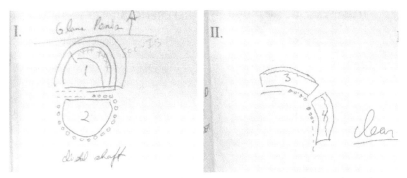

Fig. 7. Map showing orientation of tissue excised from the lesion in **Fig. 6** showing how the tissue was inked.

EMPD (86 with primary disease and 9 with recurrent disease) treated over 25 years. In this retrospective study, patients were treated with both wide local excision and MMS. Mean follow-up for patients treated with wide excision was 65 months, with a 22% recurrence rate compared with a mean follow-up following MMS of 24 months with an 8% recurrence rate. The authors recommended preoperative scouting biopsies, preoperative margin evaluation with a photodynamic evaluation, and intraoperative immunostaining with cytokeratin 7 to help aid in margin delineation. The preoperative photodynamic evaluation consisted of applying topical 20% delta-aminolevulinic acid (ALA) to the suspected area and the using a Wood lamp to delineate the tumor extent 18 hours after application of ALA. Lee and colleagues[19] presented data on 35 patients seen over a 10-year period. Mean follow-up was 62.7 months; 36.4% experienced recurrence after standard wide excision, and 18.2% of malignancies recurred following treatment with MMS. Both studies included male and female patients with genital and perigenital EMPD. Although tumor size was not discussed in these studies, dermal invasion, especially greater than 1 mm, was associated with more advanced disease and metastasis.

Nonsurgical treatments should be considered if the patient is not a surgical candidate, but they have been found to have limited utility in producing a long-term cure. These therapies are still used for remission attempts as well as a presurgical approach to decrease the extent of disease before surgical intervention. Treatment with topical 5-fluorouracil has been advocated, but disease almost invariably recurs; it may be best used as adjuvant therapy after surgery.[20] Topical 5-fluorouracil also can be used to aid in delineation of subclinical spread to surrounding skin, and it is used for this purpose for several days before surgery.[20,21] Topical photodynamic therapy (PDT) with ALA demonstrated a 37.5% relapse rate

in the 8 of 16 patients who achieved a complete response.[22] PDT may be best used in a similar adjunctive role as what was previously described for topical 5-fluorouracil.[17] Cohen and colleagues[23] reviewed case reports of EMPD treated with topical imiquimod. They reported finding some biopsy-proven complete responders, but follow-up had been short (mean of 8.5 months). Luk and colleagues[24] reported radiation therapy was associated with a 25% relapse rate in four patients treated with cutaneous only EMPD. The patient with recurrence was treated with salvage surgery. The three remaining patients were found to be disease-free at 2, 8, and 11 years of follow-up. The two additional patients with underlying carcinoma who were treated with radiation therapy died of metastasis within 15 months.

TREATMENT OF GRANULAR CELL TUMOR

Granular cell tumor (GCT) has rarely been reported to involve the penis or the perigenital region. Gardner and Goldberg reported finding only seven other cases in the literature, which were all removed by surgical excision.[25] Of eight reported

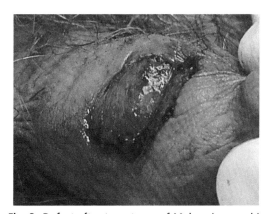

Fig. 8. Defect after two stages of Mohs micrographic surgery.

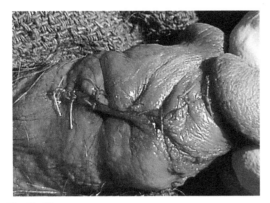

Fig. 9. Closure.

cases of penile GCT including their case, the authors reported none were reported to have recurred after an average follow-up of about 2 years. They reported that after 6 months of follow-up that their patient with a GCT located on the penis was free of evidence of recurrence and widespread disease. Dzubow and Kramer[26] reported on another case of GCT treated with MMS, but it was located on the buttocks.

In summary, MMS is a technique that provides comprehensive surgical margin evaluation and tissue sparing when used to treat penoscrotal malignancies. It provides the greatest benefits when malignancies such as SCC are superficial, small, and not contiguous with the urethra or urethral meatus. The technique is superior in reducing recurrences compared with wide excision when treating EMPD. Even with this advantage, the large areas of involvement in this condition often make MMS alone impractical unless adjunctive modalities such 5-fluorouracil, PDT, and radiation therapy are used along with MMS to increase its effectiveness.

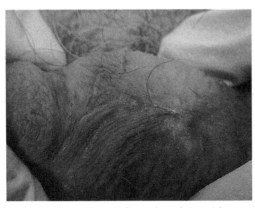

Fig. 10. Patient happy with result and no evidence of recurrence after 4-month follow-up.

REFERENCES

1. Rapini RP. Comparison of methods for checking surgical margins. J Am Acad Dermatol 1990;23: 288–94.
2. Lane JE, Kent DE. Surgical margins in the treatment of nonmelanoma skin cancer and Mohs micrographic surgery. Curr Surg 2005;62(5):518–26.
3. Gross KG, Steinman HK, Rapini RP. Mohs Surgery: fundamentals and techniques. St. Louis (MO): CV Mosby Company; 1998.
4. Mooney MA, Parry E. Mohs micrographic surgery. Available at: www.emedicine.com. Accessed August 14, 2009.
5. Minton TJ. Contemporary Mohs surgery applications. Curr Opin Otolaryngol Head Neck Surg 2008;16(4):376–80.
6. Mohs FE, Snow SN, Larson PO. Mohs micrographic surgery for penile tumors. Urol Clin North Am 1992; 19:291–304.
7. Shindel AW, Mann MW, Lev RY, et al. Mohs micrographic surgery for penile cancer: management and long-term followup. Nat Clin Pract Urol 2008; 5(7):364–5.
8. Mohs FE, Snow SN, Messing EM, et al. Microscopically controlled surgery in the treatment of carcinoma of the penis. J Urol 1985;133:961–6.
9. Brown MD, Zachary CB, Grekin RC, et al. Penile tumors: their management by Mohs micrographic surgery. J Dermatol Surg Oncol 1987; 13:1163–7.
10. Misra S, Chaturvedi A, Misra NC. Penile carcinoma: a challenge for the developing world. Lancet Oncol 2004;5(4):240–7.
11. Nash PA, Bihrle R, Gleason PE, et al. Mohs' micrographic surgery and distal urethrectomy with immediate urethral reconstruction for glanular carcinoma in situ with significant urethral extension. Urology 1996;47(1):108–10.
12. Antunes AA, Dall'Oglio MF, Srougi M. Organ-sparing treatment for penile cancer. Nat Clin Pract Urol 2007; 4(11):596–604.
13. Gibson GE, Ahmed I. Perianal and genital basal cell carcinoma: a clinicopathologic review of 51 cases. J Am Acad Dermatol 2001;45(1):68–71.
14. Nguyen H, Saadat P, Bennett RG. Penile basal cell carcinoma: two cases treated with Mohs micrographic surgery and remarks on pathogenesis. Dermatol Surg 2006;32(1):135–44.
15. Zollo JD, Zeitouni NC. The Roswell Park Cancer Institute experience with extramammary Paget's disease. Br J Dermatol 2000;142:59–65.
16. Coldiron BM, Goldsmith BA, Robinson JK. Surgical treatment of extramammary Paget's disease: a report of six cases and a re-examination of Mohs micrographic surgery compared with conventional surgical excision. Cancer 1991;67:933–8.

17. O'Connor WJ, Lim KK, Zalla MJ, et al. Comparison of Mohs micrographic surgery and wide excision for extramammary Paget's disease. Dermatol Surg 2003;29(7):723–7.

18. Zhu Y, Ye DW, Chen ZW, et al. Frozen section-guided wide local excision in the treatment of peno-scrotal extramammary Paget's disease. BJU Int 2007;100(6):1282–7.

19. Lee KY, Roh MR, Chung WG, et al. Comparison of Mohs micrographic surgery and wide excision for extramammary Paget's disease: Korean experience. Dermatol Surg 2009;35(1):34–40.

20. Goette DK. Topical chemotherapy with 5-fluorouracil. A review. J Am Acad Dermatol 1981;4:633–49.

21. Eliezri YD, Silvers DN, Horan DB. Role of preoperative topical 5- fluorouracil in preparation for Mohs micrographic surgery of extramammary Paget's disease. J Am Acad Dermatol 1987;17:497–505.

22. Shieh S, Dee AS, Cheney RT, et al. Photodynamic therapy for the treatment of extramammary Paget's disease. Br J Dermatol 2002;146:1000–5.

23. Cohen PR, Schulze KE, Tschen JA, et al. Treatment of extramammary Paget disease with topical imiquimod cream: case report and literature review. Southampt Med J 2006;99(4):396–402.

24. Luk NM, Yu KH, Yeung WK, et al. Extramammary Paget's disease: outcome of radiotherapy with curative intent. Clin Exp Dermatol 2003;28(4):360–3.

25. Gardner ES, Goldberg LH. Granular cell tumor treated with Mohs micrographic surgery: report of a case and review of the literature. Dermatol Surg 2001;27(8):772–4.

26. Dzubow LM, Kramer EM. Treatment of a large, ulcerating, granular-cell tumor by microscopically controlled excision. J Dermatol Surg Oncol 1985; 11:392–5.

Penile Cancer: Management of Regional Lymphatic Drainage

Vitaly Margulis, MD*, Arthur I. Sagalowsky, MD

KEYWORDS

- Squamous carcinoma • Penis • Urethra
- Lymph nodes • Management

Presence and magnitude of the inguinal nodal metastases are the most important determinants of oncologic outcome in patients with squamous carcinoma of the penis (SCP). At the initial presentation, clinically palpable inguinal lymphadenopathy is present in up to 60% of patients with SCP, and up to 85% of these patients will be found to harbor metastatic SCP.[1,2] By contrast, up to 30% of patients with no clinical evidence of enlarged inguinal lymph nodes are found to have occult inguinal micrometastatic disease.[1,3] Understanding of the unique features of SCP is paramount for thoughtful management of inguinal lymph nodes in patients diagnosed with penile cancer. (1) SCP demonstrates a prolonged locoregional phase, with lymphatic involvement occurring before systemic metastatic progression. (2) Metastatic lymphatic spread of SCP occurs by a predictable and well-characterized anatomic route, initially affecting the superficial inguinal nodal chain, with subsequent dissemination to deep inguinal and pelvic lymph nodes. (3) Unlike many other urologic malignancies, where lymph node dissection provides important staging and prognostic information, in patients with SCP, appropriately performed lymphadenectomy positively impacts the natural history of SCP and has a curative potential in appropriately selected patients. (4) Current clinical staging criteria (physical examination and/or radiologic imaging) are inadequate for accurate detection of micrometastatic nodal involvement and cannot be used to differentiate inflammatory nodal enlargement from metastatic involvement.

Within this framework, the ensuing discussion focuses on the management of patients with no clinical evidence of regional nodal enlargement at SCP diagnosis, individuals with clinical lymphadenopathy at the time of SCP diagnosis, and patients who develop inguinal lymphadenopathy at an interval after management of the primary lesion (**Fig. 1**).

PENILE LYMPHATIC DRAINAGE: ANATOMIC AND PROGNOSTIC CONSIDERATIONS

Lymphatic drainage of the penis has been traditionally divided into superficial and deep nodal groups of the inguinal region. The superficial nodes are located under the subcutaneous fascia and above the fascia lata within the femoral triangle. Five anatomic groups of superficial inguinal lymph nodes have been described by Daseler and colleagues:[4] (1) central nodes of the saphenofemoral junction, (2) superolateral nodes of the superficial circumflex vein, (3) superomedial nodes of the superficial external pudendal and superficial epigastric veins, (4) inferolateral nodes of the lateral femoral cutaneous vein, and (5) inferomedial nodes around the greater saphenous vein. The deep nodes lie in the region of the fossa ovalis where the greater saphenous vein drains

Department of Urology, The University of Texas Southwestern Medical Center, 5323 Harry Hines Boulevard, Dallas, TX 75390-9110, USA
* Corresponding author.
E-mail address: vitaly.margulis@utsouthwestern.edu

Urol Clin N Am 37 (2010) 411–419
doi:10.1016/j.ucl.2010.04.009
0094-0143/10/$ – see front matter © 2010 Elsevier Inc. All rights reserved.

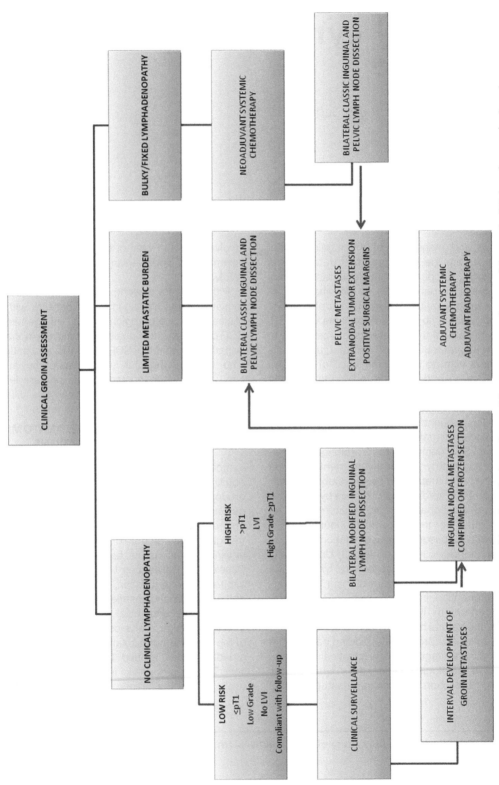

Fig. 1. Algorithm for management of the ilioinguinal lymph nodes in patients with squamous carcinoma of the penis. LVI, lymphovascular invasion.

into the femoral vein through perforating the fascia lata, mainly medial to the femoral vein.[4] The node of Cloquet represents the most cephalad extension of the deep inguinal nodal group. Finally, the lymphatic drainage proceeds cephalad to the external iliac and obturator nodal chains.

Anatomic and clinical observations support orderly and predictable metastatic spread of SCP initially to the superficial inguinal lymph nodes, followed by the deep inguinal nodal group, and subsequently to the pelvic nodal chains.[5,6] While no "skip" nodal metastases have been reported in the literature, bilateral inguinal nodal dissemination is the rule rather than the exception and has been reported in up to 80% of patients.[6]

Five-year cancer-specific survival decreases from 100% to 90% in node-negative SCP patients to roughly 60% in patients with resected inguinal nodal metastases.[7] Nonetheless, node-positive SCP patients represent a heterogeneous group and survival depends on the number of nodes involved, lymph node density, size of largest nodal deposit, presence of extranodal tumor extension, bilateral groin metastases, and involvement of the pelvic lymph nodes.[2,7–10] Cumulative data suggest that patients with minimal nodal involvement (2 or fewer lymph nodes), no evidence of extranodal extension, or pelvic disease derive the most benefit from curative inguinal lymph node dissection, with 5-year cancer-specific survival approaching 80%.[2,7–10] This figure decreases to 25% in patients with multiple (>2) lymph nodes involved or presence of extranodal disease, and to less than 10% in patients with pelvic nodal metastases.[2,7–10] It is clear that management of ilioinguinal lymph nodes in patients with clinical and pathologic features of advanced nodal disease should be evaluated in the context of a multimodality treatment paradigm, integrating surgical resection with systemic chemotherapy and/or radiation therapy approaches.

NO CLINICAL EVIDENCE OF ILIOINGUINAL LYMPHADENOPATHY
Timing of an Intervention

As previously stated, up to 30% of SCP patients with clinically negative groins will harbor micrometastatic disease. It is precisely this group of patients that derives the maximum benefit from surgical removal of their inguinal nodal metastases. Although the morbidity of the inguinal nodal dissection in the modern era has decreased, subjecting all patients with SCP and no clinical evidence of inguinal lymphadenopathy to groin dissections would result in prohibitive rates of overtreatment. There is, however, a growing body of evidence

that indicates significantly compromised survival in patients managed with clinical groin surveillance and node dissection at the time of disease progression, compared with patients treated with up-front inguinal lymph node dissection for occult nodal metastases.[11–14] In a recent report of 40 patients with clinically negative groins after management of primary SCP, the 3-year cancer-specific survival was 84% for patients who underwent immediate lymphadenectomy and were found to have nodal metastases, compared with 35% in those subjected to delayed node dissection (P = .002).[14] Consequently, a logical approach to management of SCP with clinically negative nodes centers around accurate identification of patients at a high risk of harboring occult inguinal nodal metastases, while sparing the morbidity of inguinal node dissection in patients destined to have pathologically negative nodes. Several strategies designed to address these challenges are currently in practice or are in various stages of clinical development.

Patient Selection for Surgery

Risk stratification based on the primary tumor characteristics is a widely accepted strategy to select patients at high risk of harboring occult inguinal nodal disease for inguinal node dissection. Pathologic primary tumor stage, tumor grade, and presence of lymphovascular invasion (LVI) have been demonstrated consistently to correlate with the probability of metastatic nodal egress.[3,15–17] Patients with primary tumor stage T1 or less, with no evidence of high-grade features or LVI have a less than 10% chance of metastatic nodal disease and are suitable candidates for clinical surveillance. Alternatively, presence of advanced pathologic stage (≥T2), high grade, or LVI are associated with greater than 25% risk of nodal involvement, mandating inguinal lymph node dissection. The current European Association of Urology (EAU) guidelines stratify patients into 3 risk groups according to their probability of harboring metastatic lymphadenopathy, based on stage and grade of the primary tumor: low risk: pTis, pTa grade 1 to 2, and pT1 grade 1 tumors; intermediate risk: pT1 grade 2 tumors; high risk: pT2 or higher or grade 3 tumors.[17] EAU guidelines recommend modified inguinal lymph node dissection for patients in intermediate- and high-risk categories (see **Fig. 1**). Recently, Ficarra and colleagues[18] have developed a prognostic nomogram for individualized prediction of metastatic inguinal lymphadenopathy, based on 8 clinical and pathologic variables: tumor thickness, microscopic growth pattern, grade, presence of vascular or lymphatic invasion, tumor infiltration into the corpora cavernosa, corpus spongiosum or the urethra, and the clinical stage of groin lymph nodes. The prognostic accuracy of this model (concordance index 0.876) was superior to that of EAU risk grouping (concordance index 0.697).[18]

The technique of dynamic sentinel node biopsy (DSNB) was developed and adapted for SCP, based on the concept of orderly lymphatic progression of metastatic cells from the primary tumor to the initial draining (sentinel) lymph node.[19] The group at the Netherlands Cancer Institute, which pioneered the use of DSNB for staging of SCP patients, reports cumulative false-negative rate of 5% in 75 patients managed according to their latest DSNB protocol.[20,21] Patients found to have metastatic involvement of their sentinel lymph node proceed with inguinal lymph node dissection, while patients with benign histology are spared the morbidity of a groin dissection. It should be noted that there is a significant learning curve associated with successful execution of DSNB and that this technique, so far, has been implemented only in a few centers with high volume of SCP patients.[22] Moreover, the low false-negative rate of DSNB reported by the Netherlands Cancer Institute group has not been replicated by other investigators.[23,24] Pending further standardization and independent validation, DSNB may become the cornerstone strategy for inguinal nodal staging in SCP patients without palpable lymphadenopathy.

Although traditional radiologic imaging modalities such as computed tomography (CT) or magnetic resonance imaging (MRI) are unsuitable for detection of micrometastatic nodal involvement, several evolving functional imaging strategies merit further discussion. Tabatabaei and colleagues[25] have recently reported on the utility of a nanoparticle enhanced MRI in a pilot study of 7 SCP patients, in whom they found sensitivity of 100% and specificity of 97% with a positive predictive value of 81.2% for diagnosis of metastatic involvement of the inguinal lymph nodes. Similarly, preliminary experience with ^{18}F-fluorodeoxyglucose positron emission tomography/CT in 13 patients with SCP suggested sensitivity of 80% and specificity of 100% for detection of metastatic inguinal lymph nodes.[26,27] It is clear that further prospective studies designed in the context of clinically node-negative SCP are needed to delineate the role of functional imaging in this setting.

Surgical Technique

Boundaries of classical inguinal lymph node dissection are denoted laterally by the medial edge of sartorius muscle, medially by the lateral edge of adductor muscle, inferiorly by the inferior edge of the fossa ovalis, posteriorly by the muscular floor of the femoral triangle, and superiorly by the inguinal ligament.[4,5,28] Regardless of the incision used, skin flaps are developed in the plane just below Scarpa's fascia, and the areolar tissue is dissected from the external oblique aponeurosis and the spermatic cord to the inferior border of the inguinal ligament, establishing the superior aspect of the nodal packet. The saphenous vein is identified and usually divided at the apex of the femoral triangle; however, in patients with minimal nodal burden, preservation of the saphenous vein may be feasible. The femoral artery and vein are identified at the apex of the femoral triangle (inferior aspect of the nodal packet), and dissected superiorly, controlling small perforators and dividing the saphenous vein if necessary at the saphenofemoral junction. Dissection is minimized lateral to the femoral artery to avoid injury to the femoral nerve and the profunda femoris artery. All of the lymphatic and areolar tissue overlying the femoral vessels and medial to the testicular cord is removed, including the deep inguinal nodes and the node of Cloquet at the femoral canal (**Fig. 2**). The femoral canal is closed, if necessary, by suturing Poupart's ligament to Cooper's ligament, without obstructing the femoral outflow, and the sartorius muscle is mobilized from its origin at the anterior superior iliac spine and transposed medially to cover the femoral vessels (**Fig. 3**). When pelvic lymph node dissection is indicated, an extraperitoneal approach is used and the common iliac, external iliac, and obturator lymph nodes are removed. When inguinal ligament-sparing incisions are used, care should be taken to completely remove all of the lymphatic tissue in the femoral canal,

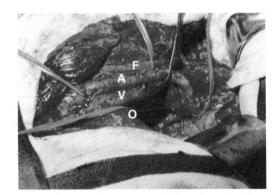

Fig. 2. Classic right ilioinguinal lymph node dissection. Inguinal ligament has been divided and external iliac/femoral artery (A), external iliac/femoral vein (V), and femoral nerve (F) are exposed. Obturator nerve (O) is seen in the right obturator fossa.

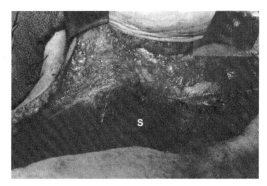

Fig. 3. Transposed sartorius muscle (S), providing coverage for the femoral vessels.

establishing continuity with the inguinal portion of the procedure.

Modified lymphadenectomy, as proposed by Catalona,[29] has replaced the classic inguinal lymph node dissection as a staging procedure in a setting of clinically negative groins. If nodal metastases are identified on frozen sections after a modified dissection, the procedure is converted to a classic dissection on the affected side. The key points of the modified groin dissection are a shorter skin incision, limitation of the dissection to nodal tissue medial to the femoral artery, preservation of the saphenous vein, and omission of the sartorius transposition (**Fig. 4**). All of the superficial nodal tissue as well the deep nodes located medial to the femoral vein, including the node of Cloquet, are removed and sent for pathologic examination.[29] There is no proven role for pelvic node dissection in the setting of pathologically benign inguinal nodes.[5] Nonetheless, the authors continue to advocate bilateral pelvic node dissection if metastatic SCP is found in the inguinal regions. Others have advocated pelvic lymph node dissection only if more than one inguinal lymph node is affected or if extranodal tumor extension is present, because the probability of pelvic involvement in these circumstances is 25% or more, compared with 0% to 5% in cases of solitary nodal metastasis.[30,31] While the debate regarding the necessity and appropriate patient selection for the pelvic lymph node dissection continues, it should be noted that the extraperitoneal pelvic lymph node dissection contributes little to the morbidity beyond that of the inguinal lymph node dissection.

Preliminary experiences with laparoscopic and robot-assisted methods of inguinal node dissection have recently been described, driven by high complication rates associated with standard inguinal lymph node dissection and by overall increasing application of minimally invasive surgical technology in urologic oncology.[32–34] Theoretical advantages of these minimally invasive surgical approaches include decreased local complication rates, and expedited patient recovery and convalescence. Tobias-Machado and colleagues[32] recently reported comparative experience in 20 and 10 clinically negative groins managed with laparoscopic and open inguinal lymph node dissections, respectively. Mean operative time was 120 minutes for the laparoscopic and 92 minutes for the open procedures. There was no statistical difference in the number of nodes removed. Complications were observed in 70% and 20% of groins managed with open and laparoscopic approaches, respectively. No recurrences have been observed at a median follow-up of 33 months.[32] With further experience, laparoscopic and/or robotic-assisted lymph node dissection undoubtedly will be incorporated into the surgical management armamentarium of SCP patients.

PALPABLE INGUINAL LYMPHADENOPATHY
Low-Volume Inguinal Lymphadenopathy

Up to 85% of SCP patients with palpable, but not fixed inguinal lymph nodes at the time of initial presentation will harbor metastatic nodal disease.[1,2] Previously a 4- to 6-week course of antibiotic therapy has been advocated to achieve resolution of infectious/inflammatory lymphadenopathy in a substantial proportion of patients. At present, a fine-needle aspiration of enlarged inguinal lymph nodes can be obtained and if positive, surgical treatment of ilioinguinal lymph nodes implemented without undue delay.[35,36] Due to the significant (5%–15%) false-negative rate associated with fine-needle biopsy, negative results should be interpreted with caution and palpable

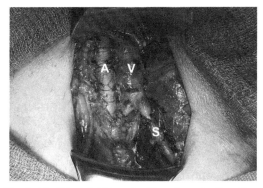

Fig. 4. Modified right inguinal lymph node dissection. Dissection lateral to the femoral artery (A) is minimized. Long saphenous vein (S) is seen is seen entering the femoral vein.

nodes after appropriate course of antibiotic therapy should be managed with inguinal lymph node dissection.[1]

The authors prefer classic inguinal lymph node dissection of the involved, grossly positive, and contralateral groins. This approach is supported by anatomic studies documenting bilateral lymphatic drainage of the penis, and by the finding of occult nodal metastases in up to 50% of clinically "negative" contralateral groins.[37] Although conclusive data on the therapeutic benefit of pelvic lymph node dissection in SCP are lacking, the authors continue to offer bilateral pelvic lymphadenectomy in a setting of positive inguinal lymph nodes. Anecdotal evidence supports curative potential associated with surgical resection of limited pelvic nodal disease, and staging information obtained by pelvic dissection may guide selection of patients for adjuvant systemic therapy.[1,30]

Bulky and/or Fixed Inguinal Lymphadenopathy

Presence of bulky or fixed inguinal lymphadenopathy uniformly signifies metastatic disease, and only a small portion of these patients will benefit from surgery as a monotherapy.[30] Presurgical systemic therapy in these patients is an attractive treatment paradigm because it allows timely delivery of therapy to treat systemic disease, results in volume-reduction of inguinal lymphadenopathy, and facilitates future surgical consolidation.[38–40] Several retrospective series using various chemotherapeutic agents report objective response rates of up to 60% and complete response rates nearing 20% in patients who underwent consolidative ilioinguinal lymph node dissections after induction systemic therapy.[30,38–40] A phase 2 clinical trial of neoadjuvant chemotherapy for patients with SCP stage Tany, N2-N3, M0 has recently completed accrual at The M.D. Anderson Cancer Center.[40] Eligible patients received 4 courses of ifosfamide, paclitaxel, and cisplatin (TIP) followed by bilateral inguinal and pelvic lymph node dissections. Preliminary analysis of data from the first 20 patients revealed an objective response rate of 55% and pathologic complete responses in 10% of the patients. No treatment-related mortality was observed.[40]

Use of external beam radiation therapy (EBRT) alone or in combination with systemic therapy has been reported to provide local palliation to inoperable patients with bulky groin disease.[41] Alternatively, a small study by investigators from Taiwan suggested that use of adjuvant EBRT after groin dissection for metastatic disease could provide additional therapeutic benefit. Chen and colleagues[42] reported regional failure rates after positive inguinal lymph node dissections in 11% (1 of 9) versus 60% (3 of 5) with and without adjuvant inguinal EBRT.

In summary, appropriate integration of systemic therapy and EBRT in patients with locally advanced nodal disease is not well delineated. However, available data suggests that select patients with bulky groin metastases benefit from induction systemic therapy, followed by aggressive surgical consolidation with or without adjuvant radiotherapy, based on extent of residual disease. The authors' current approach to this challenging patient population includes presurgical TIP, as outlined by The M.D. Anderson Cancer Center group, followed by bilateral inguinal and pelvic lymph node dissections.[40] Close collaboration with reconstructive surgeons is essential because large portions of involved inguinal skin may be resected en bloc, necessitating myocutaneous flaps for reconstruction. The authors reserve the use of adjuvant EBRT for select patients with large volume residual disease and extranodal tumor extension, or in rare cases of incomplete resection.

Development of Interval Unilateral Lymphadenopathy During Surveillance

Presentation with unilateral lymphadenopathy after a period of observation almost uniformly signifies metastatic progression. Assuming equal growth rates of metastatic groin deposits, the absence of clinical lymphadenopathy, despite prolonged observation, suggests freedom from disease on the clinically negative side. Consequently, the traditional approach in this clinical scenario has been ilioinguinal lymph node dissection of the affected side only. Nonetheless, occult contralateral nodal disease has been reported in up to 30% of patients with a bulky unilateral recurrence.[28] As a result, the authors continue to advocate adjunct contralateral modified groin dissection in patients who rapidly progress during observation trial or in patients with bulky groin disease.

MINIMIZING THE MORBIDITY OF INGUINAL LYMPH NODE DISSECTION

Classic inguinal lymph node dissection has historically been associated with high (>80%) rate of wound- and lymph-related complications, including infection, dehiscence, skin necrosis, lymphocele, and lower extremity lymphedema.[8,11,43] In addition, concerning rates of thromboembolic events, such as deep venous thrombosis (DVT) or pulmonary embolus (PE), and sensory and/or motor lower extremity neuropraxias, have been reported. Contemporary series of inguinal lymph node dissection, however, report somewhat diminished complication rates, ranging from 30% to 70%.[44–47] This section summarizes the various intra- and perioperative management strategies that may have led to the apparent decrease in groin dissection–related complications in the modern era.

Wound infection, dehiscence, and necrosis occur at a cumulative rate of up to 70% after a modified or a classic inguinal lymph node dissection.[8,11,44,46,48,49] The authors routinely stage the groin dissections to allow removal of the potentially infected primary tumor and use skin flora–specific preoperative antibiotic therapy to sterilize potentially infected groins before surgery.[50] Postoperatively, antibiotic therapy is continued until all subcutaneous drains have been removed. While there is some debate regarding the impact of the type of incision used for inguinal lymph node dissection, the single most important surgical factor essential for minimizing wound-related complications is meticulous preservation of skin flap thickness by maintaining the dissection plane below Scarpa's fascia.[29,43,44,47,51,52] Careful skin flap handling, meticulous lymphatic and vascular control, and aggressive removal of all devitalized skin and soft tissue should be uniformly employed. The authors often use myocutaneous skin flaps, harvested by the reconstructive surgeons, to achieve tension-free skin closure in situations where primary tension-free closure is not possible.[53,54]

Lymphocele formation and lower extremity lymphedema are potentially devastating complications, occurring at a cumulative rate of 2% to 15% and 10% to 30%, respectively, after an inguinal lymphadenectomy.[8,11,43–45,51,52] Consultation with a lymphedema specialist experienced in the management of postoperative lymphatic complications, and compressive stocking fitting is mandatory before surgery. In addition to meticulous lymphatic and vascular control when feasible, preservation of a saphenous vein, and intraoperative use of tissue sealants, the authors routinely employ suction groin drains until output is minimal (<30 mL/d for several consecutive days). The authors believe that these measures minimize subcutaneous fluid accumulation and promote skin flap adherence to the underlying inguinal tissues. Postoperatively, compressive stockings and early ambulation are used to prevent venous stasis, maintain appropriate limb volume, and stimulate the formation of neolymphatics.[55]

Finally, after inguinal lymphadenectomy, SCP patients are at a particularly increased risk for potentially life-threatening thromboembolic events. Immobilization, venous and lymphatic stasis, and presence of malignancy all contribute to the 5% to 10% rate of DVT/PE reported in the literature.[8,11,44] When necessary, the long saphenous vein should be ligated close to the femoral insertion, thus avoiding creation of a venous stump serving as a potential nidus for thrombus formation and propagation. Although controversial, consideration should be given to early use of anticoagulation with heparin or its low molecular weight derivatives, started before surgery, and maintained for several weeks after the procedure.[56] In addition, the authors routinely employ compression stockings and sequential compression devices along with early patient mobilization to augment venous return and prevent venous stasis.[46,56,57]

SUMMARY

Surgical removal of the inguinal lymph nodes provides an important staging and therapeutic benefit to SCP patients, while the methodology of appropriate patient selection for lymph node dissection continues to evolve. Compliant, motivated, and reliable patients with low risk of harboring metastatic inguinal lymph nodes can be managed with careful inguinal surveillance. In SCP patients whose primary tumors demonstrate pathologic features of aggressive disease, modified bilateral inguinal lymph node dissection should be performed and be converted to classic ilioinguinal lymph node dissection if metastatic disease is confirmed on frozen sections. DSNB remains an attractive staging option in select patients with clinically negative groins, but should be limited to high-volume centers fully invested in this technique. Finally, patients with bulky inguinal metastases are unlikely to be cured by surgery alone. Integration of systemic therapy, especially in a presurgical setting, is an attractive strategy for the management of patients with advanced SCP, and is currently being studied prospectively.

REFERENCES

1. Ornellas AA, Kinchin EW, Nobrega BL, et al. Surgical treatment of invasive squamous cell carcinoma of the penis: Brazilian National Cancer Institute long-term experience. J Surg Oncol 2008;97: 487–95.
2. Hegarty PK, Kayes O, Freeman A, et al. A prospective study of 100 cases of penile cancer managed

according to European Association of Urology guidelines. BJU Int 2006;98:526–31.

3. Slaton JW, Morgenstern N, Levy DA, et al. Tumor stage, vascular invasion and the percentage of poorly differentiated cancer: independent prognosticators for inguinal lymph node metastasis in penile squamous cancer. J Urol 2001;165:1138–42.

4. Daseler EH, Anson BJ, Reimann AF. Radical excision of the inguinal and iliac lymph glands; a study based upon 450 anatomical dissections and upon supportive clinical observations. Surg Gynecol Obstet 1948;87:679–94.

5. Cabanas RM. An approach for the treatment of penile carcinoma. Cancer 1977;39:456–66.

6. Leijte JA, Valdes Olmos RA, Nieweg OE, et al. Anatomical mapping of lymphatic drainage in penile carcinoma with SPECT-CT: implications for the extent of inguinal lymph node dissection. Eur Urol 2008;54:885–90.

7. Wein AJ, Kavoussi LR, Novick AC, et al. Tumors of the penis. Chapter 31. In: Wein AJ, Kavoussi LR, Novick AC, et al, editors. Campbell-Walsh urology. Philadelphia: Saunders; 2007. p. 959–92.

8. Ravi R. Morbidity following groin dissection for penile carcinoma. Br J Urol 1993;72:941–5.

9. Svatek RS, Munsell M, Kincaid JM, et al. Association between lymph node density and disease specific survival in patients with penile cancer. J Urol 2009; 182:2721–7.

10. Leijte JA, Horenblas S. Shortcomings of the current TNM classification for penile carcinoma: time for a change? World J Urol 2009;27:151–4.

11. Johnson DE, Lo RK. Management of regional lymph nodes in penile carcinoma. Five-year results following therapeutic groin dissections. Urology 1984;24:308–11.

12. McDougal WS, Kirchner FK Jr, Edwards RH, et al. Treatment of carcinoma of the penis: the case for primary lymphadenectomy. J Urol 1986;136:38–41.

13. Leijte JA, Kirrander P, Antonini N, et al. Recurrence patterns of squamous cell carcinoma of the penis: recommendations for follow-up based on a two-centre analysis of 700 patients. Eur Urol 2008;54: 161–8.

14. Kroon BK, Horenblas S, Lont AP, et al. Patients with penile carcinoma benefit from immediate resection of clinically occult lymph node metastases. J Urol 2005;173:816–9.

15. Solsona E, Iborra I, Rubio J, et al. Prospective validation of the association of local tumor stage and grade as a predictive factor for occult lymph node micrometastasis in patients with penile carcinoma and clinically negative inguinal lymph nodes. J Urol 2001;165:1506–9.

16. Ficarra V, Zattoni F, Cunico SC, et al. Lymphatic and vascular embolizations are independent predictive variables of inguinal lymph node involvement in patients with squamous cell carcinoma of the penis: Gruppo Uro-oncologico del Nord Est (Northeast Uro-oncological Group) penile cancer data base data. Cancer 2005;103:2507–16.

17. Solsona E, Algaba F, Horenblas S, et al. EAU guidelines on penile cancer. Eur Urol 2004;46:1–8.

18. Ficarra V, Zattoni F, Artibani W, et al. Nomogram predictive of pathological inguinal lymph node involvement in patients with squamous cell carcinoma of the penis. J Urol 2006;175:1700–4 [discussion: 1704–5].

19. Cabanas RM. Application of the sentinel node concept in urogenital cancer. Recent Results Cancer Res 2000;157:141–9.

20. Leijte JA, Kroon BK, Valdes Olmos RA, et al. Reliability and safety of current dynamic sentinel node biopsy for penile carcinoma. Eur Urol 2007;52:170–7.

21. Kroon BK, Horenblas S, Estourgie SH, et al. How to avoid false-negative dynamic sentinel node procedures in penile carcinoma. J Urol 2004;171:2191–4.

22. Leijte JA, Hughes B, Graafland NM, et al. Two-center evaluation of dynamic sentinel node biopsy for squamous cell carcinoma of the penis. J Clin Oncol 2009;27:3325–9.

23. Pettaway CA, Pisters LL, Dinney CP, et al. Sentinel lymph node dissection for penile carcinoma: the M. D. Anderson cancer center experience. J Urol 1995;154:1999–2003.

24. Spiess PE, Izawa JI, Bassett R, et al. Preoperative lymphoscintigraphy and dynamic sentinel node biopsy for staging penile cancer: results with pathological correlation. J Urol 2007;177:2157–61.

25. Tabatabaei S, Harisinghani M, McDougal WS. Regional lymph node staging using lymphotropic nanoparticle enhanced magnetic resonance imaging with ferumoxtran-10 in patients with penile cancer. J Urol 2005;174:923–7 [discussion: 927].

26. Scher B, Seitz M, Reiser M, et al. ^{18}F-FDG PET/CT for staging of penile cancer. J Nucl Med 2005;46: 1460–5.

27. Scher B, Seitz M, Albinger W, et al. Value of PET and PET/CT in the diagnostics of prostate and penile cancer. Recent Results Cancer Res 2008; 170:159–79.

28. Horenblas S, van Tinteren H, Delemarre JF, et al. Squamous cell carcinoma of the penis. III. Treatment of regional lymph nodes. J Urol 1993;149:492–7.

29. Catalona WJ. Modified inguinal lymphadenectomy for carcinoma of the penis with preservation of saphenous veins: technique and preliminary results. J Urol 1988;140:306–10.

30. Culkin DJ, Beer TM. Advanced penile carcinoma. J Urol 2003;170:359–65.

31. Lont AP, Kroon BK, Gallee MP, et al. Pelvic lymph node dissection for penile carcinoma: extent of inguinal lymph node involvement as an indicator for pelvic lymph node involvement and survival. J Urol 2007;177:947–52 [discussion: 952].

32. Tobias-Machado M, Tavares A, Silva MN, et al. Can video endoscopic inguinal lymphadenectomy achieve a lower morbidity than open lymph node dissection in penile cancer patients? J Endourol 2008;22:1687–91.

33. Sotelo R, Sanchez-Salas R, Clavijo R. Endoscopic inguinal lymph node dissection for penile carcinoma: the developing of a novel technique. World J Urol 2009;27:213–9.

34. Josephson DY, Jacobsohn KM, Link BA, et al. Robotic-assisted endoscopic inguinal lymphadenectomy. Urology 2009;73:167–70 [discussion: 170–1].

35. Kroon BK, Horenblas S, Deurloo EE, et al. Ultrasonography-guided fine-needle aspiration cytology before sentinel node biopsy in patients with penile carcinoma. BJU Int 2005;95:517–21.

36. Saisorn I, Lawrentschuk N, Leewansangtong S, et al. Fine-needle aspiration cytology predicts inguinal lymph node metastasis without antibiotic pretreatment in penile carcinoma. BJU Int 2006;97: 1225–8.

37. Ekstrom T, Edsmyr F. Cancer of the penis; a clinical study of 229 cases. Acta Chir Scand 1958; 115:25–45.

38. Bermejo C, Busby JE, Spiess PE, et al. Neoadjuvant chemotherapy followed by aggressive surgical consolidation for metastatic penile squamous cell carcinoma. J Urol 2007;177:1335–8.

39. Leijte JA, Kerst JM, Bais E, et al. Neoadjuvant chemotherapy in advanced penile carcinoma. Eur Urol 2007;52:488–94.

40. Pagliaro LC, Crook J. Multimodality therapy in penile cancer: when and which treatments? World J Urol 2009;27:221–5.

41. Vaeth JM, Green JP, Lowy RO. Radiation therapy of carcinoma of the penis. Am J Roentgenol Radium Ther Nucl Med 1970;108:130–5.

42. Chen MF, Chen WC, Wu CT, et al. Contemporary management of penile cancer including surgery and adjuvant radiotherapy: an experience in Taiwan. World J Urol 2004;22:60–6.

43. Ornellas AA, Seixas AL, de Moraes JR. Analyses of 200 lymphadenectomies in patients with penile carcinoma. J Urol 1991;146:330–2.

44. Bevan-Thomas R, Slaton JW, Pettaway CA. Contemporary morbidity from lymphadenectomy for penile squamous cell carcinoma: the M. D. Anderson cancer center experience. J Urol 2002;167:1638–42.

45. Coblentz TR, Theodorescu D. Morbidity of modified prophylactic inguinal lymphadenectomy for squamous cell carcinoma of the penis. J Urol 2002;168:1386–9.

46. Nelson BA, Cookson MS, Smith JA Jr, et al. Complications of inguinal and pelvic lymphadenectomy for squamous cell carcinoma of the penis: a contemporary series. J Urol 2004;172:494–7.

47. Milathianakis C, Bogdanos J, Karamanolakis D. Morbidity of prophylactic inguinal lymphadenectomy with saphenous vein preservation for squamous cell penile carcinoma. Int J Urol 2005;12: 776–8.

48. Lopes A, Hidalgo GS, Kowalski LP, et al. Prognostic factors in carcinoma of the penis: multivariate analysis of 145 patients treated with amputation and lymphadenectomy. J Urol 1996;156:1637–42.

49. Ayyappan K, Ananthakrishnan N, Sankaran V. Can regional lymph node involvement be predicted in patients with carcinoma of the penis? Br J Urol 1994;73:549–53.

50. Josephs LG, Cordts PR, DiEdwardo CL, et al. Do infected inguinal lymph nodes increase the incidence of postoperative groin wound infection? J Vasc Surg 1993;17:1077–80 [discussion: 1080–2].

51. Bouchot O, Rigaud J, Maillet F, et al. Morbidity of inguinal lymphadenectomy for invasive penile carcinoma. Eur Urol 2004;45:761–5 [discussion: 765–6].

52. Tonouchi H, Ohmori Y, Kobayashi M, et al. Operative morbidity associated with groin dissections. Surg Today 2004;34:413–8.

53. Evriviades D, Raurell A, Perks AG. Pedicled anterolateral thigh flap for reconstruction after radical groin dissection. Urology 2007;70:996–9.

54. Qi F, Gu J, Shi Y. Difficult groin reconstruction using contralateral rectus abdominis myocutaneous flap. Plast Reconstr Surg 2008;121: 147e–8e.

55. Garfein ES, Borud LJ, Warren AG, et al. Learning from a lymphedema clinic: an algorithm for the management of localized swelling. Plast Reconstr Surg 2008;121:521–8.

56. Forrest JB, Clemens JQ, Finamore P, et al. AUA best practice statement for the prevention of deep vein thrombosis in patients undergoing urologic surgery. J Urol 2009;181:1170–7.

57. Ettema HB, Kollen BJ, Verheyen CC, et al. Prevention of venous thromboembolism in patients with immobilization of the lower extremities: a meta-analysis of randomized controlled trials. J Thromb Haemost 2008;6:1093–8.

Controversies in Ilioinguinal Lymphadenectomy

P.K. Hegarty, MD[a],*, C.P. Dinney, MD[b,c],
C.A. Pettaway, MD[b,c]

KEYWORDS

- Penile carcinoma • Lymph node • Controversy
- Morbidity • Dynamic sentinel node biopsy
- Video endoscopic inguinal lymphadenectomy

Penile cancer has a predictable pattern of spread in a stepwise fashion. Initially regional inguinal lymph node metastasis occurs, followed by pelvic nodal metastasis and then distant spread.[1] Patients who are proven to have negative inguinal lymph nodes have an excellent prognosis. Furthermore, patients with small volume inguinal node involvement can often be cured by surgery alone. It seems rational then that lymphadenectomy would be standard in all patients; however, controversies arise due to the morbidity of the procedure. The difficulty in using purely clinical examination or imaging in selecting patients at risk for metastasis has led to divergent strategies such as watchful waiting versus sentinel lymph node biopsy versus limited dissections.[1] However, new techniques are evolving that aim to effectively stage the inguinal region while minimizing morbidity.[1] The prognosis for patients with advanced inguinal metastasis is dismal with surgery alone, and novel treatment strategies are clearly needed.[1,2] This article describes current controversies and challenges in managing the inguinal region for patients with squamous penile cancer.

OBJECTIVES OF LYMPHADENECTOMY

The main objective of lymphadenectomy is to provide accurate pathology-based staging and, where disease exists, to alter the natural history, clarify prognosis, and guide the future follow-up schedule. In cases with proven lymph node metastases, further therapy may be selected based on pathologic findings. Finally the provision of tissue, both from the primary tumor and from lymph nodes, is important for ongoing research.

Effect of Lymphadenectomy on Natural History of Penile Cancer

The greatest single predictor of survival in squamous cell carcinoma of the penis is the incidence and extent of lymph node involvement.[1–3] In a prospective study the 3-year disease-specific survival of men with pathologic N0 disease was 100%.[3] Also of note was that men found to have a single lymph node involved (N1 disease) had a 100% 3-year disease-specific survival without any adjuvant therapy. Presuming that the natural history of untreated micrometastatic lymph node disease become symptomatic, this result implies that surgery alone has a significant impact in early lymph node disease. Thus, a properly performed lymphadenectomy can cure some men with nodal metastasis. For more advanced nodal disease the number of positive lymph nodes predicts the 5-year overall survival as 75.6% for patients with between 1 and 3 nodes, 8.4% for 4 or 5 nodes,

[a] Department of Urology, Guy's and St Thomas' NHS Foundation Trust, Great Maze Pond, London SE1 9RT, UK
[b] Department of Urology, The University of Texas MD Anderson Cancer Center, 1515 Holcombe Boulevard, Unit 1373, Houston, TX 77030, USA
[c] Department of Cancer Biology, The University of Texas MD Anderson Cancer Center, 1515 Holcombe Boulevard, Unit 1373, Houston, TX 77030, USA
* Corresponding author.
E-mail address: Paul.hegarty@gstt.nhs.uk

Urol Clin N Am 37 (2010) 421–434
doi:10.1016/j.ucl.2010.04.005

and 0% for those with more than 5 positive nodes.[4] Other ominous features that threaten cure with surgery alone include the presence of extranodal extension and pelvic lymph node metastasis.[4] However, a pelvic dissection can at times be beneficial, as demonstrated in some reports where 16% to 20% of patients with pelvic metastasis experienced long-term survival.[5,6] Recently, a novel variable incorporating the number of positive lymph nodes/ total nodes removed, termed the lymph node density (LND[7]), was described in penile cancer. The total lymph node count captures both the extent of dissection and the degree of processing by the pathologist. In this study TNM stage was compared with LND as prognostic indices of disease-specific survival.[7] Median node counts for superficial inguinal lymph node dissection (ILND) were 8 to 10, for radical ILND 10 to 11, and for combined inguinal/ ipsilateral pelvic node dissection 22 to 25. On univariate regression analysis, disease-specific survival was associated with pathologic N3 disease, extracapsular extension, the number of positive lymph nodes, and LND. As only 18 patients died during the follow-up period, full multivariate regression analysis was not possible. However, it was possible to sequentially compare 2 indices at a time to assess their relative importance. Comparing the various indices, when LND was incorporated into the model, the other variables including TNM stage and extranodal extension lost significance. An LND of greater than 6.7% had a hazard ratio of 14.48 of disease-specific mortality compared with an LND less than 6.7%. Also, when the group of patients with positive lymph nodes had LND values broken down into increasing tertiles, the hazard ratios of mortality were 1, 4.35, and 35.54, respectively.[7] Of note, an additional finding of the study was that the number of negative lymph nodes removed among the lymph node–positive cohort was also a strong prognostic factor. This result would potentially suggest that microscopic metastases existed in this node-positive cohort and that a thorough dissection cleaned out metastases that were not detected via routine pathologic process. This novel concept requires independent validation in larger data sets to determine its routine clinical utility.

Early or Late Lymphadenectomy

The low rate of micrometastatic disease, along with the rarity of penile cancer in some countries and the morbidity of inguinal lymphadenectomy, may account for the practice of observation of men with invasive penile cancer and no palpable inguinal adenopathy. The lack of guidelines has meant that practice has varied considerably. Several articles have addressed the issue of early

lymphadenectomy versus waiting for inguinal nodes to become palpable before offering surgery. There is no randomized study of immediate ILND versus surveillance, and as such a study is neither feasible nor ethical given our current understanding from studies provided below.

McDougal[8] showed that patients who underwent lymphadenectomy for palpable disease had a 33% survival as compared with 84% for those with impalpable positive nodes. In another retrospective study from India, 28 patients underwent inguinal lymphadenectomy at either an early interval (mean of 1.7 months) or late interval (mean of 14 months) following surgery for the primary tumor.[9] Although not randomized, the groups matched well for stage and grade. The 5-year cancer-specific survival rates for early and delayed ILND groups were 90.9% and 13.3%, respectively. Those undergoing delayed ILND had a significantly higher rate of extracapsular extension.[9] One could argue, however, that these series also included patients in the "early group" whose lymph nodes were pathologically negative, and that they did not benefit from surgery but were exposed to the complications. This question was addressed in another study by Kroon and colleagues[10] from the Netherlands, who compared the disease-specific survival of 20 patients who underwent an early therapeutic dissection and had proven positive nodes versus a group that underwent surgery subsequent to recurrence. Three-year disease-specific survival in the early group was 84% versus 35% in the delayed group ($P = .0017$). This study clearly demonstrates that delayed lymphadenectomy is not a safe oncological practice for the majority of patients with clinically negative lymph nodes who exhibit "high-risk" features in their primary tumors. Further, it is now realized that the morbidity of a prophylactic dissection tends to be lower than palliative dissection performed for higher volume disease for which additional therapy is often required (ie, chemotherapy, radiation).[11]

Although early lymphadenectomy is superior to delayed lymphadenectomy, performing bilateral ILND simultaneously with surgery for the primary lesion has several disadvantages. First, it requires accurate grading of the lesion preoperatively and may demand intraoperative frozen section to stage the lesion. Second, bilateral lymphadenectomy may affect the healing of the primary lesion because of lymphedema or infection. This situation is pertinent in cases where reconstructive techniques such as glansectomy and split-skin grafting are performed. Despite technical advances that preserve shaft length and function,[12] chronic scrotal edema may lead to loss of a pendulous shaft, necessitating additional procedures (**Fig. 1**). Despite these concerns, simultaneous ILND may be indicated in

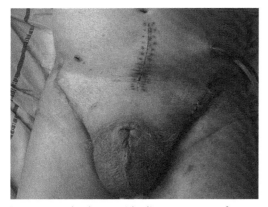

Fig. 1. Scrotal edema with disappearance of reconstructed phallus following bilateral inguinal lymph node dissection and open pelvic lymph node dissection. The patient required perineal urethrostomy.

specific cases when compliance or comorbidity is an overriding factor.

Morbidity of Lymph Node Surgery

ILND sometimes requires lengthy skin incisions, creation of skin flaps beneath Scarpa's fascia, and excision of lymphatic tissue with division of lymphatics. This procedure can have significant morbidity, and has been reviewed recently by Protzel and colleagues[13] and Spiess and colleagues.[14] The range of recorded morbidities for different approaches[11,15–27] is summarized in **Table 1**. Contemporary series show that the morbidity of ILND has decreased in recent years, with Bouchot and colleagues[25] reporting 12% overall complications. Nonetheless, many centers have higher complication rates, and this has fueled very

different strategies. The first strategy involves improving patient selection for ILND by performing dynamic sentinel node biopsy (DSNB), as described below.[28] The other strategy for reducing the morbidity of ILND uses minimally invasive laparoscopic techniques, and has been addressed by 2 pioneering groups. These laparoscopic procedures have been called video endoscopic inguinal lymphadenectomy (VEIL)[20,29] and endoscopic lymphadenectomy for penile cancer (ELPC).[21,30] This strategy has the potential to reduce skin-related morbidity substantially (see **Table 1**), although the lymphatic complications may be similar to modified or superficial dissection.

CURRENT STRATEGIES TO SELECT PATIENTS FOR PROPHYLACTIC INGUINAL STAGING/THERAPEUTIC PROCEDURES
Imaging

The clinical staging of penile cancer is inaccurate, with significant under- and overstaging of inguinal nodes. In patients with impalpable nodes who undergo prophylactic ILND, micrometastatic disease is present in about 20% to 25%, whereas between 50% and 80% of palpable inguinal nodes harbor metastases.[1,3] Radiological staging may miss micrometastatic disease. Three modalities have recently been evaluated in staging the inguinal region in patients with clinically negative nodes. Ultrasound-guided fine-needle aspiration cytology (FNAC) detected inguinal metastases in 9 of 23 (39%) patients with proven inguinal node metastases.[31] Although the sensitivity was low, the investigators used this as a staging procedure whereby patients with positive findings underwent immediate lymphadenectomy and were spared DSNB

Table 1
Range of reported morbidity

	DSNB[15–19]	VEIL/ELPC[20,21]	Superficial Modified ILND[11,21–25]	Radical ILND[11,15,25–27]
Range of patient #/series	22–92	8–10	7–118	22–234
Skin (%)	0–13	0	0–4.5	7.5–61
Infection (%)	2.6–13	0	0–14.2	7.5–14.2
DVT (%)	0	0	0	0–12.1
Seroma (%)	1.3	0	12.1–26.3	5–13.8
Edema (%)	1.1–1.7	0	3–20	14.2–22.4
Lymphocele (%)	1.7–21.7	0–23	0–30	2.5–5.2
Major (%)	0–1.3	0	0–14	5–37.5
Minor (%)	6.6–39	20–23	6.8–36.8	45–54

Data from Protzel C, Alcaraz A, Horenblas S, et al. Lymphadenectomy in the surgical management of penile cancer. Eur Urol 2009;55:1075–88.

(an estimated 11% patients were spared DSNB). Of note, FNAC has significant value among patients with palpable nodes, as Saisorn and colleagues[32] reported a sensitivity of 93% in a recent study. The initial promise regarding ^{18}F-fluorodeoxyglucose positron emission tomography/computed tomography (PET/CT) in staging the inguinal region in penile cancer[33] has been tempered by a recent report from Leijte and colleagues[34] from the Netherlands. Among 42 patients with clinically negative inguinal nodes, metastases were found in 5 but PET/CT detected only 1 of these (ie, sensitivity = 20%). Of note, size of nodal metastases missed in the study ranged from 1 to 10 mm. PET/CT did pick up metastases that ranged from 20 to 60 mm.[34] Thus its utility in detecting microscopic inguinal metastases remains unproven. PET/CT was valuable, however, in the detection of pelvic metastasis among patients with proven inguinal metastases.[35] The use of lymphotrophic nanoparticles with magnetic resonance imaging had some promise in one small study among penile cancer patients; however, as of this date this procedure remains commercially unavailable.[36]

Penile Cancer Staging Systems: Modifications to the Sixth Edition TNM Staging System

The TNM staging system is a widely accepted staging tool. However, deficiencies in the sixth

Table 2
Comparison of sixth and seventh edition TNM staging systems

Sixth Edition	Seventh Edition
T - Primary tumor	*TX* Primary tumor cannot be assessed
TX Primary tumor cannot be assessed	*T0* No evidence of primary tumor
T0 No evidence of primary tumor	*Tis* Carcinoma in situ
Tis Carcinoma in situ	*Ta* Noninvasive verrucous carcinoma (broad pushing invasion is permitted, destruction invasion is not)
Ta Noninvasive verrucous carcinoma	
T1 Tumor invades subepithelial connective tissue	*T1a* Tumor invades subepithelial connective tissue without lymphovascular invasion and is not poorly differentiated
T2 Tumor invades corpus spongiosum or cavernosum	*T1b* Tumor invades subepithelial connective tissue and either has lymphovascular invasion or is poorly differentiated
T3 Tumor invades urethra or prostate	
T4 Tumor invades other adjacent structures	*T2* Tumor invades corpus spongiosum or corpus cavernosum
	T3 Tumor invades urethra
	T4 Tumor invades other adjacent structures
N - Regional lymph nodes	*Clinical stage, based on palpation and imaging:*
NX Regional lymph nodes cannot be assessed	*cNX* Regional lymph nodes cannot be assessed
N0 No evidence of lymph node metastasis	*cN0* No palpable or visibly enlarged inguinal lymph nodes
N1 Metastasis in a single inguinal lymph node	*cN1* Palpable mobile unilateral inguinal lymph node
N2 Metastasis in multiple or bilateral superficial lymph nodes	*cN2* Palpable mobile multiple or bilateral inguinal lymph nodes
N3 Metastasis in deep inguinal or pelvic lymph nodes, unilateral or bilateral	*cN3* Palpable fixed inguinal nodal mass or pelvic lymphadenopathy, unilateral or bilateral
	Pathologic stage, based on biopsy or surgical excision:
	pNX Regional lymph nodes cannot be assessed
	pN0 No regional lymph node metastases
	pN1 Metastasis in a single superficial, inguinal lymph node
	pN2 Metastasis in multiple or bilateral superficial inguinal lymph nodes
	pN3 Metastasis in deep inguinal or pelvic lymph node(s), unilateral or bilateral
M - Distant metastases	*M0* No distant metastasis
MX Distant metastases cannot be assessed	*M1* Distant metastasis, or lymph node metastasis outside the true pelvis
M0 No evidence of distant metastases	
M1 Distant metastases	

edition TNM (**Table 2**)[37] of the American Joint Committee on Cancer (AJCC) were highlighted in a report of 513 cases treated over a 50-year interval at a single institute.[38,39] The investigators described no difference in survival between stages T2 and T3 and nodal stages N1 and N2. Based on their own data, they recommended changes in the staging system (ie, the existing sixth edition TNM) with more meaningful prognostic stratification. This modified TNM system was relevant in that the variables examined were a part of routine clinical staging, in distinction to the sixth edition TNM, which is in essence a pathologic system.[37,38]

On January 1, 2010, the seventh edition of the unified TNM staging for penile cancer became standard.[40] This edition represents consensus between representatives of the AJCC and Union Internationale Contre le Cancer (UICC). It is the first alteration in the official TNM penile cancer staging since 1987 and includes significant changes:

- T1 is subdivided into T1a and T1b, based on lymphovascular invasion (LVI) and grade. This includes the practical division of T1 into high and low risk for selecting patients for ILND, when inguinal nodes are clinically impalpable.
- Invasion of the prostate has moved from T3 to T4, with T3 denoting urethral invasion only.
- There is provision for clinical and pathologic lymph node assessment. The distinction between superficial and deep inguinal lymph nodes has been eliminated.
- In the absence of nodal or metastatic disease, the new subdivision T1b becomes Stage II, while T1a remains Stage I.
- Any lymph node–positive disease is now at least Stage III.

Clinical and pathologic staging not only determines prognosis but forms the basis of integrating multimodal therapy in the management of advanced disease. These changes aim to clarify the management of cancer, facilitate meaningful comparison between cohorts, and support multi-institutional research. Future studies should compare the prognostic value of both the seventh edition TNM[40] and that proposed by Leitje and colleagues[38] using large data sets to determine the optimal variables that best stratify patient prognosis.

Impact of Primary Tumor Histologic Features on Predicting Occult Nodal Metastasis

Patients with primary tumors exhibiting carcinoma in situ or verrucous carcinoma have little or no risk for metastasis. Only 2 cases of metastasis in association with carcinoma in situ have been reported, and none of 47 cases of penile verrucous carcinoma has been shown to metastasize.[41–43] Thus, patients with both Tis and Ta penile cancer are included in the low-risk group for inguinal metastases.[44,45]

In contrast, patients with corporal invasion (TNM stage pT2) in the penile tumor exhibit a high risk for metastasis. The average risk for inguinal metastasis among 225 patients in 7 different series was 59%.[1]

Stage T1 penile cancers exhibit involvement of the subepithelial connective tissue only and lack involvement of the corpus spongiosum, corpora cavernosa, or urethra.[37,40] Similarly staged tumors historically have been associated with a 4% to 14% incidence of nodal metastasis.[44,46,47] Theodorescu and colleagues[48] noted one exception to this relatively low rate of metastatic disease; 58% of patients (14 of 24) with pT1 primary tumors and initially negative nodes on clinical assessment subsequently developed inguinal nodal metastases. These data suggest that other variables present within the penile cancers of the cohort of patients studied (ie, tumor grade and presence of vascular invasion) may have modified the effect of tumor stage on metastasis.

Several investigators have evaluated the risk of nodal metastasis for TNM stage T1 lesions according to tumor grade.[1,44] Among 73 patients with T1, grade 1 or grade 2 primary tumors, metastasis occurred in only 5 patients (7%).[1] Recent data from Naumann and colleagues,[49] however, suggested that among stage T1 grade 2 tumors specifically, the risk of metastases could be higher than previously described. Recently, Hughes and colleagues[50] reported on a larger 2-center experience where, among 105 node-negative patients at presentation, 9 (9%) exhibited lymph node metastases at surgery or on follow-up. Thus the incidence overall was much lower in this cohort.

Ficarra and colleagues[51] developed the first penile cancer nomogram using data from 175 patients. Based on tumor thickness and growth pattern, patients with T1 grade 2 tumors exhibited metastatic rates from 5% to 20%. Thus Grade 2 tumors represent a heterogeneous group wherein the histologic criteria used to describe grade 2 and the presence or absence of other poor prognostic features ultimately determines prognosis. In this regard, the European Association of Urology Guidelines (EAU[45]) assigned patients with T1 Grade 2 tumors to the intermediate-risk category wherein the risk of lymph node metastasis is greater than 16% (low risk) and less than 68% (high risk)[45] (**Table 3**).

Table 3
Categories of risk of inguinal node involvement for cN0, according to the 2004 EAU guidelines

Group	Primary Tumor
Low risk	Tis, Ta, T1 G1
Intermediate risk	T1 G2
High risk	T1 G3, any T2 or greater

Data from Solsona E, Algaba F, Horenblas S, et al. EAU guidelines on penile cancer. Eur Urol 2004;46:1–8; and Hegarty PK, Kayes O, Freeman A, et al. A prospective study of 100 cases of penile cancer managed according to EAU guidelines. BJU Int 2006;98:526–31.

The presence of vascular invasion as a prognostic indicator of inguinal lymph node metastasis in squamous penile cancer is now evident.[6,51–54] Lopes and colleagues[6] studied the prognostic value of lymphatic invasion in 146 patients with penile cancer. In a univariate analysis, clinical nodal stage, tumor thickness, lymphatic and venous embolization, and urethral infiltration were all associated with lymph node metastasis. However, subsequent to multivariate analysis, only venous and lymphatic invasion remained significant predictors for positive lymph nodes. Data from the University of Texas M.D. Anderson Cancer Center revealed that vascular invasion was absent in all patients with T1 tumors.[53] These patients were also lymph node negative at surgery. In contrast, patients with stage pT2 primary tumors exhibited nodal metastasis in 75% of cases (15 of 20) when vascular invasion was present but in only 25% of cases (3 of 12) when it was absent.

Taking this a step further and including the variables of tumor thickness, growth pattern, grade, venous/lymphatic invasion, corpus spongiosum, or cavernosum involvement, urethral involvement, and palpable lymph nodes, Ficarra and colleagues[54] developed their nomogram predicting inguinal lymph node involvement. The most important variables were venous/lymphatic invasion and the presence of palpable nodes in multivariate analysis. The concordance index of the nomogram was very good, at 0.876. However, external validation of the nomogram is pending at this time. **Table 3** depicts variables associated with low, intermediate, and higher risks of metastasis. The International Consultation on Penile Cancer was held in Santiago, Chile in 2008. Consensus recommendations from in international panel of 38 investigators were reported (ICUD-Penile).[55] **Fig. 2** reports risk groups, metastatic rates, and management strategies from the EAU, ICUD-penile, and the literature. In general, all seem to agree that patients with clinically negative inguinal nodes in the high-risk group should have an inguinal staging procedure performed as a primary recommendation. Similarly, in the low-risk group these same patients who are felt to be compliant are offered surveillance. Among the intermediate group the

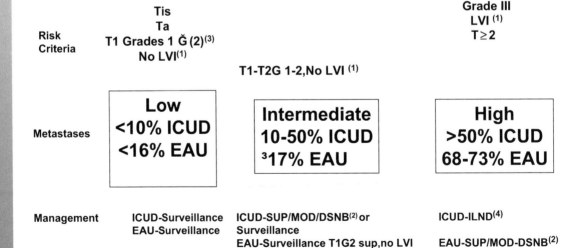

Fig. 2. Prognostic factors for inguinal lymph node metastases and recommended management strategies. Data from Refs.[1,45,50,51,54,55] (1), lymphovascular invasion; (2), superficial or modified inguinal dissection, dynamic sentinel lymph node biopsy optional in experienced centers; (3), controversy regarding whether T1 Grade 2 was in low (Refs.[1,50]) or intermediate (Ref.[49]) risk group; (4), inguinal lymph node dissection.

EAU guidelines recommend observation for those patients with T1 superficial tumors and no vascular invasion. Otherwise, with all other pathologic findings an inguinal staging procedure is recommended. The ICUD-penile panel recommended that either observation or an inguinal staging procedure is appropriate for intermediate-risk patients as long as they are informed of risks and benefits.[55]

NEW PROCEDURES TO LIMIT THE MORBIDITY OF INGUINAL STAGING: DYNAMIC SENTINEL NODE BIOPSY AND LAPAROSCOPIC INGUINAL LYMPHADENECTOMY

The concept of sentinel node was described originally in penile cancer by Cabanas in 1977.[56] Since then it has become integrated into the staging of some cancers such as breast cancer and melanoma. Despite its beginnings in penile cancer more than 30 years ago, its application in penile cancer remains highly controversial. The fundamental issue in penile cancer is that lymphadenectomy is not just for staging but has clear survival benefits. The clear advantage of DSNB strategy is the lower morbidity (see **Table 1**), with an overall complication rate of between 6% and 10% per groin in the most experienced hands.[17] Virtually all the complications associated with DSNB are minor. However, this is at the cost of a false-negative rate. Reported false-negative rates of up to 18% to 25% have previously been reported.[57,58] Innovations such as using DSNB with ultrasound-guided fine-needle aspiration have reduced the false-negative rate to 7%[59] in 2 European centers. While these results are impressive, the occurrence of a false negative is very serious and difficult to salvage. The subsequent development of nodal metastasis proved fatal in 4 of the 6 patients who had an initial negative DSNB.[60] For patients with palpable lymph nodes, DSNB is not appropriate.[61] Based on both the European Association of Urology (EAU) and the International Consultation on Penile Cancer, DSNB is an acceptable staging procedure in the hands of experienced centers where the false-negative rates are the lowest (ie, <10%).[45,55] It is, however, imperative that patients be made aware of the importance of regular follow-up and self-examination due to the possibility of false-negative findings. In all other circumstances a superficial or modified inguinal dissection should be standard.[57,62] Thus, an adequate balance between superior oncological control by superficial or modified ILND with inherently higher morbidity versus the less morbid DSNB with nonnegligible false-negative outcomes is desired. It may be that the minimally invasive laparoscopic strategies provide this balance in the future (VEIL,[20,29] ELPC[21,30]).

The laparoscopic approach to the inguinal region offers the potential for removing all the inguinal lymph nodes at risk for disease while minimizing complications. The technical details of the contemporary procedure and early results have been described by 2 groups from South America.[20,21,29,30] To date, among highly selected small series of patients the numbers of inguinal lymph nodes removed have been comparable to open series (median = 9–11 per groin). Only a single recurrence has been reported, with a 12- to 33-month follow-up, and minor complications have occurred in about 20% of patients.[14,30] Thus this approach, while promising, will require further validation with larger patient numbers and longer follow-up.

TRADITIONAL INGUINAL AND ILIOINGUINAL LYMPHADENECTOMY: ADDITIONAL CONSIDERATIONS

Should inguinal lymphadenectomy be bilateral rather than unilateral for patients presenting with unilateral adenopathy at initial presentation of the primary tumor? The answer to this question is yes. The anatomic crossover of penile lymphatics is well established, and bilateral drainage is the rule and has been proven using intraoperative lymphatic mapping studies.[28,57] The contralateral node dissection may be limited to the area superficial to the fascia lata if no histologic evidence of positive superficial nodes is found at surgery by frozen-section analysis.

Should bilateral inguinal lymphadenectomy be performed in patients who present with unilateral lymphadenopathy some time after the initial presentation and treatment of the primary tumor? It is generally believed that bilateral node dissection in this setting is not necessary. The recommendation of unilateral rather than bilateral node dissection with delayed presentation of unilateral lymphadenopathy is supported by the elapsed disease-free interval of observation on the normal side. If one assumes that nodal metastases will enlarge at the same rate, the clinical palpation of nodal metastases, if present in both groins, should appear at approximately the same time. The absence of clinical adenopathy on one side despite prolonged observation suggests freedom from disease on that side.[63] However, Horenblas and colleagues[64] noted that in patients with 2 or more unilateral metastases, contralateral occult metastases were noted in 30% of cases. Thus, in patients with a bulky unilateral recurrence, a contralateral inguinal staging procedure should be considered.

Should pelvic lymphadenectomy be performed in all patients with inguinal metastases considering its potential for added morbidity and relatively low therapeutic value? This issue remains controversial. Patients with inguinal nodal metastases are at increased risk for spread to the pelvic nodes.[65,66] However, Horenblas and colleagues[64] showed that among patients with a single inguinal lymph node involved without extracapsular extension, the incidence of pelvic metastases was rare, and recommended avoiding pelvic dissection among such patients. Zhu and colleagues[67] found that the sensitivity of CT scanning for pelvic lymph node metastasis was only 37.5%. Defining the status of Cloquet's node in predicting a positive pelvic node was only about 30% sensitive as well. Important predictors were the number of positive nodes as well as lymph node size. Two contemporary studies addressing this issue have found an incidence of 0% to 12% of pelvic lymph node metastasis when patients exhibited only 1 to 2 positive inguinal nodes, especially when extracapsular extension was absent and/or size was less than 3.5 cm. Additional factors noted in these studies included the grade of the nodal metastasis and its p53 status.[5,67] Thus, patients with only a single small lymph node metastasis discovered at the time of an inguinal dissection (ie, no extracapsular extension, not high grade) may be at very low risk for pelvic metastasis and are potentially the optimal candidates in whom pelvic lymphadenectomy could be avoided.

With respect to efficacy, the average 5-year survival for patients with positive pelvic nodes averages around 15%.[1] Although unproved, it is conceivable that patients with minimal inguinal disease who exhibit focal involvement of a pelvic node could benefit from pelvic dissection. In the series reported by Lopes and coworkers[68] among 13 patients with pathologically proven lymph nodes, 5 of 13 (38%) were alive without disease with follow-up for more than 90 months. This series is unique in that 4 of 5 survivors exhibited only a single iliac nodal metastasis and one inguinal lymph node metastasis; in fact, one patient with iliac metastases had no inguinal disease. This series is clearly the exception, but reveals that selected patients with minimal inguinal and pelvic disease may be cured with surgery alone.[68]

Thus, in patients undergoing inguinal lymphadenectomy for curative intent (ie, in whom preoperative studies reveal no pelvic adenopathy), pelvic lymphadenectomy should be considered in most patients with positive nodes because it can serve as an effective staging tool for identifying those patients who should receive adjuvant combination chemotherapy or radiation.[5,69] It also adds to local-regional control and provides little additional morbidity to the simultaneous inguinal procedure being performed. Alternatively, if pelvic nodal metastases are proven before lymphadenectomy, consideration should be given to neoadjuvant chemotherapeutic strategies followed by surgery in those patients who respond.[69–71]

INTEGRATION OF THERAPY TO IMPROVE SURVIVAL
Chemotherapy

Although overall cancer-specific survival rates of over 80% to 90% in early-stage penile cancer have been reported with surgery alone, higher-stage disease (ie, bilateral inguinal metastases, extranodal extension, pelvic nodal metastases) requires additional treatment to achieve potential cure. Three contemporary series have shown that selected patients can benefit from induction chemotherapy. Corral and colleagues[70] reported on the long-term follow-up of a prospective group of patients treated with bleomycin, methotrexate, and cisplatin. Objective responses were noted in 12 (57%) including 2 of 5 with distant metastases. Six patients in the group (28.5%) achieved disease-free status with either CT alone (2) or surgery (3) or RT (1) with a median survival of 27.8 months. This period was significantly longer than that of those not achieving disease-free status (6.7 months, $P = .004$). Thus, this prospective study showed that a multidisciplinary approach to achieve disease-free status could prolong survival.

Subsequently, Leijte and colleagues[18] from the Netherlands Cancer Institute reviewed their experience with neoadjuvant CT in patients with initially unresectable penile cancer. The series included 20 patients treated with 5 different regimens, including (1) single-agent bleomycin; (2) bleomycin, vincristine, methotrexate; (3) cisplatin, 5-fluorouracil; (4) bleomycin, cisplatin, methotrexate; and (5) cisplatin, irinotecan. The objective responses were evaluable in 19 (one patient died due to bleomycin toxicity after 2 weeks) with 12 responses (63%; 2 complete, 10 partial). Among 12 responders only 9 went to surgery, as 2 died of bleomycin-related complications while the third was deemed unfit for surgery. Eight of 9 responding patients taken to surgery (2 were pT0) were free of disease at their last assessment, with a median follow-up of 20 months. This result is in contrast to 3 nonresponders who went to surgery for palliative intent. All 3 died within 4 to 8 months due to locoregional recurrence. The implications from this study indicate that response to CT together with an aggressive surgical procedure provides the optimal scenario for significant palliation or potential cure.

In a separate study, Bermejo and colleagues[71] described the surgical considerations and complications among 10 patients who had either a response or stable disease after combination CT followed by surgery. The regimens used included (1) bleomycin, methotrexate, cisplatin; (2) paclitaxel, ifosfamide, cisplatin (TIP); or (3) paclitaxel, carboplatin. This cohort of patients exhibited bulky inguinal or pelvic metastases, with the only exclusions being patients with fixed pelvic masses or complete encasement of the femoral vessels. Among 5 patients exhibiting an objective response, 3 were alive and disease-free at 48, 50, and 73 months. Two other patients died (one of disease at 30 months, another of unknown causes at 21 months). Among the 5 remaining patients with stable disease, 3 were dead of disease within 7 months while 1 patient treated with bleomycin died of "failure to thrive" at 8 months. However, another patient treated with paclitaxel and carboplatin achieving only stable disease was alive and disease-free at 84 months. These data appear to reinforce the concept that response to systemic CT before surgery enhances the chance for long-term survival among those undergoing surgical resection. Regarding systemic therapy, the investigators reported that the TIP regimen was well tolerated and all 3 pT0 responses at surgery were among patients treated with TIP. This result provided the rationale for the prospective phase 2 study of 30 patients (registered on the National Institute of Health clincaltrials.gov Web site as NCT00512096). This cohort has completed therapy with final results pending. Preliminary analysis of data of the first 20 patients describes an objective response rate of 55% and a pathologic complete response in 10% (2 patients).[72]

In the United Kingdom, a multicenter non-randomized trial has been opened examining the role of neoadjuvant docetaxel, cisplatin, and 5-fluorouracil (TPF) chemotherapy in patients with locally advanced or metastatic penile cancer. Primary outcome is to assess the efficacy of the regimen. The secondary outcomes are to assess the number of cases rendered operable by chemotherapy, to evaluate safety and tolerability of the regime, and to report outcomes in terms of disease-free and overall survival.

Palliative Surgical Procedures

There are other benefits to regional oncological control. Untreated inguinal nodes may develop foul-smelling and painful ulcers. These nodes may also erode into the adjacent vessels and lead to catastrophic hemorrhage. Therefore control of the regional nodes has quality of life issues. Advanced cases may require vascular replacement. A series of 5 patients with metastatic inguinal nodes involving the femoral artery underwent extra-anatomic transobturator bypass with either Dacron graft or autologous saphenous vein graft.[73] In this series all 5 cases had good pulses following the procedure. Four of the 5 patients died between 8 and 20 months following surgery, due to pulmonary metastases in 3 and an acute myocardial infarction in 1. The fifth case was alive at 8 months follow-up, undergoing palliative adjuvant chemotherapy. Thus no case had prosthetic or hemorrhagic complications, with patients eventually succumbing to distant disease. Other options include use of an endovascular stent[74] or ligation of the femoral artery with major excisions such as hemipelvectomy or hind quarter/lower extremity amputation.[75] Locally advanced cases may require plastic surgical techniques to achieve coverage. A well-vascularized pedicled graft hastens healing and can allow adjuvant radiotherapy if necessary.[76] The steps in the mobilization and placement of a vertical rectus abdominis myocutaneous (VRAM) flap are shown in **Fig. 3**.

Radiotherapy

The literature is particularly sparse in the area of radiotherapy as a treatment modality for advanced penile cancer. One of the largest series demonstrating a benefit of radiotherapy for lymph node metastases and/or distant metastases from penile cancer was published by Ravi and associates in 1994.[77] Pertinent to the advanced disease presentation setting, 33 patients were treated with preoperative radiotherapy at 40 Gy over 4 weeks and subsequently had inguinal lymphadenectomy. Of note, after radiotherapy and surgery only 8% had evidence of extranodal extension (ENE) and 3% recurred within the groin. This result is relevant, as in a prior report within a contemporary time frame the incidence of ENE was 33% among patients treated with surgery alone and groin recurrence was noted in 19%. The difference for both ENE and local recurrence were statistically lower ($P = .01$ and .03, respectively). The data are strongly suggestive but not definitive that preoperative radiotherapy for nodes 4 cm or larger without skin fixation improved local control. The 5-year survival among the latter group was 70%.

FORMULATION OF FOLLOW-UP STRATEGY

The object of follow-up is to detect recurrence at an earlier and hopefully more treatable stage. A recent article from 2 European centers describes

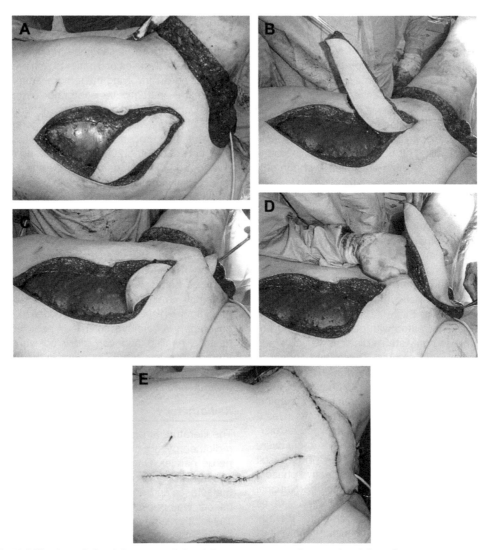

Fig. 3. Mobilization of the right rectus abdominis myocutaneous flap on the right inferior epigastric artery to achieve coverage following extirpation of locoregionally advanced penile cancer. (*A*) Right rectus muscle and overlying skin is delineated, with posterior sheath intact. (*B*) Mobile flap on inferior blood supply. (*C*) Flap is passed posterior to skin bridge. (*D*) Superior portion is applied laterally. (*E*) Flap is sutured in place and the donor site closed primarily.

the recurrence pattern of 700 patients treated between 1956 and 2007.[78] These centers have excellent, albeit retrospective, follow-up data with follow-up of up to 30 years in some patients, providing several interesting results. First, all distant recurrences occurred within 16 months and were universally fatal. All regional recurrences occurred within 50 months of treatment of the primary and all 87% of local recurrences happened within 5 years. Thus, recurrences after 5 years were all local. A local recurrence rate (LRR) of 18.6% was noted and driven by penile-preserving procedures (LRR = 27% vs amputation LRR = 5.3%). Of concern was that those who were staged as pN0 on ILND had a 2% regional recurrence, as compared with a 2.8% regional recurrence for those staged as N0 on DSNB. Theoretically if all first-echelon nodes are removed and negative, one would expect virtually no regional recurrences as noted by Spiess and colleagues[57] following DSNB and completion superficial dissection. The investigators also noted that three-fourths of all recurrences (local, regional, and distant) occurred in the first 2 years. Based on these retrospective data, they recommend increased follow-up during the initial 2 years using the following protocol.

Table 4
Penile cancer follow-up recommendations

	Monthly Interval			
	Year 1–2	Year 3	Year 4	Year 5
Low-risk primary lesion: G1–2, Tis, Ta, T1, no vascular invasion	3	4	6	12
High-risk primary lesion: G3, T2–3, vascular invasion	2	3	6	12
Pathologically N0	4	6	12	12
Pathologically node positive	3[a]	4[a]	6[a]	12[a]

[a] Includes: Ultrasound with fine-needle aspiration cytology (US-FNAC), computed tomography (CT), chest radiograph (CXR).
Data from Heyns C, Fleshner N, Sangar V, et al. Management of the lymph nodes in penile cancer. In: Pompeo ACL, Heyns CF, Abrams P, editors. International consultation on penile cancer. Montreal: Societe Internationale d'Urologie; 2009. p. 161.

Surveillance cases, penile preservation, and pN+: every 3 months for 2 years, 6 monthly for years 3 to 5. For pN0 cases: every 6 months for 2 years; annually for years 3 to 5. Discharge from follow-up after 5 years. Based on the 13% of local recurrences beyond 5 years the authors would differ slightly in recommending yearly follow-up as well as patient self-examination. An alternative follow-up strategy was recently recommended by the International Consultation on Urologic Diseases Penile Cancer Subcommittee, and is included in **Table 4**.[55]

FUTURE CHALLENGES

The surgical management of the inguinal region in penile cancer remains controversial in earlier-stage disease where increasing cure rates must be accompanied by decreasing morbidity. Lymphadenectomy has probably reached a plateau as a monotherapeutic option in the setting of advanced disease. The optimal integration of surgery with other therapies such as chemotherapy and radiotherapy along with our evolving knowledge of molecular pathways (ie, human papillomavirus, receptor tyrosine kinase pathways) in penile cancer carcinogenesis and progression are the next frontier to be conquered.[79–81] A case can certainly be made for referral of penile cancer patients to cancer centers with expertise in these strategies, so as to support innovation. This development is nicely illustrated currently in the United Kingdom, where super-regional centers exist that serve a population of 4 million each and see a minimum of 25 cases per year.[82] Collaboration between such centers could significantly benefit expansion of knowledge, basic research, and treatment paradigms.

SUMMARY

Lymphadenectomy has clear survival benefits for patients when applied to those at risk for and with lymph node metastasis. However, the current morbidity of the standard technique of lymphadenectomy is an impediment to its universal application, and innovative strategies to reduce the morbidity of staging/treatment that do not compromise oncologic control must be developed and standardized. The optimal integration of multimodality therapy to improve survival in advanced disease will only occur through collaborative studies between centers with significant patient volume. A plea is made for the development of regional referral centers to accomplish this objective.

REFERENCES

1. Pettaway C, Lynch D, Davis J. Tumors of the penis. In: Wein AJ, Kavoussi LR, Novick AC, et al, editors. Campbell-Walsh urology. 9th edition. St Louis (MO): WB Saunders; 2007. p. 959–92, Chapter 31.
2. Ornellas AA, Kinchin EW, Nobrega BL, et al. Surgical treatment of invasive squamous cell carcinoma of the penis: Brazilian National Cancer Institute long-term experience. J Surg Oncol 2008;97: 487–95.
3. Hegarty PK, Kayes O, Freeman A, et al. A prospective study of 100 cases of penile cancer managed according to EAU guidelines. BJU Int 2006;98: 526–31.

4. Pandey D, Mahajan V, Kannan RR. Prognostic factors in node-positive carcinoma of the penis. J Surg Oncol 2006;93(2):133–8.

5. Lont AP, Kroon BK, Gallee MP, et al. Pelvic node dissection for penile carcinoma: extent of inguinal lymph node involvement as an indicator for pelvic lymph node involvement and survival. J Urol 2007; 177:947–52 [discussion: 952].

6. Lopes A, Hidalgo GS, Kowalski LP, et al. Prognostic factors in carcinoma of the penis: multivariate analysis of 145 patients treated with amputation and lymphadenectomy. J Urol 1995;156:1637–42.

7. Svatek RS, Munsell M, Kincaid JM, et al. Association between lymph node density and disease specific survival in patients with penile cancer. J Urol 2009; 182:2721–7.

8. McDougal WS. Carcinoma of penis: improved survival by early lymphadenectomy based on histological grade and depth of invasion of primary lesion. J Urol 1995;154:1364–6.

9. Gulia AK, Mandhani A, Muruganandham K, et al. Impact of delay in inguinal lymph node dissection in patients with carcinoma of penis. Indian J Cancer 2009;46:214–8.

10. Kroon BK, Horenblas S, Lont AP, et al. Patients with penile carcinoma benefit from immediate resection of clinically occult lymph node metastases. J Urol 2005;173:816–9.

11. Bevan-Thomas R, Slaton JW, Pettaway CA. Contemporary morbidity from lymphadenectomy for penile squamous cell carcinoma: the M.D. Anderson Cancer Center Experience. J Urol 2002;167:1638–42.

12. Hegarty PK, Shabbir M, Hughes B, et al. Penile preserving surgery and surgical strategies to maximize penile form and function in penile cancer: recommendations from the United Kingdom experience. World J Urol 2009;27:179–87.

13. Protzel C, Alcaraz A, Horenblas S, et al. Lymphadenectomy in the surgical management of penile cancer. Eur Urol 2009;55:1075–88.

14. Spiess PE, Hernandez MS, Pettaway CA. Contemporary inguinal lymph node dissection: minimizing complications. World J Urol 2009;27(2):205–12.

15. Perdona S, Autorino R, De Sio M, et al. Dynamic sentinel node biopsy in clinically node-negative penile cancer versus radical inguinal lymphadenectomy: a comparative study. Urology 2005;66: 1282–6.

16. Hadway P, Smith Y, Corbishley C, et al. Evaluation of dynamic lymphoscintigraphy and sentinel lymph-node biopsy for detecting occult metastases in patients with penile squamous cell carcinoma. BJU Int 2007;100:561–5.

17. Leijte JAP, Kroon BK, Valdes Olmos RA, et al. Reliability and safety of current dynamic sentinel node biopsy for penile carcinoma. Eur Urol 2007;52: 170–7.

18. Leijte JAP, Kerst JM, Bais E, et al. Neoadjuvant chemotherapy in advanced penile carcinoma. Eur Urol 2007;52:488–94.

19. Heyns CF, Theron PD. Evaluation of dynamic sentinel lymph node biopsy in patients with squamous cell carcinoma of the penis and palpable inguinal nodes. BJU Int 2008;102:305–9.

20. Tobias-Machado M, Tavares A, Silva MN, et al. Can video endoscopic inguinal lymphadenectomy achieve a lower morbidity than open lymph node dissection in penile cancer patients? J Endourol 2008;22:1687–91.

21. Sotelo R, Sánchez-Salas R, Carmona O, et al. Endoscopic lymphadenectomy for penile carcinoma. J Endourol 2007;21:364–7.

22. d'Ancona CA, de Lucena RG, Querne FA, et al. Long-term follow up of penile carcinoma treated with penectomy and bilateral modified inguinal lymphadenectomy. J Urol 2004;172:498–501 [discussion: 501].

23. Jacobellis U. Modified radical inguinal lymphadenectomy for carcinoma of the penis: technique and results. J Urol 2003;169:1349–52.

24. Milathianakis C, Bogdanos J, Karamanolakis D. Morbidity of prophylactic inguinal lymphadenectomy with saphenous vein preservation for squamous cell penile carcinoma. Int J Urol 2005;12: 776–8.

25. Bouchot O, Rigaud J, Maillet F, et al. Morbidity of inguinal lymphadenectomy for invasive penile carcinoma. Eur Urol 2004;45:761–6 [discussion: 765–6].

26. Ravi R. Morbidity following groin dissection for penile carcinoma. BJU Int 1993;72:941–5.

27. Nelson BA, Cookson MS, Smith JA Jr, et al. Complications of inguinal and pelvic lymphadenectomy for squamous cell carcinoma of the penis: a contemporary series. J Urol 2004;172:494–7.

28. Horenblas S, Jansen L, Meinhardt W, et al. Detection of occult metastasis in squamous cell carcinoma of the penis using a dynamic sentinel node procedure. J Urol 2000;163:100–4.

29. Tobias-Machado M, Tavares A, Ornellas AA, et al. Video endoscopic inguinal lymphadenectomy: a new minimally invasive procedure for radical management of inguinal nodes in patients with penile squamous cell carcinoma. J Urol 2007;177: 953–7.

30. Sotelo R, Sanchez-Salas R, Clavijo R. Endoscopic inguinal lymph node dissection for penile carcinoma: the development of a novel technique. World J Urol 2009;27:213–9.

31. Kroon BK, Horenblas S, Deurloo EE, et al. Ultrasonography-guided fine-needle aspiration cytology before sentinel node biopsy in patients with penile carcinoma. BJU Int 2005;95(4):517–21.

32. Saisorn I, Lawrentschuk N, Leewansangtong S, et al. Fine-needle aspiration cytology predicts

inguinal lymph node metastasis without antibiotic pretreatment in penile carcinoma. BJU Int 2006; 97(6):1225–8.

33. Scher B, Seitz M, Reiser M, et al. 18F-FDG PET/CT for staging of penile cancer. J Nucl Med 2005; 46(9):1460–5.

34. Leijte JA, Graafland NM, Valdes Olmos RA, et al. Prospective evaluation of hybrid 18F-fluorodeoxyglucose positron emission tomography/computed tomography in staging clinically node-negative patients with penile carcinoma. BJU Int 2009; 104(5):640–4.

35. Graafland NM, Leijte JAP, Valdes Olmos RA, et al. Scanning with 18F-FDG-PET/CT for detection of pelvic nodal involvement in inguinal node-positive penile carcinoma. Eur Urol 2009;56:339–45.

36. Tabatabaei S, Harisinghani M, McDougal WS. Regional lymph node staging using lymphotropic nanoparticle enhanced magnetic resonance imaging with ferumoxtran-10 in patients with penile cancer. J Urol 2005;174:923–7 [discussion: 927].

37. Greene FL, Compton CC, Fritz AG, et al. In penis. American Joint Committee on Cancer: staging atlas. New York: Springer; 2006. p. 287–92.

38. Leijte JA, Gallee M, Antonini N, et al. Evaluation of current TNM classification of penile carcinoma. J Urol 2008;180:933–8 [discussion: 938].

39. Leitje JA, Horenblas S. Shortcomings of the current TNM classification for penile carcinoma: time for a change? World J Urol 2009;27:151–4.

40. Edge SB, Byrd DR, Compton CC, et al. AJCC cancer staging manual. 7th edition. New York: Springer; 2009. p. 447–56.

41. Eng TY, Petersen JP, Stack RS, et al. Lymph node metastasis from carcinoma in situ of the penis: a case report. J Urol 1995;153:432–4.

42. Johnson DE, Lo RK, Srigley J, et al. Verrucous carcinoma of the penis. J Urol 1985;133:216–8.

43. Seixas ALC, Ornellas AA, Marota A, et al. Verrucous carcinoma of the penis: retrospective analysis of 32 cases. J Urol 1994;152:1476–9.

44. Solsona E, Iborra I, Ricos JV, et al. Corpus cavernosum invasion and tumor grade in the prediction of lymph node condition in penile carcinoma. Eur Urol 1992;22:115–8.

45. Solsona E, Algaba F, Horenblas S, et al. EAU guidelines on penile cancer. Eur Urol 2004;46:1–8.

46. Villavicencio H, Rubio-Briones J, Regalado R, et al. Grade, local stage and growth pattern as prognostic factors in carcinoma of the penis. Eur Urol 1997;32: 442–7.

47. Hall MC, Sanders JS, Vuitch F, et al. Deoxyribonucleic acid flow cytometry and traditional pathologic variables in invasive penile carcinoma: assessment of prognostic significance. Urology 1998;52:111–6.

48. Theodorescu D, Russo P, Zhang ZF, et al. Outcomes of initial surveillance of invasive squamous cell carcinoma of the penis and negative nodes. J Urol 1996;155:1626–31.

49. Naumann CM, Alkatout I, Al-Najar A, et al. Lymph node metastasis in intermediate-risk squamous cell carcinoma of the penis. BJU Int 2008;102:1102–6.

50. Hughes BE, Leijte JAP, Kroon B, et al. Lymph node metastasis in intermediate-risk penile squamous cell cancer: a two-centre experience. Eur Urol 2010; 57:688–92.

51. Ficarra V, Zattoni F, Cunico SC, et al. Lymphatic and vascular embolizations are independent predictive variables of inguinal lymph node involvement in patients with squamous cell carcinoma of the penis. Gruppo Uro-Oncologico del Nord Est (Northeast Uro-Oncological Group) Penile Cancer data base. Cancer 2005;103:2507–16.

52. Cubilla AL. The role of pathologic prognostic factors in squamous cell carcinoma of the penis. World J Urol 2009;27:169–77.

53. Slaton JW, Morgenstern N, Levy DA, et al. Tumor stage, vascular invasion and the percentage of poorly differentiated cancer: independent prognosticators for inguinal lymph node metastasis in penile squamous cancer. J Urol 2001;165:1138–42.

54. Ficarra V, Zattoni F, Artibani W, et al. Nomogram predictive of pathological inguinal lymph node involvement in patients with squamous cell carcinoma of the penis. J Urol 2006;175:1700–4 [discussion: 1704–5].

55. Heyns C, Fleshner N, Sangar V, et al. Management of the lymph nodes in penile cancer. In: Pompeo ACL, Heyns CF, Abrams P, editors. International Consultation on Penile Cancer. Montreal: Societe Internationale d'Urologie; 2009. p. 161.

56. Cabanas RM. An approach for the treatment of penile carcinoma. Cancer 1977;39:456–66.

57. Spiess PE, Izawa JI, Bassett R, et al. Preoperative lymphoscintigraphy and dynamic sentinel node biopsy for staging penile cancer: results with pathological correlation. J Urol 2007;177(6):2157–61.

58. Kroon BK, Horenblas S, Estourgie SH, et al. How to avoid false-negative dynamic sentinel node procedures in penile carcinoma. J Urol 2004;171(6 Pt 1): 2191–4.

59. Leijte JA, Hughes B, Graafland NM, et al. Two-center evaluation of dynamic sentinel node biopsy for squamous cell carcinoma of the penis. J Clin Oncol 2009;27:3325–9.

60. Kroon BK, Horenblas S, Meinhardt W, et al. Dynamic sentinel node biopsy in penile cancer: evaluation of 10 years experience. Eur Urol 2005;47:601–6.

61. Hungerhuber E, Schlenker B, Frimberger D, et al. Lymphoscintigraphy in penile cancer: limited value of sentinel node biopsy in patients with clinically suspicious lymph nodes. World J Urol 2006;24:319–24.

62. Colberg JW, Andriole GL, Catalona WJ. Long-term follow-up of men undergoing modified inguinal

lymphadenectomy for carcinoma of the penis. Br J Urol 1997;79:54–7.

63. Ekstrom T, Edsmyr F. Cancer of the penis: a clinical study of 229 cases. Acta Chir Scand 1958;115: 25–45.

64. Horenblas S, van Tinteren H, Delemarre JF, et al. Squamous cell carcinoma of the penis. III. Treatment of regional lymph nodes. J Urol 1993;149: 492–7.

65. Ravi R. Correlation between the extent of nodal involvement and survival following groin dissection for carcinoma of the penis. Br J Urol 1993;72: 817–9.

66. Srinivas V, Morse MJ, Herr HW, et al. Penile cancer: relation of extent of nodal metastasis to survival. J Urol 1987;137:880–2.

67. Zhu Y, Zhang SH, Ye DW, et al. Predicting pelvic lymph node metastasis in penile cancer patients: a comparison of computed tomography, Cloquets's node, and disease burden of the inguinal lymph nodes. Onkologie 2008;31:37–41.

68. Lopes A, Bezerra AL, Serrano SV, et al. Iliac nodal metastases from carcinoma of the penis treated surgically. BJU Int 2000;86:690–3.

69. Pizzocaro G, Piva L, Bandieramonte G, et al. Up-to-date management of carcinoma of the penis. Eur Urol 1997;32:5–15.

70. Corral DA, Sella A, Pettaway CA, et al. Combination chemotherapy for metastatic or locally advanced genitourinary squamous cell carcinoma: a phase II study of methotrexate, cisplatin and bleomycin. J Urol 1998;160(5):1770–4.

71. Bermejo C, Busby JE, Spiess PE, et al. Neoadjuvant chemotherapy followed by aggressive surgical consolidation for metastatic penile squamous cell carcinoma. J Urol 2007;177:1335–8.

72. Pagliaro L, Williams D, Daliani D, et al. Neoadjuvant paclitaxel, ifosfamide, and cisplatin chemotherapy prior to inguinal/pelvic lymphadenectomy for stage Tany, N2-3, M0 squamous carcinoma of the penis [abstract #602]. J Urol 2006;175:195.

73. Ferreira U, Reis LO, Ikari LY, et al. Extra-anatomical transobturator bypass graft for femoral artery involvement by metastatic carcinoma of the penis: report of five patients. World J Urol 2008;26:487–91.

74. Link RE, Soltes GD, Coburn M. Treatment of acute inguinal hemorrhage from metastatic penile carcinoma using an endovascular stent graft. J Urol 2004;172:1878–9.

75. Block NL, Rosen P, Whitmore WF Jr. Hemipelvectomy for advanced penile cancer. J Urol 1973; 110(6):703–7.

76. Kayes OJ, Durrant CA, Ralph D, et al. Vertical rectus abdominis flap reconstruction in patients with advanced penile squamous cell carcinoma. BJU Int 2007;99:37–40.

77. Ravi R, Chaturvedi HK, Sastry DV. Role of radiation therapy in the treatment of carcinoma of the penis. BJU Int 1993;74:646–51.

78. Leijte JAP, Kirrander P, Antonini N, et al. Recurrence patterns of squamous cell carcinoma of the penis: recommendations for follow-up based on a two-centre analysis of 700 patients. Eur Urol 2008;54: 161–9.

79. Krustrup D, Jensen HL, van der Brule AJ, et al. Histological characteristics of human papillomavirus-positive and -negative invasive and in situ squamous cell tumours of the penis. Int J Exp Pathol 2009;90:182–9.

80. Muneer A, Kayes O, Ahmed HU, et al. Molecular prognostic factors in penile cancer. World J Urol 2009;27:161–7.

81. Pagliaro LC, Osai W, Tamboli P, et al. Epidermal growth factor receptor expression in and targeted therapy for metastatic squamous cell carcinoma of the penis [meeting abstracts]. J Clin Oncol 2007; 25:14045.

82. National Institute for Clinical Excellence. Guidance on cancer services. Improving outcomes in urological cancers - the manual. London: NICE; 2002. p. 83–5. Available at: http://www.nice.org.uk/nicemedia/live/10889/28771/28771.pdf. Accessed June 2, 2010.

Radiation Therapy for Cancer of the Penis

Juanita Crook, MD, FRCPC

KEYWORDS
- Penile cancer • Penile conservation • Radiation therapy
- Brachytherapy • Advanced penile cancer

Carcinoma of the penis is relatively rare but the incidence shows wide geographic variation. It occurs in about 1 per 100,000 men in North America and Western Europe where it represents less than 1% of cancers in men, but has an incidence as high as 10 to 20 per 100,000 men in parts of Asia, Africa, and South America.[1] Socioeconomic and cultural factors play a role in this disparity. As a rare tumor, most published reports span several decades and often represent experience from a single center, during which time staging systems and management policies have evolved. Apart from the investigation of systemic agents for advanced disease, randomized trials are essentially nonexistent.

Primary surgical management is effective in localized disease but traditional extirpative surgery often results in profound psychosexual consequences.[2,3] Radiotherapeutic approaches and newer surgical techniques strive to conserve penile function and morphology. Whenever possible, management should be centralized to tertiary referral centers with collective expertise, including expert pathologists, urologists, and radiation and medical oncologists, to deliver a cooperative multidisciplinary approach from the outset. Such an approach should include psychosocial support and counseling. Sexual consequences of treatment should be discussed with the patient and his partner during the decision-making phase.

CAUSE

Incidence increases with increasing age, being most common in the sixth decade, but earlier where the incidence is higher. Human papillomavirus types (HPV) 16 and 18 are most frequently associated with invasive squamous cell carcinomas. Amplification of DNA by polymerase chain reaction (PCR) can demonstrate viral DNA in about 40% to 45% of tumors, especially those of the basaloid variety but less frequently in squamous or verrucous types.[4] Premalignant conditions including bowenoid papulosis, Bowen disease, and erythroplasia of Queryat show a high incidence of HPV positivity in penile intraepithelial neoplasia, whereas lichen sclerosis is associated with non-HPV variants.[5] The presence of HPV does not confer a worse prognosis whereas p53 positivity, detected in 41% to 75% of invasive cancers, is associated in multivariate analysis with the presence of lymph node metastases.[6,7]

Circumcision is protective when performed in infancy and is associated with a 3-fold decrease in the risk of penile carcinoma. However, circumcision is not 100% protective and subsequent infection with genital condylomas in adulthood (overall 3–5 times increased risk), presumably in conjunction with oncogenic HPV strains, has been reported to be associated with subsequent development of squamous carcinoma[8] in circumcised men. Lack of circumcision is believed to play a role through association with poor hygiene and chronic infection, with phimosis being a factor in as many as 50% of cases in some series.[9] However, infant circumcision is no longer recommended on these grounds alone; rather the emphasis is on education, hygiene, and correction of phimosis.[10]

Smoking is an additional causal factor that may play a role as a promoter in conjunction with other oncogenic factors.[9]

Conflict of interest statement: There are no conflicts of interest in the preparation of this manuscript.
British Columbia Cancer Agency, Cancer Center for the Southern Interior, Department of Radiation Oncology, 399 Royal Avenue, Kelowna, British Columbia V1Y 5L3, Canada
E-mail address: jcrook@bccancer.bc.ca

Urol Clin N Am 37 (2010) 435–443
doi:10.1016/j.ucl.2010.04.004

STAGING

Staging systems have evolved in recent decades. The 3 commonly encountered systems, Jackson,[11] TNM 1978,[12] and TNM 1987[13] are shown in **Box 1**. The Jackson system is purely anatomically based with stage 1 tumors limited to the prepuce and glans, stage 2 involving the shaft, and stage 3 confined to the shaft but with malignant operable nodes. Although somewhat simplistic, this system is practical and clinically useful as decisions on management are often made on this basis. In contrast, TNM 1978 was based on tumor size, distinguishing T stages by less than 2 cm, 2 to 5 cm, and greater than 5 cm.

Box 1
Staging systems for carcinoma of the penis

Jackson Classification[11]

Primary tumor:

1. Limited to the glans or prepuce
2. Extending into the shaft or corpora but without nodal involvement
3. Confined to the shaft but with malignant lymph nodes considered operable
4. Invading beyond the shaft, with inoperable lymph nodes or distant metastases

TNM Staging UICC 1978[12]

Tis: Carcinoma in situ

T1: ≤2 cm

T2: >2 cm and ≤5 cm

T3: >5 cm or deep invasion including urethra

T4: Invades adjacent structures

Positive inguinal lymph nodes

N1: Unilateral

N2: Bilateral

N3: Fixed

TNM Staging UICC 1987–2009[13]

Tis: Carcinoma in situ

Invasive tumor involving:

T1: Subepithelial connective tissue

T2: Corpus spongiosum or cavernosum

T3: Urethra/prostate

T4: Other adjacent structures

Positive lymph nodes

N1 1 superficial inguinal

N2 Multiple/bilateral superficial inguinal

N3 Deep inguinal or pelvic

Again this system had clinical usefulness because tumor size influences the choice of treatment approach and suitability for penile conservation. The current TNM system has not changed in the past 2 decades and is based on final surgical pathology, distinguishing T1 from T2 by depth of invasion into the erectile tissue. This information, unfortunately, is often not available when planning a penile-conserving approach.

One of the difficulties in determining tumor stage in the current TNM system is that diagnostic biopsies are often superficial, with only enough tissue to establish the diagnosis of malignancy, but not enough to determine the depth of invasion, or to reliably determine grade or rule out lymphovascular invasion (LVI).[14] In 1 study, 30% of tumors were upgraded on final pathology compared with biopsy, and only 1/8 of biopsies correctly identified LVI. Imaging such as ultrasound (US) or magnetic resonance imaging with prostaglandin-induced artificial erection may help to distinguish invasion of the corpora when clinical examination is uncertain.[15–17]

Evaluation of lymph nodes is important as nodal involvement is the strongest predictor of survival. Although clinical examination of the inguinal regions may be sufficient for Tis-T1, grade 1 to 2 lesions, for G3 lesions or T2 disease, computed tomography (CT) staging should be performed as an initial step; US-guided fine-needle aspiration cytology is useful for nodes that are clinically suspicious.[18] For tumors that are less than well differentiated, showing LVI, or higher than stage T2, surgical staging is recommended with either modified inguinal lymph node dissection or dynamic sentinel lymph node mapping, which uses a gamma probe after intradermal injection of technetium 99m around the primary tumor. Centers with expertise report low false-negative rates, ranging from 2% to 11%, suggesting that this is an adequate substitute for groin dissection in experienced hands.[19–22]

PATHOLOGIC PROGNOSTIC FACTORS

Tumor differentiation, stage (or depth of invasion), the presence of lymphovascular invasion and p53 positivity are the most important predictors of outcome. These may be difficult to assess on biopsy as many biopsies are too superficial to assess the depth of invasion and may miss other important prognostic features.[14] Lymph node involvement has been reported in 30% of well-differentiated tumors and 81% of moderately or poorly differentiated tumors.[23] Similarly G3 lesions with invasion of the corpora had a 78% rate of lymph node positivity after inguinal dissection, whereas for G1 to G2 T1, the rate of nodal involvement was only 4%.[24,25]

EARLY DISEASE

A 2001 survey of practice confirmed the preference for amputative surgery for distal lesions that is still prevalent in many centers.[26–28] European Association of Urology guidelines[29] direct urologists away from amputative surgery toward penile conservation whenever possible. A penile-sparing approach is recommended for Ta-T1, grade 1 to 2 tumors. For grade 3 T1 or grade 1 to 2 T2, penile sparing may be considered provided the lesion takes up less than half the glans and the patient is reliable for follow-up. This represents a significant change in philosophy away from traditional surgical approaches involving partial or total penectomy.[26] The literature contains reports of suicide or attempted suicide following surgery,[30] and although some men may be willing to sacrifice their sexual function for a treatment that may offer a better chance of survival, the converse is also true.[3] The sexual sequelae of partial penectomy are almost as severe as for total penectomy and although the capacity for erection of the penile stump and orgasm may be retained, only one-third of men continue to enjoy the same frequency and quality of sexual encounters as before surgery.[31]

PENILE CONSERVATION
Surgical

The first steps are to obtain a biopsy for diagnosis and to perform a circumcision to permit full exposure of the lesion and prevent complications such as radiation balanitis and phimosis if a radiotherapeutic approach is chosen. Because more than one-third of penile cancers involve the prepuce, with or without involvement of the glans, circumcision also removes a portion of the tumor.

Several surgical approaches exist for penis conservation. Mohs surgery involves removal of successive thin layers of tissue until microscopically verified clear margins are obtained.[32] Generally tumors that involve the corpora, urethra, or urethral meatus are not considered suitable for Mohs surgery.[33] Other options for superficial disease (Tis, T1) include carbon dioxide or neodymium-yttrium-aluminum-garnet laser resection.[34,35] Results are poor for T2 disease and long-term close follow-up is required because 30% of recurrences occur between 6 and 10 years and 15% after 10 years.[36] Glansectomy and reconstruction can be considered as a limited partial penectomy but with a better functional result and preservation of penile length.[37,38] The traditional surgical approach requiring a 2-cm margin does not leave much of an option for functional preservation, but recent reports of successful outcomes with margins of 1 cm or less have challenged the old dogma.[39,40] Closer margins, however, do impart a higher risk of local recurrence and necessitate closer follow-up.

Radiation

Radiation is an organ-conserving modality that can be delivered by an external beam approach (EBRT) or as interstitial brachytherapy (BT). Both are locally effective and spare amputation in a significant proportion of cases (**Tables 1** and **2**). The choice of modality depends on patient selection factors and the availability of expertise. Either modality must be preceded by a full circumcision.

External Radiotherapy

EBRT has the advantage of being widely available and does not require the specific technical expertise of brachytherapy. Small superficial lesions (Tis) can be treated using superficial electrons or kilovoltage radiation with a fractionation scheme typical of that for skin cancer (35–40 Gy/10 fractions over 2 weeks). However, most lesions referred for consideration of radiotherapy are more advanced and are not suitable for superficial radiation. Because of the uncertainty in assessing the depth of invasion, treatment to the full thickness of the penis with full dose to the skin surface is required. Larger tumors and those with extension onto the shaft can be better handled by EBRT than BT.

Treatment with EBRT requires a setup that positions the penis for access by the radiation beams without incidental irradiation to adjacent normal tissue and overcomes the skin-sparing nature of megavoltage radiation. This is accomplished by constructing a 10 × 10 cm block out of tissue-equivalent material, bivalving it, and fashioning a central cylindrical chamber to house the penis. A tissue-equivalent "cork" is required to close the open end of the cylindrical space. The patient is positioned supine on the treatment table, with the penis encased in the block and supported in an upright position. The block can be constructed of material such as wax or Perspex. If wax is used, the block is single-use, constructed for the individual case. The position of the penis within the wax cannot be visually verified so the fit has to be snug or the penis may slump within the wax, resulting in treatment to a lesser length than planned. Because the radiation reaction peaks during the 6-week course of treatment, the central chamber may have to be enlarged to

Table 1
Summary of reported brachytherapy results

Author	Year	No. of Patients	Dose (Gy)	Follow-up, Months (Range)	5-Year Local Control[a]	5-Year Cause-Specific Survival[a]	Necrosis/ Stenosis	Penile Preservation
Chaudhery et al[41]	1999	23	50	21 (4–117)	70% (8 y)	—	0/9%	70% (8 y)
Crook et al[42]	2009	67	60	48 (6–194)	87% 72% (10 y)	83.6%	12%/9%	88% (5 y) 67 (10 y)
DeCrevoisier et al[43]	2009	144	65	68 (6–348)	80% (10 y)	92% (10 y)	26%/29%	72 (10 y)
Delannes et al[44]	1992	51	50–65	65 (12–144)	86% crude	85%	23%/45%	75%
Kiltie et al[45]	2000	31	64	61.5	81%	85.4%	8%/44%	75%
Mazeron et al[46]	1984	50	60–70	36–96	78% crude	—	6%/19%	74%
Rozan et al[47]	1995	184	59	139	86%	88%	21%/45%	78%
Sarin et al[30]	1996	102	61–70	111	77%	72%	Not stated	72% (6 y)

[a] Five years unless stated otherwise.

accommodate penile edema, and the setup may become uncomfortable. If Perspex is used instead of wax, a set of preconstructed blocks can be available in the department with central cylindrical chambers of varying sizes. A different size can be chosen to accommodate edema during treatment. Perspex also has the advantage of being transparent so that the penile position can be verified before each treatment, and the blocks can be sterilized for re-use. The fractionation scheme most commonly used consists of 2-Gy daily fractions for a total dose of 60–66 Gy in 6 to 6.5 weeks using 2 opposed beams.

Brachytherapy (Interstitial Radiation)

There is considerable worldwide experience with brachytherapy for penile cancer, with reports from several European countries, Canada, and India. The penis lends itself well to interstitial brachytherapy. Lesions can be encompassed using 2 to 3 parallel planes of needles held in position with predrilled Lucite templates, with geometry and dose prescription following the rules of the Paris system (**Fig. 1**). Needles and planes are equidistant with typical spacing of 12 to 18 mm and should be positioned such that the prescription isodose covers about a 10-mm lateral margin on

Table 2
Summary of reported results for external beam radiation

Author	Year	No. of Patients	Dose (Gy)	Follow-up, Months (Range)	5-Year Local Control	5-year Cause-Specific Survival	Complications
Gotsadze et al[56]	2000	155	40–60	4 decades	65%	86%	1% necrosis 7% stenosis
McLean et al[57]	1993	26	35/10 to 60/25	116 (84–168)	61.5%	69%	28% unspecified
Neave et al[58]	1993	20	50–55	36 mo minimum	69.7%	58%	10% stenosis
Ozsahin et al[27]	2006	33	52	62 (6–450)	44%	—	10% stenosis
Sarin et al[30]	1997	59	60/30	62 (2–264)	55%	66%	3% necrosis 14% stenosis
Zouhair et al[59]	2001	23	45–74	12 (5–139)	41%	—	10% stenosis

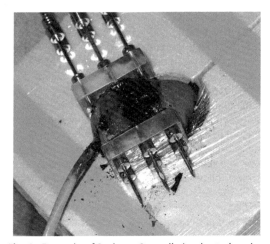

Fig. 1. Example of 2-plane, 6-needle implant, showing Lucite templates and Styrofoam collar.

visible or palpable tumor and at least 10 mm on the deep aspect. A dose of 60 Gy can be delivered in 4 to 5 days, with the patient hospitalized for the duration. A classic low dose rate (LDR) implant can be performed using iridium192 wires or ribbons after-loaded manually into the needles, or using automated after-loading with a pulse dose rate (PDR) machine programmed to deliver hourly pulses from a high-activity iridium 192 source. The 2 approaches are radiobiologically equivalent and aim to deliver an hourly dose rate of 50 to 65 cGy. On the contrary, high dose rate brachytherapy (HDR) requires compensation in total dose because of the increased dose rate, fraction size, and much smaller number of fractions. Suggested fractionation schemes for HDR brachytherapy for penile cancer have not been published.

Penile brachytherapy can be performed under general or local anesthesia, taking about 45 minutes. Ideal lesions should be less than 4 cm in maximum diameter and with no extension onto the shaft (**Fig. 2**A). Technical considerations of brachytherapy for meatal or unilateral lesions have been described.[48] At completion, a Styrofoam or sponge collar is fashioned to support the penis in a vertical position to distance the distally located sources from adjacent normal tissues. If preservation of spermatogenesis is an issue, a thin layer of lead can be added to the supporting collar to reduce the testicular dose. The needles are surprisingly well tolerated, with patients generally requiring minimal analgesia. Implant removal can occur at the bedside after premedication with a narcotic analgesic.

ACUTE AND LATE REACTIONS

Moist desquamation develops in the irradiated area, peaking midway through the course of EBRT and about 3 weeks after BT. Healing occurs in 6 to 8 weeks after EBRT and in 2 to 3 months after BT (see **Fig. 2**B). Adhesions may form acutely in the distal urethra causing a deviated or divided urinary stream and should be separated using either a meatal dilator or by inserting the tip of an 18 Fr Foley catheter a few centimeters into the urethra. Intercourse can be resumed when the patient is comfortable, although additional water-based lubrication is recommended to protect the

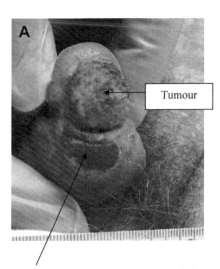

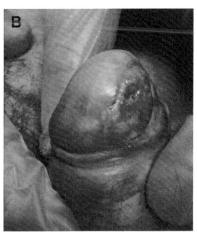

Fig. 2. (*A*) Typical case selected for brachytherapy, before circumcision. (*B*) Moist desquamation healing 8 weeks after implant.

fragile new epithelium in the treated area. More deeply invasive tumors leave a crater that takes take longer to re-epithelialize. Local hygiene is important with frequent soaks in baking soda and water, a loose telfa protective dressing, and the use of antibiotic and/or vitamin E ointment.

The 2 most common late complications are meatal stenosis and nonhealing soft-tissue ulceration or necrosis. Both can occur with either type of radiotherapy but are more common after brachytherapy (see **Tables 1** and **2**). Soft-tissue ulceration may take weeks to heal. Hygiene, control of infection, and protection from trauma are important. Deep or painful areas may respond well to a course of hyperbaric oxygen therapy, and if this is available it should be tried before resorting to amputation. Soft-tissue necrosis is reported in up to 23% of cases and in severe cases may require amputation of a tumor-free penis. Peak onset is at 7 to 18 months and may be provoked by trauma or cold exposure. Treatment- and tumor-related factors include T3 disease, larger tumors or larger implant volumes (>30 cm^3), and doses more than 60 Gy.[46,47]

Meatal stenosis is reported in 10% to 45% and occurs later than soft-tissue ulceration but usually before 3 years. Meatal stenosis can usually be managed with intermittent dilatation and may be prevented by providing the patient with a meatal dilator shortly after the procedure that can be used as required. Meatal stenosis is more common after EBRT if a hypofractionated regimen is used,[49] and after BT if central planes are close to the urethra.[47] Use of PDR after-loading allows dose optimization to reduce the urethral dose when central planes are required.

Although long-term cosmesis is generally very good, other sequelae include pigmentation change in the irradiated area and telangiectasia formation. There may be some tissue loss at sites of deep invasion. Retention of erectile function depends on the length of penile shaft irradiated, and although many series do not report on postraradiotherapy potency, it seems to be well maintained after brachytherapy because the erectile tissue of the penile shaft has been spared from unnecessary irradiation.[30,44,46,50]

EFFICACY OF RADIATION

A summary of reported results is presented in **Table 1** (BT) and **Table 2** (EBRT). As can be seen, both forms of radiation can be effective in penile conservation, although BT seems to be more successful than EBRT. Five-year penile preservation rates with BT are 70% to 88% and with EBRT 36% to 66%. No longer-term results are reported for EBRT but for BT, 10-year results indicate actuarial penile preservation of 67% to 72%.[42,43] Recurrences can occur several years after treatment. In a report on 67 patients, Crook and colleagues[42] found that local failure had a bimodal distribution, with two-thirds occurring in the first 2 years and the remainder after 5 years. De Crevoisier and colleagues[43] reported that 20% of local recurrences occurred after 8 years. Given the extremely long interval since treatment, these may represent new primaries, but certainly prolonged follow-up is required. As surgical salvage is highly effective in these cases, there is no decrease in cause-specific survival between 5 and 10 years, being 83.6% at both time points in Crook and colleagues's[42] series and 92% at 10 years for de Crevoisier and colleagues[43] Surgical salvage usually requires either partial or total penectomy, depending on the length of unirradiated penile shaft, which is usually greater with BT compared with EBRT.

ADVANCED DISEASE

Patients presenting with a small primary tumor but concurrent resectable adenopathy can still be offered a penile-conserving approach. Although tumor grade is strongly prognostic of lymph node involvement and cause-specific survival, it does not adversely affect control rates with BT. Bilateral groin dissection can be undertaken concurrently with BT or shortly afterwards. A surgical approach, however, is appropriate for those with a locally advanced disease greater than 4 cm or extending onto the penile shaft and concurrent resectable adenopathy. Partial penectomy is possible when the tumor involves the distal shaft if the length of penile remnant is sufficient for the patient to direct the urinary stream. Otherwise, total penectomy and perineal urethrostomy is required.

The role of postoperative radiotherapy is not clearly defined in the literature; however, studies on squamous cell cancers of other sites, such as the anal canal and vulva, that drain primarily to the inguinal regions would suggest that postoperative radiotherapy to the groin should be considered when there are multiple positive nodes or evidence of extracapsular spread.[51] If the status of the deep pelvic nodes is unknown, the pelvis should be included but if pelvic nodes are known to be histologically negative, radiotherapy can be limited to the inguinal region delivering a dose of 45 to 50 Gy over 5 weeks at an appropriate depth, with a boost if necessary for known extracapsular disease.

For unresectable nodal disease, radiotherapy alone can provide palliation. If the patient's general condition permits, neoadjuvant chemotherapy may render the nodes resectable. Postoperative radiation may be indicated depending on the final pathology. If the response after chemotherapy is insufficient to proceed with surgery, radiotherapy can consolidate the response and prolong the palliative effect.

Various combinations of chemotherapy have been tried. Intraarterial chemotherapy for locally advanced or recurrent penile cancer using cisplatin, methotrexate, and bleomycin (CMB)[52] or CMB plus 5-fluorouracil and mitomycin C[53] have shown promise. The Southwest Oncology Group[54] has reported a trial using CMB in locally advanced or metastatic penile cancer in 40 men with a response rate of 32.5%. An ongoing trial of neoadjuvant paclitaxol, ifosfamide, and cisplatin at the MD Anderson Cancer Center has reported a response rate of 55% in the first 20 patients.[55]

SUMMARY

Squamous cell carcinoma of the penis is a rare malignancy that can be successfully managed with acceptable morbidity in its early stages but is fatal if neglected. Penile-conserving approaches should be tried when possible for localized disease but the patient must be compliant with extended follow-up. Advanced disease has a high fatality rate and should be managed in a multidisciplinary setting.

REFERENCES

1. Parkin DM, Muir CS. Cancer incidence in five continents. Comparability and quality of data. IARC Sci Publ 1992;120:45–173.

2. Opjordsmoen S, Waehre H, Aass N, et al. Sexuality in patients treated for penile cancer: patients' experience and doctors' judgement. Br J Urol 1994;73:554–60.

3. Opjordsmoen S, Fossa SD. Quality of life in patients treated for penile cancer. A follow-up study. Br J Urol 1994;74:652–7.

4. Cubilla AL, Reuter VE, Gregoire L, et al. Basaloid squamous cell carcinoma: a distinctive human papilloma virus-related penile neoplasm: a report of 20 cases. Am J Surg Pathol 1998;22:755–61.

5. Porter WM, Francis N, Hawkins D, et al. Penile intraepithelial neoplasia: clinical spectrum and treatment of 35 cases. Br J Dermatol 2002;147:1159–65.

6. Lopes A, Bezerra AL, Pinto CA, et al. P53 as a new prognostic factor for lymph node metastasis in penile carcinoma: analysis of 82 patients treated with amputation and bilateral lymphadenectomy. J Urol 2002;168:81–6.

7. Zhu Y, Zhou XY, Yao XD, et al. The prognostic significance of p53, ki-67, epithelial cadherin and matrix metalloproteinase-9 in penile squamous cell carcinoma treated with surgery. BJU Int 2007;100:204–8.

8. Saibishkumar EP, Crook J, Sweet J. Neonatal circumcision and invasive squamous cell carcinoma of the penis: a report of 3 cases and a review of the literature. Can Urol Assoc J 2008;2:39–42.

9. Daling JR, Madeleine MM, Johnson LG, et al. Penile cancer: importance of circumcision, human papillomavirus and smoking in in situ and invasive disease. Int J Cancer 2005;116:606–16.

10. Lerman SE, Liao JC. Neonatal circumcision. Pediatr Clin North Am 2001;48:1539–57.

11. Jackson S. The treatment of carcinoma of the penis. Br J Surg 1966;53:33–5.

12. Harmer M. Penis (ICD-0187). In: Harmer MH, editor. TNM classification of malignant tumours. 3rd edition. Geneva: UICC; 1978.

13. Hermanek P. Sobin LH. Penis. (ICD-0 187) In: Hermanek P, Sobin LH, editors. TNM classification of malignant tumours. 4th edition. Berlin: Springer-Verlag; 1987. p. 130–2.

14. Velazquez EF, Barreto JE, Rodriguez I, et al. Limitations in the interpretation of biopsies in patients with penile squamous cell carcinoma. Int J Surg Pathol 2004;12:139–46.

15. Scardino E, Villa G, Bonomo G, et al. Magnetic resonance imaging combined with artificial erection for local staging of penile cancer. Urology 2004;63:1158–62.

16. Lont AP, Besnard AP, Gallee MP, et al. A comparison of physical examination and imaging in determining the extent of primary penile carcinoma. BJU Int 2003;91:493–5.

17. Petralia G, Villa G, Scardino E, et al. Local staging of penile cancer using magnetic resonance imaging with pharmacologically induced penile erection. Radiol Med 2008;113:517–28.

18. Kochhar R, Taylor B, Sangar V. Imaging in primary penile cancer: current status and future directions. Eur Radiol 2009.

19. Jensen JB, Jensen KM, Ulhoi BP, et al. Sentinel lymph-node biopsy in patients with squamous cell carcinoma of the penis. BJU Int 2009;103:1199–203.

20. Heyns CF, Theron PD. Evaluation of dynamic sentinel lymph node biopsy in patients with squamous cell carcinoma of the penis and palpable inguinal nodes. BJU Int 2008;102:305–9.

21. Hadway P, Smith Y, Corbishley C, et al. Evaluation of dynamic lymphoscintigraphy and sentinel lymph-node biopsy for detecting occult metastases in patients with penile squamous cell carcinoma. BJU Int 2007;100:561–5.

22. Crawshaw JW, Hadway P, Hoffland D, et al. Sentinel lymph node biopsy using dynamic lymphoscintigraphy combined with ultrasound-guided fine needle aspiration in penile carcinoma. Br J Radiol 2009; 82:41–8.

23. Theodorescu D, Russo P, Zhang ZF, et al. Outcomes of initial surveillance of invasive squamous cell carcinoma of the penis and negative nodes. J Urol 1996;155:1626–31.

24. McDougal WS. Carcinoma of the penis: improved survival by early regional lymphadenectomy based on the histological grade and depth of invasion of the primary lesion. J Urol 1995;154:1364–6.

25. McDougal WS, Kirchner FK Jr, Edwards RH, et al. Treatment of carcinoma of the penis: the case for primary lymphadenectomy. J Urol 1986;136:38–41.

26. Harden SV, Tan LT. Treatment of localized carcinoma of the penis: a survey of current practice in the UK. Clin Oncol (R Coll Radiol) 2001;13:284–7 [quiz: 288].

27. Ozsahin M, Jichlinski P, Weber DC, et al. Treatment of penile carcinoma: to cut or not to cut? Int J Radiat Oncol Biol Phys 2006;66:674–9.

28. Sacoto CD, Marco SL, Solchaga GM, et al. Cancer de pene. Nuestra experiencia en 15 anos. Acta Urol 2009;33:143.

29. Solsona E, Algaba F, Horenblas S, et al. EAU guidelines on penile cancer. Eur Urol 2004;46:1–8.

30. Sarin R, Norman AR, Steel GG, et al. Treatment results and prognostic factors in 101 men treated for squamous carcinoma of the penis. Int J Radiat Oncol Biol Phys 1997;38:713–22.

31. Romero FR, Romero KR, Mattos MA, et al. Sexual function after partial penectomy for penile cancer. Urology 2005;66:1292–5.

32. Mohs FE, Snow SN, Larson PO. Mohs micrographic surgery for penile tumors. Urol Clin North Am 1992; 19:291–304.

33. Shindel AW, Mann MW, Lev RY, et al. Mohs micrographic surgery for penile cancer: management and long-term followup. J Urol 2007;178:1980–5.

34. Schlenker B, Gratzke C, Seitz M, et al. Fluorescence-guided laser therapy for penile carcinoma and precancerous lesions: long-term follow-up. Urol Oncol 2009. [Epub ahead of print].

35. Meijer RP, Boon TA, van Venrooij GE, et al. Long-term follow-up after laser therapy for penile carcinoma. Urology 2007;69:759–62.

36. Windahl T, Andersson SO. Combined laser treatment for penile carcinoma: results after long-term followup. J Urol 2003;169:2118–21.

37. Smith Y, Hadway P, Biedrzycki O, et al. Reconstructive surgery for invasive squamous carcinoma of the glans penis. Eur Urol 2007;52:1179–85.

38. Palminteri E, Berdondini E, Lazzeri M, et al. Resurfacing and reconstruction of the glans penis. Eur Urol 2007;52:893–8.

39. Minhas S, Kayes O, Hegarty P, et al. What surgical resection margins are required to achieve oncological control in men with primary penile cancer? BJU Int 2005;96:1040–3.

40. Hoffman MA, Renshaw AA, Loughlin KR. Squamous cell carcinoma of the penis and microscopic pathologic margins: how much margin is needed for local cure? Cancer 1999;85:1565.

41. Chaudhary AJ, Ghosh S, Bhalavat RL, et al. Interstitial brachytherapy in carcinoma of the penis. Strahlenther Onkol 1999;175:17–20.

42. Crook J, Ma C, Grimard L. Radiation therapy in the management of the primary penile tumor: an update. World J Urol 2009;27:189.

43. de Crevoisier R, Slimane K, Sanfilippo N, et al. Long-term results of brachytherapy for carcinoma of the penis confined to the glans (N- or NX). Int J Radiat Oncol Biol Phys 2009;74:1150–6.

44. Delannes M, Malavaud B, Douchez J, et al. Iridium-192 interstitial therapy for squamous cell carcinoma of the penis. Int J Radiat Oncol Biol Phys 1992;24:479–83.

45. Kiltie AE, Elwell C, Close HJ, et al. Iridium-192 implantation for node-negative carcinoma of the penis: the Cookridge Hospital experience. Clin Oncol (R Coll Radiol) 2000;12:25–31.

46. Mazeron JJ, Langlois D, Lobo PA, et al. Interstitial radiation therapy for carcinoma of the penis using iridium 192 wires: the Henri Mondor experience (1970–1979). Int J Radiat Oncol Biol Phys 1984;10:1891–5.

47. Rozan R, Albuisson E, Giraud B, et al. Interstitial brachytherapy for penile carcinoma: a multicentric survey (259 patients). Radiother Oncol 1995;36:83–93.

48. Crook J, Jezioranski J, Cygler JE. Penile brachytherapy: technical aspects and postimplant issues. Brachytherapy 2009.

49. Duncan W, Jackson SM. The treatment of early cancer of the penis with megavoltage x-rays. Clin Radiol 1972;23:246–8.

50. Crook J, Grimard L, Tsihlias J, et al. Interstitial brachytherapy for penile cancer: an alternative to amputation. J Urol 2002;167:506–11.

51. Katz A, Eifel PJ, Jhingran A, et al. The role of radiation therapy in preventing regional recurrences of invasive squamous cell carcinoma of the vulva. Int J Radiat Oncol Biol Phys 2003;57:409–18.

52. Huang XY, Kubota Y, Nakada T, et al. Intra-arterial infusion chemotherapy for penile carcinoma with deep inguinal lymph node metastasis. Urol Int 1999;62:245–8.

53. Roth AD, Berney CR, Rohner S, et al. Intra-arterial chemotherapy in locally advanced or recurrent

carcinomas of the penis and anal canal: an active treatment modality with curative potential. Br J Cancer 2000;83:1637–42.

54. Haas GP, Blumenstein BA, Gagliano RG, et al. Cisplatin, methotrexate and bleomycin for the treatment of carcinoma of the penis: a Southwest Oncology Group study. J Urol 1999;161:1823–5.

55. Pagliaro LC, Crook J. Multimodality therapy in penile cancer: when and which treatments? World J Urol 2009;27:221–5.

56. Gotsadze D, Matveev B, Zak B, et al. Is conservative organ-sparing treatment of penile carcinoma justified? Eur Urol 2000;38:306–12.

57. McLean M, Akl AM, Warde P, et al. The results of primary radiation therapy in the management of squamous cell carcinoma of the penis. Int J Radiat Oncol Biol Phys 1993;25:623–8.

58. Neave F, Neal AJ, Hoskin PJ, et al. Carcinoma of the penis: a retrospective review of treatment with iridium mould and external beam irradiation. Clin Oncol (R Coll Radiol) 1993;5: 207–10.

59. Zouhair A, Coucke PA, Jeanneret W, et al. Radiation therapy alone or combined surgery and radiation therapy in squamous-cell carcinoma of the penis? Eur J Cancer 2001;37:198–203.

Surgery for Urethral Cancer

R. Jeffrey Karnes, MD*, Rodney H. Breau, MD, FRCSC,
Deborah J. Lightner, MD

KEYWORDS

• Urethral cancer • Surgery • Male • Female

Primary urethral cancers represent less than 1% of genitourinary malignancy. Given this is an uncommon disease, there are limited data to guide diagnostic and treatment strategies. Surgical extirpation remains the standard for most patients, with the addition of chemotherapy and radiation therapy in select patients. The surgical approach to urethral cancer depends largely on the location and extent of the tumor.

SURVIVAL

Survival in men and women depends on the stage (**Fig. 1**). See Appendix for TNM staging.

MALE URETHRAL CANCER

The diagnosis of urethral cancer can be elusive. Although most urethral cancers are associated with symptoms (ie, bleeding, lower urinary tract symptoms),[1,2] concomitant disease may delay diagnosis. In men, urethral cancer is commonly associated with stricture disease, sexually transmitted disease, immunosuppression, or previous urethral surgery or radiation therapy.[1–5] The mean age at presentation is approximately 60 years.[1–6]

Anatomic Considerations

The typical epithelial neoplasms in the male urethra are squamous cell carcinoma (SCC), adenocarcinoma, and urothelial carcinoma (UC). Overall, SCC represents the most common histology.[1–6] Other variant malignancies, such as villous adenocarcinoma are rare (**Fig. 2**).[7]

Historically, primary cancers of the urethra have been divided into 2 regions: anterior and posterior. Anterior is more common than posterior. Some investigators have described distal urethral cancers to differentiate those from within the bulb or other more proximal locations. In general, distal cancers or penile urethral cancers are diagnosed at an earlier stage and are potentially more amenable to local treatment (organ-preserving). Correspondingly, survival has been more favorable for patients with anterior tumors compared with posterior tumors. A possible explanation for lower stage at diagnosis is that anterior tumors may be more obstructive because of a smaller caliber distal urethral or, associated with signs (ie, a palpable mass). The surgical approach to urethral cancers is dependent on stage and location with less importance on grade and histopathologic type.

Historical Perspective

Thiaudierre is credited with the first description of a male urethral cancer case in 1834.[8] In 1951, McCrea and Furlong reviewed more than 200 patients.[9] The investigators noted that no patient lived more than 10 months from the time of diagnosis without definitive treatment. A follow-up article in the same era reported 5 cases requiring penile amputation and 2 that required radical cystectomy for male urethra carcinoma.[10] These investigators commented that when they reviewed the literature they were "unable to arrive at any decision regarding the value of any specific type of treatment." Unfortunately, since that time, there have been few data to allow consensus on how to best manage primary male urethral cancer.

In the 1960s, Kaplan and colleagues[11] reported a median survival of only 3 months and the longest

Department of Urology, Mayo Clinic, 200 1st Street SW, Rochester, MN 55905, USA
* Corresponding author.
E-mail address: karnes.r@mayo.edu

Urol Clin N Am 37 (2010) 445–457
doi:10.1016/j.ucl.2010.04.011

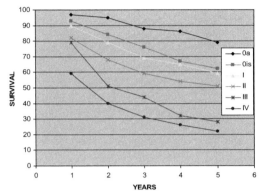

Fig. 1. Overall survival of patients with urethral cancers stratified by AJCC stage/prognostic groups. (*Data from* Edge SB, Byrd DR, Compton CC, et al. AJCC cancer staging manual. 7th edition. New York: Springer; 2010. p. 507–10.)

survival of 15 months in 46 men who had only palliation or no treatment at all. This report did conclude that radical surgery could be effective and that in most cases adequate local control of the disease would translate into improved survival. In another series of posteriorly located tumors, 5-year cancer-specific survival (CSS) was 30% following radical surgery and 3% without treatment.[12]

In the early 1980s, urologists from MD Anderson Cancer Center (MDACC) and Memorial Sloan-Kettering Cancer Center (MSKCC) detailed the types of exenterative surgery they believed necessary to provide local control of these cancers.[13,14] The report from MSKCC had more than 50% CSS when neoadjuvant radiation was added to radical excision including inferior pubectomy. Around the same time, Bracken[15] reported on 3 posterior urethral cancers and described a 2-stage procedure that involved an ileal conduit and then an anterior exenteration and total emasculation with en bloc pubectomy. In this report, the men were free of disease at 18 to 60 months follow-up and it was concluded that, "no less radical treatment seems appropriate." Although not debating the paramount importance of local control, to equate a local recurrence with lethality based on these historic reports does not justify such exenterative surgery in all cases of urethral cancer in the modern era.

Contemporary Series

A MDACC series describes the presentation and treatment of 23 men with urethral cancer between 1979 and 1990[2] and was a follow-up from their previous report.[13] The overall survival (OS) for this group was 52% at a mean follow-up of 50

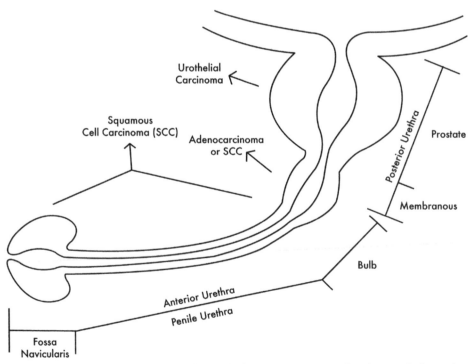

Fig. 2. The anatomic regions of the male urethra with the typical corresponding histopathology. The average male urethral length is 22 cm.

months (range 5–156 months). Approximately two-thirds of the patients had tumors in the distal anterior urethra and one-third within the bulb region. The investigators observed that survival was dependent on stage, grade, and location; for instance, patients with fossa navicularis lesions and all grade I tumors were associated with 100% survival at last follow-up. Patients with penile urethral tumors had 60% CSS at a mean follow-up of 48 months and patients with bulbomembranous urethral tumors had 29% CSS at a mean follow-up of 31 months. This report also demonstrated that radiation therapy alone did not provide local disease control and that chemotherapy may be beneficial for patients who present with metastatic disease. Based on the investigators' experience, they concluded that tumors in the fossa navicularis and penile urethra should be treated with distal urethrectomy and partial penectomy; and tumors in the bulbomembranous urethra should be treated with en bloc resection of the penis, scrotum, prostate, bladder and inferior pubic rami. This was a similar conclusion that had been made in the previous issue of *Urologic Clinics of North America* on this topic in 1992.[16]

MSKCC has provided the largest and longest single institution series to date of 46 men with primary urethral cancers from 1958 to 1996.[1] Median follow-up was 125 months. Very similar to the MDACC survival data, MSKCC reported 5-year CSS was approximately 50% and the OS was 42%. Location of the lesion was associated with outcome as 26% survival was observed for patients with bulbar tumors compared with 69% for patients with distal anterior urethral tumors. Not surprisingly tumor stage was also associated with outcome as patients with noninvasive lesions (<T1) had 83% OS compared with 36% for invasive lesions ($\geq$T1). Disease-free survival was 38% for patients with distal tumors compared with 14% for patients with tumors in the bulb. As with most series, treatment was not standardized in all patients. A somewhat alarming finding within their study was that survival rates appeared unchanged when they compared 1975 and before with 1976 and after. Any meaningful conclusions are hard to draw from this observation given the relatively small numbers and lack of balance of stage/grade/location distributions within these time periods. Furthermore, these large series from MDACC and MSKCC and others perhaps do not reflect how all men with urethral cancers present, are treated, and their outcomes. There is an inherent bias in these types of reporting as cases sent to tertiary care cancer centers are probably different and more advanced than the cases that are handled within the community.

Nonetheless, like the MDACC series, most of the MSKCC series was composed of symptomatic SCCs. There was an obvious difference with the MSKCC series in that two-thirds of cases were located within the bulb and only one-third within the distal anterior urethra, which was the opposite in the MDACC series. Of the 46 cases at MSKCC, 40 underwent surgery alone and 6 had preoperative radiation. It is not clear whether these 6 men had planned resection after radiation or whether they required a salvage surgery. The men who did receive radiation were typically of higher stage (n = 3 for T3 and n = 3 for T4) and did not seem to fare as well. In additionally, Zeidman and colleagues[16] summarized the ineffective results of radiation alone on male urethral cancers. A second primary malignancy was discovered in 9 men during the follow-up, which might be explained by concurrent (n = 10) or previous smoking history (n = 31). Within this report, it is difficult to detail how many if any received postoperative chemotherapy but it seems none received it preoperatively despite concluding that the locally advanced cases should be treated aggressively with preoperative chemotherapy and radiation. When present (n = 14), the distant metastatic site most commonly involved was the lung. This report concluded that newer treatment strategies are needed and the investigators proposed that locally advanced cases should be managed with neoadjuvant chemoradiation followed by penectomy for distal anterior urethral lesions and with the addition of an anterior exenteration for more proximal (posterior) lesions.

Another series by Gheiler and colleagues[6] from 1980 to 1996 described the Wayne State experience for 11 men with a mean follow-up of 40 months. Distal lesions and lower-stage lesions fared better than proximal and higher-stage lesions. In particular, with this study, 4 men (T3–4, N0–2) underwent neoadjuvant chemoradiation followed by surgical resection and 2 of the 4 were disease-free at follow-up. The investigators acknowledged that the numbers were small but their findings suggested that the addition of this neoadjuvant regimen might result in better survival. They also suggested that Ta-T2N0 cases could be managed surgically perhaps without multimodal therapy but their series on which this statement was based also included about half women.

Another combined (male/female) series from 1958 to 1998 that included 8 men showed that those with higher-stage lesions (T2M1, T3, and T4) were dead of their disease at 10, 56, and 4 months, respectively.[17] With the lower-stage lesions (T1–2) no metastasis developed; 2 underwent transurethral resection alone (TUR) and 1 a wide local excision. Although not the first series to report on organ/penile preservation, perhaps there are cases that definitely do not require a more radical excision. It is not clear that this is true only for the lower-stage lesions but potentially with the inclusion of other modalities, penile preservation can be accomplished. A European study from Mainz, Germany, described the management of male urethral cancers (n = 9) between 1986 and 2006.[4] As expected various treatments (only 2 requiring penectomy) were provided for the anteriorly located cancers (n = 6) and the 3 that involved the prostatic urethra (minimal details provided) involved a TUR alone. With a median follow-up of 20 months all but 1 were disease free. Although the follow-up is short most would believe that survival rates are improving in the current era and 4 of the 6 men had penile-preserving surgery. Most would agree that penile-preserving surgery can be accomplished for the properly selected urethral cancer case.

Penile-preserving Surgery

In the previous Urologic Clinics of North America, Zeidman and colleagues[16] presented 7 series of conservatively managed male urethral cancers. Of the 19 men, cases were handled by either local excision, fulguration, or TUR (surgical details without precision). Seven were SCCs and 7 were transitional cell cancers (TCCs). Eleven were in the distal urethra and 6 were in the bulb and all were free of disease at follow-up. Within this series, Mandler and Pool[18] had 3 men whom were managed with local excision in the distal urethra (1 SCC, 2 TCC, grade and T stage not provided) and follow-up was not short at 2, 10, and 20 years. In 3 of the more modern series provided,[1,2,6] conservatively managed patients (ie, penile-preserving) were performed at MSKCC (n = 13), MDACC (n = 2), and Wayne State (n = 4), and all had disease-free status at follow-up. Nonetheless, these are probably highly selected cases and this is not an endorsement for penile-preserving surgery for all cases of urethral cancer. A low-grade and low-stage distal urethral cancer might be properly suited for distal urethrectomy and partial or radical penectomy in terms of local control but could definitely constitute over treatment and the sequelae of penile loss. On the other hand, in the properly evaluated and motivated patient with urethral cancer, penile-preserving surgery could be doable without compromising cancer control. Most of these cases outlined earlier have involved lower-stage and probably lower-grade lesions; however, further discussion

focuses more on advanced stages as well as a series of penile-preserving cases.

Baskin and Turzan[19] first reported on a case involving neoadjuvant chemoradiation for SCC of the anterior urethra in 1992. The patient then underwent a distal urethrectomy and had a pT0 response. The rationale and regimen of neoadjuvant chemoradiation for SCC of the penis or urethra, which has paralleled other anatomic sites such as the anus, is outlined elsewhere in this issue.

Bird and Coburn[20] described 3 men with invasive SCC urethral cancers (T3, corporal cavernosa invasion) located within the bulb and/or penile urethra who did not want emasculation. Neither neoadjuvant or adjuvant therapy was provided. Within this case report, the surgical approach is described for phallus preservation along with the glans penis with a subcutaneous penectomy/urethrectomy. No local recurrences were seen but distant progression was present during follow-up. These lesions were also away from the glans and not fixed to the skin. On this later note outlined by these investigators, such a surgery could still be accomplished even if a wide ellipse of skin is taken. This article also clearly showed that the glans penis can survive via the vascular tributaries within the penile skin. Given that such a phallus is nonfunctional, it is not known if patients would be better served with this approach or have a penectomy and go onto phallic reconstruction as detailed elsewhere in the issue.

Davis and colleagues[21] report on their series of conservatively managed penile and urethral carcinomas. There was only 1 case of male urethral cancer (SCC) who underwent a urethrectomy alone for a T2 lesion within the bulb. The patient eventually succumbed to the disease without local recurrence 2 years later as a result of progression that started with pelvic lymphadenopathy. This case also highlights the need to potentially manage lymph node drainage prophylactically as a node dissection was not performed or detailed in this report.

Kent and colleagues[22] presented successful management of a case of urethral TCC with squamous differentiation in the distal urethra diagnosed as a T1 by initial TUR and was also N+. MVAC chemotherapy was provided as well as salvage chemotherapy and the patient was rendered pT0 and was free of recurrence locally and systemically at 39 months. This case and those outlined earlier highlight that metastasis still drives survival and that management of the primary should take this into account and not subject the patient to surgery on the primary lesion that may have little effect on the CSS.

These cases involved the distal anterior urethra. The next case involves an invasive SCC of the bulb.[23] Penile preservation was accomplished and surgery was a complete urethrectomy along with a nerve-sparing radical prostatectomy. The bladder was left in situ and bladder neck closure was performed with a Mitrofanoff reconstruction. Surgical pathology revealed a T4 secondary to involvement of testicular tunica and surgery also required an orchiectomy. Adjuvant pelvic chemoradiation was provided and at 15 months the patient was disease-free. This case shows that the native bladder can often be used as it is frequently unaffected by bulb lesions or primary male urethral cancers in general. It also highlights the resourcefulness of the surgeons. Cadaveric tensor fascia lata was used to reconstruct the tunica of the ventral corpora cavernosal bodies in their attempt to preserve erectile functioning and efforts to maintain adequate surgical margins. The surgical approaches are obviously evolving from earlier recommendations of emasculation and anterior exenteration along with inferior pubectomy and other attempts at organ preservation.

The largest series to date, and the most contemporary, on penile-preserving surgery for distal urethral cancers without preoperative treatment comes from the United Kingdom.[5] The presentation and outcome of 18 men treated consecutively is outlined for a 5-year time period. The median follow-up was only 21 months. A surgical treatment and reconstruction algorithm was created and presented within this report based on the exact location of the lesions. There have been no local recurrences to date, 6 of the men did have nodal disease, and there have been 2 cancer-related deaths. Obviously such a series will need to withstand the test of time over a longer follow-up but it underscores the point that most of the time any systemic component of cancer will drive survival. An additional highlight of this report is the issue of what constitutes appropriate surgical margins in urethral cancer. Former dogmatic teaching in the surgical management of penile cancer was a 2 cm margin but this was not based on high-level evidence and more recent studies have questioned the necessity of such a margin.[24,25] In this study by Smith and colleagues, 8 men had margins less than 5 mm but it is hard to know exactly where the margin was taken. When it comes to urethral cancer, there is really a vacuum of recommendations. Penile cancer margins are primarily based on the skin; however, this does not readily apply to urethral cancer. Margins in urethral cancer encompass the proximal and distal urethral segments as well as the dorsally located corpora cavernosa bodies

and ventrally the penile skin. This article also highlighted the usefulness of magnetic resonance imaging (MRI) for surgically planning in penile cancer or with management in general, and its potential applicability in urethral cancer.[26,27]

Although not a pure surgical series, Cohen and colleagues[3] have presented their series from the Lahey Clinic of 18 men with invasive urethral cancer treated between 1991 and 2006 with the same concurrent chemoradiation protocol. Half of the tumors were located in the penile urethra and the other half in the bulbomembranous urethra. Ninety-five percent of the cases were SCC. A complete response (CR) was seen in 15/18 or 83% and the reported 5-year OS was 60% and a CSS of 83%. In the 3 nonresponders to the chemoradiation, salvage surgery (details not provided) was performed but all died of their disease. There was a reported local recurrence rate of 30% or 5/15 who had an initial CR and 4 of these underwent salvage surgery. Thus, 10 of 18 men had a durable CR and of these 10, 3 required a complex urethral reconstruction. All the men essentially required posttreatment management of treatment-related stricture disease with most having cystoscopic intervention (except for the cases requiring salvage surgery and the 3 having a complex urethral reconstruction). This center kept the same treatment algorithm for this rare malignancy during this time period and provides these unique data. There is no doubt that surgery alone cannot be curative in some locally advanced lesions of the urethra. Unfortunately, the timing and/or the exact role of the other treatment modalities is not precisely known. Furthermore, the nature of the biopsies are not described in this study; for instance, did they debulk the lesions endoscopically or perform an open local excision or just take the biopsy before the chemoradiation?

When a surgeon is considering a penile-preserving operation for cancer of the urethra, the first step is assessing the primary lesion and whether it is amenable to such an operation. An examination along with cystoscopy and retrograde urethrography is essential and at times an MRI scan can be useful. **Fig. 3** illustrates the potential use of MRI. A biopsy should be performed to determine the histologic subtype especially if neoadjuvant chemotherapy is considered. The biopsy, usually done endoscopically, can also help determine the grade and potential stage/local depth.

During consideration of a penile-preserving operation, there is a balance between oncologic principles (local control), functionality (ability to void standing and erectile function), and the

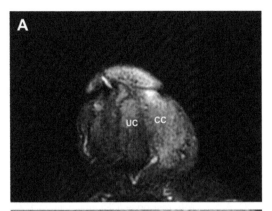

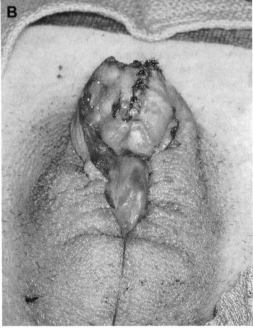

Fig. 3. A 60-year-old man presented with a history of subcoronal hypospadias and underwent a urethroplasty later in life. A subsequent neomeatus stricture required multiple procedures to stay open and a biopsy revealed invasive SCC and he was referred for a penile-sparing treatment. (*A*) MRI demonstrating close proximity to the corpora cavernosum and potential invasion. UC, urethral carcinoma; CC, left corpus cavernosum. (*B*) A glansectomy and distal urethrectomy/penectomy was performed secondary to the proximity to the cavernosum. Pathology revealed a pT2 SCC. Further details on partial penectomy and radical penectomy can be found elsewhere in this issue.

patient's desires along with his comorbidity and the rest of his metastatic work-up. In cases that cannot be managed with penile preservation, consideration should be given to a preoperative plastic surgery consultation along with evaluation by psychiatry for body image changes.

Furthermore, for those cases managed conservatively, the exact nature of the surveillance timing or methods are not known. The obvious choices are cystoscopy and cytology along with examination and potentially the incorporation of imaging. **Figs. 4** and **5** are examples of penile preservation.

Lymph Node Management

The role of lymph node dissection in the management of urethral cancers is even less clear than how to manage the primary. The management of lymphatic drainage and controversies in ilioinguinal lymphadenectomy as well as imaging of the groins are highlighted in different articles in this issue. Prophylactic groin dissection for urethral cancers was felt to be controversial dating back to the 1960s.[18] On the other hand, MDACC reports demonstrated that cures are possible with limited lymph node disease.[2,13] The biology of urethral SCC can mirror that of penile SCC; thus, lymph node dissection should be considered for limited nodal disease or neoadjuvant chemotherapy incorporated for cN2 disease or higher. A prophylactic node dissection could be planned for high-grade T1 lesions or higher. Lesions involving the fossa and penile urethra typically involve the groin nodes primarily; however, lesions in the bulb and posterior urethra can also involve the pelvic lymph nodes so surgery should take this into account.

Primary Prostatic Urethral Cancer

Primary cancers involving the prostatic urethra are even more rare than those involving the anterior urethra. In the previous issue of *Urologic Clinics of North America*, Zeidman and colleagues[16] presented survival data on 16 prostatic urethral cancers with an estimated 5-year survival rate of 25%. Further details are not known. Cheville and colleagues[28] presented Mayo Clinic data on 50 prostate UCs or TCCs but approximately two-thirds had a history of bladder cancer. Noninvasive prostatic urethral disease along with disease involving only the ducts or acini had a 5-year CSS of 100%. On the other hand, prostate TCC stromal involvement had a 5-year CSS of 45%. Palou and colleagues[29] recently reviewed urothelial carcinomas of the prostate as part of a consensus conference. Primary cancers are rare without a history of or concomitant bladder cancer. This type of cancer can be frequently understaged and usually requires an extensive TUR along with bladder interrogation to determine its exact involvement and consideration of a transrectal ultrasound-guided biopsy of the prostate. Primary noninvasive prostatic urethral cancer could be managed in the same way as noninvasive

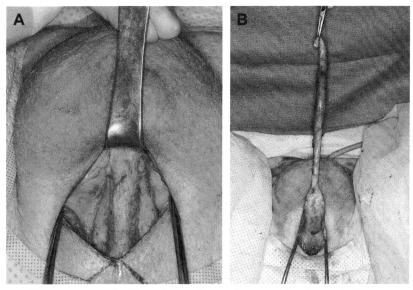

Fig. 4. A 55-year-old man presented with a history of a penile urethral stricture. A biopsy was performed for recurrent bleeding and palpable disease at the stricture site. The biopsy revealed a high-grade SCC but appeared confined to the urethra/corpus spongiosum. He refused all treatment other than urethrectomy with a proximal urinary continent catheterizable stoma. (*A*) Perineal exposure with proximal mobilization of the urethra off the corpora cavernosal bed. (*B*) Complete urethrectomy facilitated by penile eversion through the perineal incision. Pathology revealed a pT2 SCC.

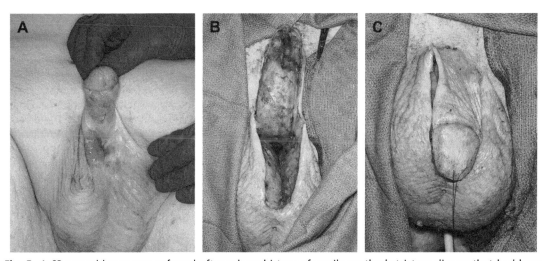

Fig. 5. A 63-year-old man was referred after a long history of penile urethral stricture disease that had been managed more than 20 years ago by the creation of a penile-scrotal neomeatus. He had developed marked pain and irritation in the neomeatus region and a biopsy confirmed invasive SCC. He had erectile dysfunction but was motivated for a penile-sparing operation. After management of the primary lesion, a prophylactic lymph node dissection was recommended and performed 6 weeks later and despite negative imaging, 2 positive nodes were found during the right groin dissection. Adjuvant chemotherapy was advocated. (*A*) Preoperative picture showing the biopsy-proved SCC along with associated biopsy-induced inflammation about his neomeatus, adjacent scrotal skin, and the ventral penile skin that was in contact with these regions. (*B*) Resection: a wide local excision was performed en bloc along with distal urethrectomy and intraoperative frozen-section monitoring. (*C*) Reconstruction: the dorsal penile skin and edge of the glans was sewn to the scrotal skin and a perineal urethrostomy was created. Eventually local scrotal skin flaps will be created for the ventral surface of the penis as he has been free of cancer recurrence for 6 months.

bladder cancer. On the other hand, there are no data supporting any optimal treatment or support for a radical prostatectomy or radical cystoprostatectomy for the rare, invasive, organ-confined, primary cancer of the prostatic urethra. The surgical approach needs to be geared to the stage of the cancer (see Appendix for TNM stage).

Summary

Surgery plays an instrumental role in the management of male urethral cancers. At times it might be enough for a cure and at other times it might not. Exactly which cases benefit from chemotherapy and/or radiation therapy is unresolved. Even in cases that are managed exclusively with chemoradiation, the urologist plays a role in establishing the diagnosis but is also involved in the morbidity of the treatment on the urethra. Overall, the urologist should involve colleagues within medical and radiation oncology when it comes to invasive lesions. Given the rarity of these lesions, clinical trials or guidelines have not been established. The outcomes seem most dependent on the stage and grade at presentation as well as the location along the male urethra. The first step in the process should be assessment of the primary in terms of stage and extent as well as a metastatic work-up. There is no doubt that over time radiographic imaging and reconstructive surgery efforts have improved. With proper selection, penile-preserving surgery should be considered in the management of male urethral cancers. In addition, surgical management of lymph node drainage should be considered for those cases involving invasive lesions and should parallel those of penile SCC.

FEMALE URETHRAL CANCER

Primary female urethral cancer is an unusual cancer, presenting in the postmenopausal or aging female. More commonly, involvement of the female urethra by malignancy is by direct extension from malignancy within a urethral diverticulum,[30–32] from adjacent organs, such as the vaginal or bladder, or rarely by metastases.[33] The National Cancer Institute Surveillance, Epidemiology and End Results (SEER) database reported 540 case of primary female urethral cancer in the United States from 1973 to 2002,[34] only half the number reported for men.

The highest incidence of female urethral cancer was in the 75- to 84-year-old age group, with primary TCC the most common type overall at 3.7 cases per million, versus SCC at 2.9 per million and adenocarcinoma at 1.6 per million. The incidence of adenocarcinoma was more common in the age group less than 64 years, and in African American women,[35,36] than other cell types, with a steady increase in the incidence of TCCs and SCCs in the those older than 65 years. Primary urethral malignant melanoma is rarer still, accounting for only 0.2% of all melanomas[37] and for only 11 cases of the 63 female urethral malignancies seen at Mayo Clinic Rochester between 1950 and 1999[38,39] Case reports of granular cell tumor,[40] clear cell variants of adenocarcinoma,[41] and childhood urethral sarcoma[42] underscore the extremely rare nature of some other cell types.

The overall prevalence of primary female urethral cancer seems to be decreasing over the decades, with the incidence dropping by half for all cell types between 1973 to 1977 and 1998 to 2002.[34] Analyses, especially those using large diagnosis-coded databases, may have historically over reported urethral cancer as a positive urethral biopsy is more commonly associated with contiguous spread from another primary site, such as vulvar and vaginal SCC, bladder TCC, or urethral diverticular adenocarcinoma cancers. Miscoding of secondary urethral involvement as a primary may erroneously over inflate the incidence of these cancers in women. Hence, previous reports might be erroneous in suggesting that female urethral cancer is more common than male urethral cancer.[43]

Essentially all urethral cancers are symptomatic.[44] However, the presenting symptoms of female urethral cancer may be mistaken for the wider range of common benign urethral diseases, such as a caruncle, prolapse or diverticulum, thereby risking a delay in diagnosis. Urethral bleeding, mass or irritative voiding symptoms are the most commonly associated symptoms; urinary retention has also been reported.[45–47] The diverse differential requires that women with irritative or obstructive voiding symptoms undergo pelvic examination, with careful attention to the meatus. It is unfortunately common that during the pelvic examination, if performed, the meatus is not visually inspected and the length of the urethra is not palpated. Furthermore, the common practice of rigid cystoscopy of the female urethra using the obturator rather than direct urethral inspection from the meatus proximally to the bladder neck can miss pathologic lesions. A diverticular opening is more likely visualized with fluid inflowing toward it; the strictured urethral appearance associated with urethral mass is not attributed to cystoscope trauma. Palpation of the urethra against the cystoscope can reveal masses and induration unsuspected during the nonintubated examination. Lesions may not be palpable; 48% of patients in the Wayne State series had no appreciable urethral mass.[6]

Of palpable lesions of the urethra, a urethral diverticulum is the most common, distantly followed by leiomyoma, ectopic ureters, and vaginal cancers.[48] A visual meatal lesion is most likely to be a caruncle, a soft highly vascularized protrusion occurring in the inferior quadrants of the urethral meatus; however, distal malignancies can have a similar appearance. A high index of suspicion, therefore, is necessary to appropriately stage and manage the rarer malignant lesions. Proximal lesions present at a later stage presumably because of delays in diagnosis.[6] In an older series, increasing size was associated with poorer prognosis; lesions greater than 4 cm were associated with 5-year survival of 13% versus 60% for lesions less than 2 cm.[49]

In the presence of urethral pathology, imaging of the urethra for evaluation and staging may be performed by ultrasound and computed tomography scanning, but urethral MRI is rapidly accomplished, supplies fine anatomic detail, and identifies local tissue extension as reported by multiple investigators.[41,50–52] On axial T2-weighted MRI images, the normal 4-cm urethra has a distinct 4-layered target appearance: a low signal intensity outer ring of the striated muscle surrounds a higher intensity inner ring of smooth muscle, then a low signal ring of the submucosa and then a bright high-intensity central ring of the mucosa.[53] Gadolinium-enhanced T1-weighted images also present a target appearance of these 4 layers. Thin-section thickness (3–5 mm) and a small intersection gap between images of 1 to 2 mm is appropriate for imaging this narrow organ.[54] Differentiation of the primary as arising from the urethra or from a urethral diverticulum can be improved with MRI imaging.[41]

Imaging for metastatic disease should concentrate on inguinal and pelvic lymphadenopathy, chest and liver involvement. Positron emission tomography (PET) scanning may be helpful in identifying nodal disease, with rare reports of its use in female urethral cancers.[55] Cystoscopic examination is mandatory in all but widely disseminated disease. Voided urine cytology has not proved reliable in the diagnosis of urethral cancer.[56]

Biopsy is necessary to determine the appropriate management of these rare but diverse malignancies. Chemotherapeutic regimes differ based on the tissue type of the primary, which include lymphoma,[57–59] SCC,[46,60,61] adenocarcinoma,[62–64] TCC.[38] and melanoma,[65] Urethral melanoma been reported as amelanontic.[66] However, histology of adenocarcinoma, TCC or SCC was not a predictor of outcome,[38,44] using multimodal therapies. In contrast, melanoma had poor oncologic outcomes; the local recurrence rate was 60% at 1 year, and the OS and CSS at 3 years was 27% and 38%, respectively.[39]

Most recent reports of malignancy arising in a urethral diverticulum are adenocarcinoma, consistent with the presumptive origin of a diverticulum from the paraurethral glands,[30–32,67–70] These tumors may stain positively for prostate-specific antigen (PSA)[67] (suggestive of Skene gland homology) and immunoreactivity for the prostate marker, P504S.[32] They may show mucin production and neuroendocrine differentiation.[67] However, all adenocarcinomas in a recent archival study of adenocarcinomas stained positively for mAbDas1, an antibody developed against colonic metaplasia.[70] Rarely is SCC associated with a diverticulum.[71,72]

Investigation of nodal status should be performed with consideration of the primary site of lymphatic drainage. The anterior/distal female urethra drains primarily to the inguinal nodes; the mid and proximal urethra drain to the external iliac and deep pelvic lymph nodes.[73] Although under studied, sentinel node imaging and biopsy may be preferable to prophylactic lymphadenectomy, but lymphadenectomy is advocated for grossly positive nodes in the setting of bulky or radiation/chemoresistant tumor; chemoradiation therapy has been reported to occasionally sterilize inguinal nodal disease from squamous cell urethral cancer.[60,74]

A rare malignancy is unlikely to be treated in a uniform fashion, but standardization of management[44] would likely clarify many issues. Many articles suggest that treatment "remain individualized," a code for no clear standard. The literature is poor; most are case reports. Many reports have inadequate staging of the primary, antiquated or commingled surgical, radiation, and chemotherapy techniques. Many also have short nonstandardized follow-up.

Discussing specifically the few published series of the last 20 years for treatment of female urethral cancer, Dalbagni and colleagues[44] showed that primary stage, nodal status, and site of disease were independent predictors of survival in 72 female patients with 5-year survival of 83% for low-stage tumors and 33% for high-stage tumors. Local control was poor with 5-year local recurrence-free survival of 46%, and uninfluenced by the primary treatment with radiation, surgical therapy, or both in the Dalbagni series. Even local control of anterior urethra (distal) cancer remained poor at 5 years in 53% when extirpative surgery was used in 27 of the 42 patients. Survival after recurrence was poor, with 71% of women dying of cancer at 5 years after their recurrence.[38]

Surgical management of the primary is often not described. The radical urethral extirpation should resect all of the periurethral soft tissues from the bulbocarvernosis muscles bilaterally and distally, encompassing a cylinder of all adjacent soft tissue up to the pubic symphysis and up to the bladder neck, and posteriorly including the anterior vaginal wall. Local recurrences rates appeared lower in patients treated with this, a radical urethrectomy.[38]

Small exophytic distal tumors have been treated with distal urethrectomy alone with frozen section to ensure a clear margin,[43] however, achievement of a 2-cm tumor-free margin in the urethra is oncologically difficult without disrupting sphincteric and conduit function. Distal sleeve resection of greater than 2 cm of urethra is associated with a 42% rate of secondary urinary sphincteric weakness and incontinence,[38] requiring reconstructive repair. There is scant literature on the treatment of small distal cancers with ablative techniques including TUR or laser,[43] but partial urethrectomy or transurethral resection was associated with urethral recurrence in 4 out of 25 and cancer death in 50% of those so treated.[38] Poor local failure is highly associated with metastases, but local control does not necessarily improve survival.[75]

The addition of radiation therapy and/or chemotherapy would seem wise in higher-grade and -stage lesions after treatment with extirpation. Higher-stage lesions and lesions greater than 2 cm likely have higher local control rates with radiation therapy and extirpative surgery,[76] but any advantage in local control or cancer-free survival with adjunctive therapy is theoretic given the paucity of well-described cases. Bulky disease should be treated aggressively. A recent case report of T4 SCC would suggest that chemotherapy with paclitaxel, ifosfamide, and cisplatin followed by consolidative therapy with radiation therapy and cisplatin can provide tumor-free survival.[46]

Distal tumors tend to fare better than those more proximal,[77] but the lower stages of the distal tumors (6 out of 9 distal in this series were stage I or II) as reported by others[6] may negate that association if sufficient case numbers existed to sufficiently power such an analysis. The length of the urethral involvement, a surrogate for tumor volume, was also an independent prognostic factor in patients treated for curative intent with radiation therapy, but the type of radiation therapy, external beam versus brachytherapy did not.[35] In this large series of 97 women treated at MDACC, local radiation failure occurred early; more than 95% of failures occurred in the first 2 years, with 5-year local control of 64%.

Nodal control is difficult. In the MDACC series, 1 of 3 patients with pelvic nodal disease treated with radiation therapy remained free of disease. Inguinal nodal disease was treated with lymphadenectomy after radiation therapy to the primary; of 4 positive dissections, 1 patient recurred at the primary site (radiation failure), 1 recurred in the inguinal nodal area (surgical failure), and 1 recurred in the pelvic nodes. Only 1 remained free of disease. Of the 73 women whose nodes were clinically negative at radiation treatment of the primary, 9 subsequently developed nodal disease; only 2 were survivors,[35] underscoring not only the importance of nodal surveillance, but the need to study prophylactic treatment of the clinically negative nodal sites.

Surgical complications are more commonly related to the risks of inguinal lymphadenectomy, or to the abdominal complications of diversion. Radical urethrectomy, as described in the Mayo Clinic series, with bladder neck closure and proximal diversion through an appendico-vesicostomy for distal lesions is theoretically associated with fistula from the bladder neck closure. Local control with this radical extirpation was excellent with no local or bladder recurrences in 7 patients so treated. Only 1 was transitional cell histology, and she remains with no evidence of disease with the bladder in situ after 58 months. Primary radiation therapy is associated with dose-related local complications, with severe local morbidity and loss of urethral function in 8 of 97 patients.[35] Higher-stage tumors, T3 and T4, should likely not be treated with any single modality. Certainly, high-grade disease treated with surgery or radiation alone leads almost invariably to metastatic disease and death.[17,38,43] The Mayo series included 35 clinical T3/T4 lesions with 1 survivor at 14 years after radical surgery alone. Analysis of survival using multimodal therapies are difficult at this time because of the low number of reported series and the nonparametric data.

Should a low-stage T1 or T2 primary be treated surgically, with deep pelvic node dissection and radiation therapy to the inguinal nodes? Should the primary be treated with radiation therapy, and an early local recurrence treated then with surgical extirpation? Is chemotherapy primary[46,58] or an adjunct to radiation therapy for bulky disease,[74,78] or should it be used in a neoadjuvant fashion for this difficult malignancy? Many of the questions regarding the individual and collective roles of surgical extirpation, nodal treatment, local control with radiation therapy versus surgery and of the systemic chemotherapy remain unanswered. Clinical trials are needed for this disease.

A high index of suspicion when evaluating the older female for new onset of lower urinary tract signs and symptoms would likely improve detection at lower stages when the disease is still amenable to as yet undefined standardized regimes.

REFERENCES

1. Dalbagni G, Zhang ZF, Lacombe L, et al. Male urethral carcinoma: analysis of treatment outcome. Urology 1999;53:1126–32.
2. Dinney CP, Johnson DE, Swanson DA, et al. Therapy and prognosis for male anterior urethral carcinoma: an update. Urology 1994;43:506–14.
3. Cohen M, Triaca V, Billmeyer B, et al. Coordinated chemoradiation therapy with genital preservation for the treatment of primary invasive carcinoma of the male urethra. J Urol 2008;179:536–41.
4. Gillitzer R, Hampel C, Wiesner C, et al. Single-institution experience with primary tumours of the male urethra. BJU Int 2007;101:964–8.
5. Smith Y, Hadway P, Ahmed S, et al. Penile-preserving surgery for male distal urethral carcinoma. BJU Int 2007;100:82–7.
6. Gheiler E, Tefilli M, Tiguert R, et al. Management of primary urethral cancer. Urology 1998;52:487–93.
7. Lieber M, Malek R, Farrow G, et al. Villous adenocarcinoma of the male urethra. J Urol 1983;83:1191–3.
8. Thiaudierre PD. Bull Gen De Therap 1834;240.
9. McCrea LE, Furlong JH Jr. Primary carcinoma of the male urethra. Urol Surv 1951;1:30.
10. Hotchkiss RS, Amelar RD. Primary carcinoma of the male urethra. J Urol 1954;72:1181.
11. Kaplan GW, Bulkey GJ, Grayhack JT. Carcinoma of the male urethra. J Urol 1967;98:365–71.
12. Farrer JH, Lupu AN. Carcinoma of deep male urethra. Urology 1984;24:527–31.
13. Bracken RB, Henry R, Ordonez N. Primary carcinoma of the male urethra. South Med J 1980;73:1003–5.
14. Klein FA, Whitmore WF, Herr HW, et al. Inferior pubic rami resection with en bloc radical excision for invasive proximal urethral carcinoma. Cancer 1983;51:1238–42.
15. Bracken RB. Exenterative surgery for posterior urethral cancer. Urology 1982;19:248–51.
16. Zeidman EJ, Desmond P, Thompson M. Surgical treatment of the male urethra. Urol Clin North Am 1992;19:359–72.
17. Eng TY, Naguib M, Galang T, et al. Retrospective study of the treatment of urethral cancer. Am J Clin Oncol 2003;26(6):558–62.
18. Mandler JL, Pool TL. Primary carcinoma of the male urethra. J Urol 1966;96:67–72.
19. Baskin LS, Turzan C. Carcinoma of male urethra: management of locally advanced disease with combined chemotherapy, radiotherapy, and penile-preserving surgery. Urology 1992;39:21–5.
20. Bird E, Coburn M. Phallus preservation for urethral cancer: subcutaneous penectomy. J Urol 1997;158:2146–8.
21. Davis J, Schellhammer P, Schlossberg S. Conservative surgical therapy for penile and urethral carcinoma. Urology 1999;53:386–92.
22. Kent D, Gee J, Amato R, et al. Successful management of metastatic urethral cancer with organ preservation. J Urol 2001;166:2308.
23. Christopher N, Arya M, Brown R, et al. Penile preservation in squamous cell carcinoma of the bulbo-membranous urethra. BJU Int 2002;89:464–5.
24. Hoffman MA, Renshaw AA, Loughlin KR. Squamous cell carcinoma of the penis and microscopic pathologic margins: how much margin is needed for local cure? Cancer 1999;85:1565–8.
25. Minhas S, Kayes O, Hegarty P, et al. What surgical resection margins are required to achieve oncological control in men with primary penile cancer? BJU Int 2005;96:1040–3.
26. Lont AP, Besnard AP, Gallee MP, et al. A comparison of physical examination and imaging in determining the extent of primary penile carcinoma. BJU Int 2003;91:493–5.
27. Scardino E, Villa G, Bonomo G, et al. Magnetic resonance imaging combined with artificial erection for local staging of penile cancer. Urology 2004;63:1158–62.
28. Cheville J, Dundore P, Bostwick D, et al. Transitional cell carcinoma of the prostate. Cancer 1998;82:703–7.
29. Palou J, Baniel J, Klotz L, et al. Urothelial carcinoma of the prostate. J Urol 2006;69:50–61.
30. Ghoniem G, Khater U, Hairston J, et al. Urinary retention caused by adenocarcinoma arising in recurrent urethral diverticulum. Int Urogynecol J Pelvic Floor Dysfunct 2004;15(5):363–5.
31. Thomas AA, Rackley RR, Lee U, et al. Urethral diverticula in 90 female patients: a study with emphasis on neoplastic alterations. J Urol 2008;180(6):2463–7.
32. Lang EK, Sethi E, Ordonez A, et al. Adenocarcinoma of suburethral diverticulum. J Urol 2008;179(2):728.
33. Noorani S, Rao AR, Callaghan PS. Urethral metastasis: an uncommon presentation of a colonic adenocarcinoma. Int Urol Nephrol 2007;39(3):837–9.
34. Swartz MA, Porter MP, Lin DW, et al. Incidence of primary urethral carcinoma in the United States. Urology 2006;68(6):1164–8.
35. Garden AS, Zagars GK, Delclos L. Primary carcinoma of the female urethra. Results of radiation therapy. Cancer 1993;71(10):3102–8.
36. Meis JM, Ayala AG, Johnson DE. Adenocarcinoma of the urethra in women. A clinicopathologic study. Cancer 1987;60(5):1038–52 [erratum appears in: Cancer 1987;60(12):2900].

37. Kim CJ, Pak K, Hamaguchi A, et al. Primary malignant melanoma of the female urethra. Cancer 1993;71(2):448–51.

38. DiMarco DS, DiMarco CS, Zincke H, et al. Surgical treatment for local control of female urethral carcinoma. Urol Oncol 2004;22(5):404–9.

39. DiMarco DS, DiMarco CS, Zincke H, et al. Outcome of surgical treatment for primary malignant melanoma of the female urethra. J Urol 2004;171(2 Pt 1):765–7.

40. Yokoyama H, Kontani K, Komiyama I, et al. Granular cell tumor of the urethra. Int J Urol 2007;14(5):461–2.

41. Takeuchi M, Matsuzaki K, Nishitani H. Clear cell adenocarcinoma of the female urethra: magnetic resonance imaging. J Comput Assist Tomogr 2009; 33(1):142–4.

42. Liu AX, Zhou JH, Jin HM, et al. Primary rhabdomyosarcoma of urethra in a 5-year-old girl: case report and literature review. Urology 2007;69(6):1208. e17–9.

43. Narayan P, Konety B. Surgical treatment of female urethral carcinoma. Urol Clin North Am 1992;19(2): 373–82.

44. Dalbagni G, Zhang ZF, Lacombe L, et al. Female urethral carcinoma: an analysis of treatment outcome and a plea for a standardized management strategy. Br J Urol 1998;82(6):835–41.

45. Kobashi KC, Hong TH, Leach GE. Undiagnosed urethral carcinoma: an unusual cause of female urinary retention. Urology 2000;55(3):436.

46. Nicholson S, Tsang D, Summerton D. Aggressive combined-modality therapy for squamous cell carcinoma of the female urethra. Nat Clin Pract Urol 2008; 5(10):574–7.

47. Filipkowski LA, Barker MA, Karram MM. Primary genitourinary melanoma presenting as voiding dysfunction. Int Urogynecol J 2009;20(9):1141–3.

48. Blaivas JG, Flisser AJ, Bleustein CB, et al. Periurethral masses: etiology and diagnosis in a large series of women. Obstet Gynecol 2004;103(5 Pt 1): 842–7.

49. Bracken RB, Johnson DE, Miller LS, et al. Primary carcinoma of the female urethra. J Urol 1976; 116(2):188–92.

50. Foster RT, Amundsen CL, Webster GD. The utility of magnetic resonance imaging for diagnosis and surgical planning before transvaginal periurethral diverticulectomy in women. Int Urogynecol J 2007; 18(3):315–9.

51. Kawashima A, Sandler CM, Wasserman NF, et al. Imaging of urethral disease: a pictorial review. Radiographics 2004;24(Suppl 1):S195–216.

52. Neitlich JD, Foster HE, Glickman MG, et al. Detection of urethral diverticula in women: comparison of a high resolution fast spin echo technique with double balloon urethrography. J Urol 1998;159(2): 408–10.

53. Hricak H, Secaf E, Buckley DW, et al. Female urethra: MR imaging. Radiology 1991;178(2):527–35.

54. Ryu J, Kim B. MR imaging of the male and female urethra. Radiographics 2001;21(5):1169–85.

55. Short S, Hoskin P, Wong W. Ovulation and increased FDG uptake on PET: potential for a false-positive result. Clin Nucl Med 2005;30(10):707.

56. Touijer AK, Dalbagni G. Role of voided urine cytology in diagnosing primary urethral carcinoma. Urology 2004;63(1):33–5.

57. Dell'Atti C, Missere M, Restaino G, et al. Primary lymphoma of the female urethra. Rays 2005;30(3): 269–72.

58. Inuzuka S, Koga S, Imanishi D, et al. Primary malignant lymphoma of the female urethra. Anticancer Res 2003; 23(3C):2925–7.

59. Vapnek JM, Turzan CW. Primary malignant lymphoma of the female urethra: report of a case and review of the literature. J Urol 1992;147(3):701–3.

60. Hara I, Hikosaka S, Eto H, et al. Successful treatment for squamous cell carcinoma of the female urethra with combined radio- and chemotherapy. Int J Urol 2004;11(8):678–82.

61. Tran LN, Krieg RM, Szabo RJ. Combination chemotherapy and radiotherapy for a locally advanced squamous cell carcinoma of the urethra: a case report. J Urol 1995;153(2):422–3.

62. Miller J, Karnes RJ. Primary clear-cell adenocarcinoma of the proximal female urethra: case report and review of the literature. Clin Genitourin Cancer 2008;6(2):131–3.

63. Cimentepe E, Bayrak O, Unsal A, et al. Urethral adenocarcinoma mimicking urethral caruncle. Int Urogynecol J 2006;17(1):96–8.

64. Nagano M, Hasui Y, Ide H, et al. Primary adenocarcinoma arising from a paraurethral cyst in a female patient. Urol Int 2002;69(3):244–6.

65. Yoshizawa T, Kawata N, Sato K, et al. Primary malignant melanoma of the female urethra. Urology 2007; 70(6):1222.e13–6.

66. Nakamoto T, Inoue Y, Ueki T, et al. Primary amelanotic malignant melanoma of the female urethra. Int J Urol 2007;14(2):153–5.

67. Kato H, Kobayashi S, Islam AM, et al. Female para-urethral adenocarcinoma: histological and immunohistochemical study. Int J Urol 2005;12(1): 117–9.

68. von Pechmann WS, Mastropietro MA, Roth TJ, et al. Urethral adenocarcinoma associated with urethral diverticulum in a patient with progressive voiding dysfunction. Am J Obstet Gynecol 2003;188(4): 1111–2.

69. Awakura Y, Nonomura M, Itoh N, et al. Adenocarcinoma of the female urethral diverticulum treated by multimodality therapy. Int J Urol 2003;10(5):281–3.

70. Murphy DP, Pantuck AJ, Amenta PS, et al. Female urethral adenocarcinoma: immunohistochemical

evidence of more than 1 tissue of origin. J Urol 1999; 161(6):1881–4.

71. Young D, Bilello S, Gomelsky A. Squamous cell carcinoma in situ in a female urethral diverticulum. South Med J 2007;100(5):537–9.

72. Shalev M, Mistry S, Kernen K, et al. Squamous cell carcinoma in a female urethral diverticulum. Urology 2002;59(5):773.

73. Carroll PR, Dixon CM. Surgical anatomy of the male and female urethra. Urol Clin North Am 1992;19(2):339–46.

74. Licht MR, Klein EA, Bukowski R, et al. Combination radiation and chemotherapy for the treatment of squamous cell carcinoma of the male and female urethra. J Urol 1995;153(6):1918–20.

75. Dalbagni G, Donat SM, Eschwege P, et al. Results of high dose rate brachytherapy, anterior pelvic exenteration and external beam radiotherapy for carcinoma of the female urethra. J Urol 2001;166(5): 1759–61.

76. Grigsby PW, Corn BW. Localized urethral tumors in women: indications for conservative versus exenterative therapies. J Urol 1992;147(6):1516–20.

77. Thyavihally YB, Wuntkal R, Bakshi G, et al. Primary carcinoma of the female urethra: single center experience of 18 cases. Jpn J Clin Oncol 2005;35(2):84–7.

78. Lee KC. Carcinoma of the female urethra responsive to moderate dose chemoradiotherapy. J Urol 2000; 163(3):905–6.

APPENDIX: STAGING

Definitions of TNM

Primary tumor (T) (male and female)

TX Primary tumor cannot be assessed

T0 No evidence of primary tumor

Ta Noninvasive papillary, polypoid, or verrucous carcinoma

Tis Carcinoma in situ

T1 Tumor invades subepithelial connective tissue

T2 Tumor invades any of the following: corpus spongiosum, prostate, periurethral muscle

T3 Tumor invades any of the following: corpus cavernosum, beyond prostatic capsule, anterior vagina, bladder neck

T4 Tumor invades other adjacent organs

Regional lymph nodes (N)

NX Regional lymph nodes cannot be assessed

N0 No regional lymph node metastasis

N1 Metastasis in a single lymph node 2 cm or less in greatest dimension

N2 Metastasis in a single node more than 2 cm in greatest dimension, or in multiple nodes

Distant metastasis (M)

M0 No distant metastasis

M1 Distant metastasis

Anatomic stage/prognostic groups

Stage 0a	Ta	N0	M0
Stage 0is	Tis	N0	M0
	Tis pu	N0	M0
	Tis pd	N0	M0
Stage I	T1	N0	M0
Stage II	T2	N0	M0
Stage III	T1	N1	M0
	T2	N1	M0
	T3	N0	M0
	T3	N1	M0
Stage IV	T4	N0	M0
	T4	N1	M0
	Any T	N2	M0
	Any T	Any N	M1

Urothelial (transitional cell) carcinoma of the prostate

Tis pu Carcinoma in situ, involvement of the prostatic urethra

Tis pd Carcinoma in situ, involvement of the prostatic ducts

T1 Tumor invades urethral subepithelial connective tissue

T2 Tumor invades any of the following: prostatic stroma, corpus spongiosum, periurethral muscle

T3 Tumor invades any of the following: corpus cavernosum, beyond prostatic capsule, bladder neck (extraprostatic extension)

T4 Tumor invades other adjacent organs (invasion of the bladder)

From AJCC cancer staging manual, Urethra, 7th edition, 2010; with permission.

Carcinoma of the Urethra: Radiation Oncology

Bridget F. Koontz, MD*, W. Robert Lee, MD, MS, MEd

KEYWORDS

- Urethra • Radiotherapy • Chemoradiation
- Combined modality therapy

Primary urethral cancer is a rare diagnosis in men and women, presenting most commonly with bleeding or obstruction. The most common histologic finding is squamous cell carcinoma, although adenocarcinoma and transitional cell carcinoma also occur.[1]

Anatomically, the urethra in men can be divided into 3 sections: the penile (or pendulous) urethra, the bulbomembranous urethra, and the prostatic urethra. In women, the distal half of the urethra is considered the anterior urethra and the proximal half is considered the posterior urethra. Lymphatic drainage patterns follow the surrounding organs and are different for the 3 regions of the urethra. Initial drainage patterns for the penile urethra include the superficial and deep inguinal nodes. The bulbomembranous urethra is drained by the internal and external iliac nodes. Sites of drainage for the prostatic urethra include the internal and external iliacs, the obturator, and the presacral nodal beds.[1,2]

Historically, urethral cancer carries a poor prognosis, and location and stage affect outcome. Distal lesions have a similar outcome as penile cancer of the same stage and are often treated with similar techniques. Early distal lesions have a very good prognosis with primary excision (70%–100% disease-free survival [DFS]).[3–6] Prostatic lesions behave and are treated in the same way as bladder carcinoma. Bulbomembranous urethral cancers are more often locally advanced and difficult to manage with surgical techniques; this location carries the worst prognosis (25% DFS).[4–7]

ROLE OF RADIATION IN EARLY-STAGE URETHRAL CANCERS

For small early-stage cancers, a single modality treatment may offer a good chance of control and may limit overall morbidity of therapy. Primary management of urethral cancers in men is most often surgical. In women, radiotherapy is more often the primary modality because of the morbidity associated with surgical management. Radiotherapy, using external beam radiotherapy (EBRT), brachytherapy (BT), or a combination of the two, seems to have equivalent results as surgery, given that all results have been reported in case review form (**Table 1**).

A review from MD Anderson Cancer Center, including 5 women with early-stage urethral cancer, reported excellent local control with 4 out of 5 patients without evidence of disease at a median follow-up of 4 years. Treatment included BT in 4 patients (60 Gy using radium or iridium needles) and a combination of EBRT and BT in 1 patient (70 Gy).[8] Moinuddin Ali and colleagues[9] reported on 3 women with early-stage urethral cancers who were treated with EBRT (40–50 Gy) with a BT boost dose of 28 to 30 Gy. All the 3 patients remained disease free at follow-up periods of 20, 30, and 30 months, respectively.

Radiotherapy alone may be the most optimal treatment in early-stage tumors involving only the distal urethra. In a series from the University of Maryland, 3 women with distal urethral cancers had local control at extended follow-up; disease

Financial disclosure: None.
Department of Radiation Oncology, Duke University Medical Center, Box 3085, Durham, NC 22710, USA
* Corresponding author.
E-mail address: bridget.koontz@duke.edu

Urol Clin N Am 37 (2010) 459–466
doi:10.1016/j.ucl.2010.04.007

Table 1
Results of treatment for early-stage urethral cancer

| | | Gender | Number of Patients | Treatment, (#) Indicates Number of Patients Receiving Treatment | | | Mean Follow-up (mo) | OS (%) | CSM (%) | DFS (%) | LC (%) |
				Neoadjuvant	Primary	Adjuvant					
Eng et al[12]	2003	M/F	10		Surgery (9); CRT (1)		189	70[a]	0[a]	70[a]	100[a]
Dalbagni et al[5]	1999	M	10		Surgery		125	83[b]			
Gheiler et al[3]	1998	M/F	9	CRT (2)	Surgery	RT (1)	42			89[a]	
Moinuddin et al[9]	1988	F	3	40 Gy (1)	Surgery		118	67[a]	0[a]	33[a]	67[a]
Farrer and Lupu[31]	1984	M	2	45 Gy (1)	Surgery		102	100[a]	0[a]	100[a]	100[a]
Dinney et al[6]	1994	M	6		Surgery (5); CRT (1)		55	83[a]	83[a]	83[a]	83[a]
Moinuddin et al[9]	1988	F	3		EBRT+BT		27	67[a]	0[a]	67[a]	100[a]
Johnson and O'Connell[8]	1983	F	5		BT ± EBRT		41	80[a]	0[a]	60[a]	60[a]
Prempree et al[10]	1984	F	7		BT ± EBRT		ns			71[b]	71[b]

Crude OS equals number of patients alive at last follow-up divided by total number of patients.
CSM equals number of patients dead because of the disease divided by total number of patients.
DFS equals number of patients alive without disease divided by total number of patients.
LC equals number of patients with local control divided by total number of patients.
Abbreviations: CRT, chemoradiation; CSM, cause-specific mortality; CT, chemotherapy; F, female; LC, local control; M, male; ns, not stated; OS, overall survival; RT, radiotherapy.
[a] Crude rate.
[b] Five-year actuarial data.

was controlled only half of the time in 4 women with early-stage tumors involving the proximal urethra.[10] Weghaupt and colleagues[11] confirm this finding in an institutional review of 62 women from the University of Vienna. Five-year overall survival was 71% for women with anterior lesions and 50% for women with distal lesions (outcome was not otherwise evaluated by stage, although most patients were node negative).

Dinney and colleagues[6] reported excellent survival and local control for early-stage urethral cancers of men treated in 5 out of 6 cases by partial penectomy or urethrectomy. One more patient with a stage B bulbomembranous lesion refused surgery and was treated with 66 Gy and concurrent chemotherapy; this patient was disease free at 30 months of follow-up. A series of 9 low-stage distal cancers in both genders found that 83% of patients treated with surgery alone (5 of 6) and 100% of those treated with combination therapy (2 with neoadjuvant chemo-radiation and 1 with adjuvant radiation) remained disease free with a mean follow-up of 49 months.[3]

ROLE OF RADIATION IN ADVANCED-STAGE URETHRAL CANCERS

For more advanced lesions, a multidisciplinary approach is frequently recommended. Although no rigorous comparisons have been published, there seems to be improved local control and cure rates in patients treated with a multidisciplinary approach when compared with surgery alone. In one series, patients treated with combination therapy had improved DFS rate compared with patients managed with surgery alone (45 vs 23 months).[12] Many series reporting outcomes of advanced disease after surgery or radiation therapy as the sole modality showed poor outcomes (**Table 2**). Concurrent chemotherapy with definitive radiation doses seems more promising, with 80% to 100% complete response rates and 60% to 80% crude DFS rates (**Table 3**).

Adjuvant Radiotherapy

In patients treated with surgical resection, local recurrence is common and associated with significant morbidity and increased cancer-specific deaths. Local control in penile lesions can be reasonably achieved with surgery in node-negative penile lesions (89% in one series[6]) but is low in bulbomembranous lesions treated surgically (38% in the same series[6]).

Local recurrence is associated with cancer-related death. In a study in 72 women, Dalbagni and colleagues[13] reported a 10-year disease-specific survival (DSS) rate of 68% versus 18%

based on the presence of local recurrence. Adjuvant radiotherapy has been proposed for locally advanced lesions with the goal of reducing recurrence risk and thereby affecting survival. Narayan and Konety[14] reported an overall survival difference between cohorts of women with locally advanced urethral cancer who did or did not receive radiotherapy in addition to surgery (5% vs 34%).[14]

One case report described 4 men with locally advanced penile squamous cell carcinoma treated with cisplatin and 5-fluorouracil (5-FU), in which all had partial responses. One patient went on to receive surgical resection (including inguinal nodal dissection) and adjuvant radiotherapy, whereas the 3 remaining patients received adjuvant radiotherapy only. Although all the patients eventually died of their disease, 2 were able to achieve disease-free intervals of 18 months.[15]

Adjuvant radiotherapy is complicated by the healing tissues within the potentially contaminated surgical bed. External radiation in this situation must be performed with care respecting the tolerance of critical structures, particularly bowel. BT has been used to reduce the exposure of bowel and other structures to radiation, while allowing a high dose to the surgical bed. This technique can be performed using interstitially placed catheters to hold either high-dose or low-dose rate temporary sources, or can be accomplished intraoperatively, which allows the normal structures to be physically moved and/or shielded. Successful intraoperative high-dose rate BT has been reported, with competitive local control (crude rate 67% at 21-month mean follow-up).[13]

Neoadjuvant Radiotherapy

Dalbagni and colleagues[16] reported an improvement in local relapse–free survival with the use of neoadjuvant radiotherapy. In a review of 30 patients, none of the 10 patients receiving radiotherapy had disease recurrence compared with 15 of 20 patients treated only with excision (actuarial 5-year local recurrence–free survival [LRFS] 37%). Although retrospective, the investigators reported similar staging between the 2 cohorts. No overall survival difference was seen based on the use of preoperative radiotherapy. A small series of men treated to between 20 and 60 Gy followed by surgery reported an absolute locoregional failure rate of 29%.[17]

Gheiler and colleagues[3] published a small series on men and women with primary urethral cancer. Of the 12 patients with advanced-stage (all proximal/bulbomembranous) cancer, 2 patients treated with surgery alone failed, whereas 57%

Table 2
Results of treatment for advanced-stage urethral cancer

| | | Number of Patients | Treatment, (#) Indicates Number of Patients Receiving Treatment | | | Mean Follow-up (mo) | OS (%) | CSM (%) | DFS (%) | LC (%) |
	Gender		Neoadjuvant	Primary	Adjuvant					
Moinuddin et al[9] 1995	F	3		Surgery		19	67[a]	33[a]	0[a]	33[a]
Dalbagni et al[5] 1999	M	36		Surgery (30), RT (6)		125	45[b]			
Dalbagni et al[13] 2001	F	6	CT (4)	Surgery	EBRT+BT	21	50[a]	50[a]	33[a]	67[a]
Dalbagni et al[16] 1998	F	ns	RT	EBRT ± BT or surgery		85	22[b]	67[b]		
Dinney et al[6] 1994	M	14		Surgery (13), CRT (1)	CT (6)	55	50[a]	36[a]	43[a]	71[a]
Gheiler et al[3] 1998	M/F	12		Surgery (3), CRT (9)	CT (1)	42			42[a]	
Farrer et al[31] 1984	M	8		Surgery (6), CRT (2)	RT (1), CT (2)	18	0[a]	88[a]	0[a]	88[a]
Moinuddin et al[9] 1995	F	4	20–30 Gy	Surgery		35	75[a]	25[a]	25[a]	50[a]
Johnson and O'Connell[8] 1983	F	7	50 Gy	Surgery		6	71[a]	29[a]	43[a]	43[a]
Johnson and O'Connell[8] 1983	F	6		BT ± EBRT		26	67[a]	17[a]	67[a]	83[a]
Kuettel et al[27] 1997	F	4		EBRT+BT (66–70 Gy)		29	25[a]	50[a]	25[a]	100[a]
Prempree et al[10] 1984	F	7		BT ± EBRT		ns			71[b]	86[b]

Crude OS equals number of patients alive at last follow-up divided by total number of patients.
CSM equals number of patients dead because of the disease divided by total number of patients.
DFS equals number of patients alive without disease divided by total number of patients.
LC equals number of patients with local control divided by total number of patients.
Abbreviations: CSM, cause-specific mortality; CT, chemotherapy; F, female; LC, local control; M, male; OS, overall survival; RT, radiotherapy; ns, not stated.
[a] Crude rate.
[b] Five-year actuarial data.

Table 3
Results of definitive chemoradiation

		Gender	Number of Patients	Treatment Chemotherapy	Radiation Dose	Adjuvant	Mean Follow-up	OS	CSS	LC
Cohen et al[26]	2008	M	18	MMC/5-FU	45–55 Gy			60%[b]	72%[b]	56%[a]
Gheiler et al[3]	1998	M/F	10	CDDP/5-FU or MVAC	70–75 Gy	Surgery (7)	32			72%[a]
								ANED	AWD	DWD
Oberfield et al[32]	1996	M	2	MMC/5-FU	45 Gy		34	2		
Tran et al[24]	1995	F	1	MMC/5-FU	55.8 Gy		66	1		
Shah et al[23]	1985	F	1	MMC/5-FU	30 Gy		30	1		
Licht et al[22]	1995	M/F	4	MMC/5-FU	30–50 Gy		61	3		
Lutz and Huang[25]	1995	M	1	MMC/5-FU	51.2 Gy		16	1	1	1
Baskin and Turzan[21]	1992	M	1	MMC/5-FU	40 Gy	Surgery	ns	1		
Hussein et al[15]	1990	M	4	CDDP/5-FU	45–54 Gy	Surgery (1)	11	4		
Farrer and Lupu[31]	1984	M	1	CTX/5-FU	60 Gy		7			1
Total			15					13	1	2
								0.87		

LC equals number of patients with local control divided by total number of patients.
Abbreviations: 5-FU, 5-fluorouracil; AWD, alive with disease; ANED, alive no evidence of disease; CDDP, cisplatin; CSS, cause-specific survival; CTX, cyclophosphamide; DWD, dead with disease; F, female; LC, local control; M, male; MMC, mitomycin C; ns, not stated; OS, overall survival.
[a] Crude rate.
[b] Five-year actuarial data.

of the patients treated with chemoradiation, either pre- or postoperatively, remained disease free at a mean follow-up of 32 months. One of the 3 patients treated with definitive chemoradiation remained cancer free.

Definitive Radiotherapy

In locally advanced cancers, definitive radiation monotherapy shows poor results. Dalbagni and colleagues[16] reported on 29 patients who underwent primary radiotherapy with surgery for salvage; LRFS was similar for patients who were initially treated surgically. However, another report on 42 women suggested that radiotherapy results in better local control than surgery alone.[18]

Some evidence exists suggesting that higher doses provided by a combination of EBRT and BT are more effective. Milosevic and colleagues[19] reported that in a multivariate analysis taking stage, location, and tumor extension to adjacent structures into account, patients treated with only external radiation (received median 50 Gy) were 4.2 times more likely to fail locally than patients who received BT as part of their treatment.

Garden and colleagues[20] reported on 84 women with urethral cancer treated at MD Anderson Cancer Center between 1955 and 1989. Although women of all stages were included in the analysis, most were women with larger tumors involving the entire urethra. Patients were treated with either BT, EBRT, or both, depending on the size and location of the tumor. Local control and cause-specific survival rates were 64% and 49%, respectively, at 5 years, and the overall survival rate was 41%. The length of urethral involvement was independently prognostic for both outcomes; women with only partial involvement had a local control rate of 74% compared with 55% for those with cancer involving the entire urethra.

Definitive Chemoradiation

The combination of chemotherapy with primary radiotherapy may allow for sufficient tumor regression to allow for less extensive surgical procedures or reserve surgery for salvage. Multiple investigators have put forth case reports showing good response to combined chemotherapy and radiation (see **Table 3**).[3,7,21–25] Some of these studies used mitomycin C (MMC) and 5-FU based on anal squamous cell carcinoma, whereas other studies used cisplatin and 5-FU. For transitional cell cancers, a bladder-based regimen such as methotrexate, vinblastine, doxorubicin, and cisplatin (MVAC) is the most appropriate agent.

Cohen and colleagues[26] described 18 patients treated on a protocol of definitive external radiotherapy combined with MMC and 5-FU. Patients received between 45 and 55 Gy to the pelvis, with gross disease boosted an additional 12 to –15 Gy. MMC was given 10 mg/m^2 by bolus intravenous injection on days 1 and 29, and 5-FU was given as a 24-hour continuous infusion from days 1 to 4 and 29 to 32. Surgery was reserved for salvage. Despite a significant proportion of advanced disease (55% T3–4, 32% N+), DSS rate at 5 years was 72%. Of the 15 complete responders, 10 remained disease free and did not require disfiguring surgery. The investigators noted that all patients eventually did develop urethral stricture requiring dilation or reconstructive surgery.

Gheiler and colleagues[3] tabulated the outcome of these case reports to find a crude rate of disease control of 70% with a mean follow-up of 43 months. Half of the 20 patients reported did not have any attempt at resection, and 6 remained disease free at the last follow-up.

TECHNIQUE

Traditional external beam fields have included a 2-field whole pelvic therapy treating bilateral common, internal, and external iliacs and, depending on the location, inguinal lymph nodes. Nodal drainage patterns closely follow penile tissue for penile urethral lesions, so coverage of bilateral inguinal regions is recommended for distal urethral cancers. Using traditional methods, inguinal dose could be entirely from the photon fields (a wide anterior to posterior parallel pair technique) or boosted with superficially penetrating electrons (wide-AP narrow-PA technique). Initial fields should be taken to 45 Gy in 25 fractions.

Boosting gross primary disease can be performed using a perineal field or interstitial therapy. A perineal field is most effective for women with superficial tumors. Low-dose rate iridium Ir 192 sources can be used with a template or urethral catheter,[27] if the tissue depth is less than 5 mm. A vaginal cylinder helps to push posterior vaginal tissues out of the high-dose region.

Recently, intensity-modulated radiation therapy (IMRT) has been used more often in treating anal cancer and gynecologic malignancies for the primary and boost treatment.[28,29] IMRT in this region has reduced both acute and late toxicities without losing efficacy. When using IMRT, the radiation oncologist must take care to adequately define areas at risk for microscopic disease extension with appropriate expansions for motion and setup error.

TOXICITY

Severe complication rates for definitive radiotherapy are reported between 16% and 20%.[19,20,30] The most common severe toxicity is fistula development, which is more likely with advanced tumors eroding into the vagina, bladder, or rectum. Fistula formation can be associated with recurrent disease. In the setting of organ-sparing treatment, urethral stricture is common, although it is usually effectively treated with balloon dilation. Cystitis or bladder hemorrhage can also occur.

Grigsby[30] reported the Mallinckrodt Institute experience for women with urethral cancer treated by surgical or radiation means. Severe complications were observed in 19% of women treated with radiation therapy. These included rectovaginal fistula formation and vaginal or rectal stricture. All complications occurred when tumor dose was at or more than 70 Gy. Care must be taken with larger lesions involving the vagina or other nearby structures, because fistula formation is more likely in this setting.

Another review of 55 patients with local control after definitive radiation found that cumulative dose was related to risk of complication. The risk of toxicity was reduced with doses of 60 Gy or less; in fact, no severe complication occurred at less than 65 Gy.[20]

SUMMARY

Early lesions can be effectively treated with excision or radiotherapy depending on the preference for organ preservation. Combined chemoradiation seems to be more effective than traditional surgery with adjuvant or neoadjuvant radiotherapy for advanced-stage urethral cancers.

REFERENCES

1. Mansur DB, Chao KSC. Penis and male urethra. In: Perez CA, Brady LW, Halperin EC, et al, editors. Principles and practice of radiation oncology. 4th edition. Philadelphia: Lippincott Williams and Wilkins; 2004. p. 1785–99.

2. Rouviere H. Anatomy of the human lymphatic system. Ann Arbor (MI): Edward Brothers, Inc; 1938.

3. Gheiler EL, Tefilli MV, Tiguert R, et al. Management of primary urethral cancer. Urology 1998;52(3):487–93.

4. Konnak JW. Conservative management of low grade neoplasms of the male urethra: a preliminary report. J Urol 1980;123(2):175–7.

5. Dalbagni G, Zhang ZF, Lacombe L, et al. Male urethral carcinoma: analysis of treatment outcome. Urology 1999;53(6):1126–32.

6. Dinney CP, Johnson DE, Swanson DA, et al. Therapy and prognosis for male anterior urethral carcinoma: an update. Urology 1994;43(4):506–14.

7. Ray B, Canto AR, Whitmore WF. Experience with primary carcinoma of the male urethra. J Urol 1977;117(5):591–4.

8. Johnson DE, O'Connell JR. Primary carcinoma of female urethra. Urology 1983;21(1):42–5.

9. Moinuddin Ali M, Klein FA, Hazra TA. Primary female urethral carcinoma. A retrospective comparison of different treatment techniques. Cancer 1988;62(1):54–7.

10. Prempree T, Amornmarn R, Patanaphan V. Radiation therapy in primary carcinoma of the female urethra. II. An update on results. Cancer 1984;54(4):729–33.

11. Weghaupt K, Gerstner GJ, Kucera H. Radiation therapy for primary carcinoma of the female urethra: a survey over 25 years. Gynecol Oncol 1984;17(1):58–63.

12. Eng TY, Naguib M, Galang T, et al. Retrospective study of the treatment of urethral cancer. Am J Clin Oncol 2003;26(6):558–62.

13. Dalbagni G, Donat SM, Eschwege P, et al. Results of high dose rate brachytherapy, anterior pelvic exenteration and external beam radiotherapy for carcinoma of the female urethra. J Urol 2001;166(5):1759–61.

14. Narayan P, Konety B. Surgical treatment of female urethral carcinoma. Urol Clin North Am 1992;19(2):373–82.

15. Hussein AM, Benedetto P, Sridhar KS. Chemotherapy with cisplatin and 5-fluorouracil for penile and urethral squamous cell carcinomas. Cancer 1990;65(3):433–8.

16. Dalbagni G, Zhang ZF, Lacombe L, et al. Female urethral carcinoma: an analysis of treatment outcome and a plea for a standardized management strategy. Br J Urol 1998;82(6):835–41.

17. Klein FA, Whitmore WF Jr, Herr HW, et al. Inferior pubic rami resection with en bloc radical excision for invasive proximal urethral carcinoma. Cancer 1983;51(7):1238–42.

18. Foens CS, Hussey DH, Staples JJ, et al. A comparison of the roles of surgery and radiation therapy in the management of carcinoma of the female urethra. Int J Radiat Oncol Biol Phys 1991;21(4):961–8.

19. Milosevic MF, Warde PR, Banerjee D, et al. Urethral carcinoma in women: results of treatment with primary radiotherapy. Radiother Oncol 2000;56(1):29–35.

20. Garden AS, Zagars GK, Delclos L. Primary carcinoma of the female urethra. Results of radiation therapy. Cancer 1993;71(10):3102–8.

21. Baskin LS, Turzan C. Carcinoma of male urethra: management of locally advanced disease with combined chemotherapy, radiotherapy, and penile-preserving surgery. Urology 1992;39(1):21–5.

22. Licht MR, Klein EA, Bukowski R, et al. Combination radiation and chemotherapy for the treatment of squamous cell carcinoma of the male and female urethra. J Urol 1995;153(6):1918–20.

23. Shah AB, Kalra JK, Silber L, et al. Squamous cell cancer of female urethra. Successful treatment with chemoradiotherapy. Urology 1985;25(3):284–6.

24. Tran LN, Krieg RM, Szabo RJ. Combination chemotherapy and radiotherapy for a locally advanced squamous cell carcinoma of the urethra: a case report. J Urol 1995;153(2):422–3.

25. Lutz ST, Huang DT. Combined chemoradiotherapy for locally advanced squamous cell carcinoma of the bulbomembranous urethra: a case report. J Urol 1995;153(5):1616–8.

26. Cohen MS, Triaca V, Billmeyer B, et al. Coordinated chemoradiation therapy with genital preservation for the treatment of primary invasive carcinoma of the male urethra. J Urol 2008; 179(2):536–41 [discussion: 541].

27. Kuettel MR, Parda DS, Harter KW, et al. Treatment of female urethral carcinoma in medically inoperable patients using external beam irradiation and high dose rate intracavitary brachytherapy. J Urol 1997; 157(5):1669–71.

28. Kidd EA, Siegel BA, Dehdashti F, et al. Clinical outcomes of definitive intensity-modulated radiation therapy with fluorodeoxyglucose-positron emission tomography simulation in patients with locally advanced cervical cancer. Int J Radiat Oncol Biol Phys 2009. [Epub ahead of print].

29. Salama JK, Mell LK, Schomas DA, et al. Concurrent chemotherapy and intensity-modulated radiation therapy for anal canal cancer patients: a multicenter experience. J Clin Oncol 2007;25(29):4581–6.

30. Grigsby PW. Carcinoma of the urethra in women. Int J Radiat Oncol Biol Phys 1998;41(3):535–41.

31. Farrer JH, Lupu AN. Carcinoma of deep male urethra. Urology 1984;24(6):527–31.

32. Oberfield RA, Zinman LN, Leibenhaut M, et al. Management of invasive squamous cell carcinoma of the bulbomembranous male urethra with co-ordinated chemo-radiotherapy and genital preservation. Br J Urol 1996;78(4):573–8.

Chemotherapy for Penile and Urethral Carcinoma

Edouard J. Trabulsi, MD[a,*], Jean Hoffman-Censits, MD[b]

KEYWORDS

• Penile carcinoma • Urethral carcinoma • Chemotherapy

Systemic therapy for carcinoma of the penis and urethra is considered for locally advanced disease as part of a multimodal treatment regimen, or for suspected or proven metastatic disease. The mainstay of systemic therapy for these conditions has traditionally been cytotoxic chemotherapeutic agents, but may incorporate small-molecule targeted agents in the future as their use widens with other solid tumors. The field is limited, however, by the relative rarity of the disease in the Western world, and the lack of robust, large clinical trials to date. This article reviews the systemic therapy agents and data available for these conditions in the neoadjuvant or adjuvant setting as well as for metastatic disease, and highlights the importance of stage and histology for these categories.

PENILE SQUAMOUS CELL CARCINOMA

Penile carcinoma is a rare tumor in the Western world, with only 1290 cases expected in the United States in 2009.[1] Unfortunately, because of the disease site, patient reluctance, and social mores, patients commonly present with advanced disease.[2,3] Therefore, effective systemic therapies are necessary and are commonly incorporated into multimodal treatment regimens. These strategies are palliative, to debulk advanced tumors in an attempt at local control, as well as potentially curative for lesser burdens of disease.

Neoadjuvant Chemotherapy for Bulky/ Unresectable Disease

Patients presenting with locally advanced penile tumors with clinically negative inguinal lymph nodes are typically treated surgically initially, with chemotherapy considered in the adjuvant setting for high-risk patients. If patients have unresectable locally advanced penile tumors, or bulky inguinal nodal disease, neoadjuvant chemotherapy before surgical consolidation can be considered. Multiple cytotoxic agents have been reported to be active for penile carcinoma, either as single agent or in combination, including methotrexate, bleomycin, cisplatin, and 5-fluorouracil (5-FU).

Small, retrospective, single-institution studies have investigated neoadjuvant chemotherapy for unresectable disease. Leijte and colleagues[4] reported on a 33-year experience from Amsterdam of 20 patients with unresectable inguinal lymphadenopathy, with a total of 5 different chemotherapy regimens used neoadjuvantly during that time period. In this series, single-agent bleomycin was used until 1985; from 1985 to 1999 combination bleomycin, vincristine, and methotrexate (VBM) were administered; cisplatin and 5-FU were given from 1999 to 2001; and since 2001 a 3-drug regimen of cisplatin, bleomycin, and methotrexate has been used, with 1 patient receiving cisplatin and irinotecan on a separate protocol. There was an overall response rate of 63%, and 5-year survival of 32%. There was

a Department of Urology, Kimmel Cancer Center, Thomas Jefferson University, 1015 Walnut Street, Suite 1102, Philadelphia, PA 19107, USA
b Department of Medical Oncology, Kimmel Cancer Center, Thomas Jefferson University, 834 Chestnut Street, Suite 314, Philadelphia, PA 19107, USA
* Corresponding author.
E-mail address: edouard.trabulsi@jefferson.edu

Urol Clin N Am 37 (2010) 467–474
doi:10.1016/j.ucl.2010.04.010

marked difference in survival between chemotherapy responders and nonresponders: 56% 5-year survival in responders versus all nonresponders died within 9 months. Of the responders, 9 underwent consolidative surgical resection, with 8 of these patients achieving durable long-term survival. The chemotherapy regimens did carry significant toxicity, however, with 3 toxic deaths and cessation of chemotherapy because of toxicity in 1 patient. Using a similar VBM regimen, investigators from Milan reported a small pilot neoadjuvant and adjuvant study of 17 patients, including 5 patients receiving neoadjuvant therapy.[5] Of these 5 patients with bulky unresectable inguinal nodal disease, 3 (60%) had a partial response to VBM, allowing consolidative surgery with durable disease-free responses; the 2 nonresponders died within 1 year of diagnosis.

In a another study from Texas, Bermejo and colleagues[6] reported on the MD Anderson experience with surgical resection after neoadjuvant chemotherapy for unresectable penile squamous cell carcinoma from 1985 to 2000 in 10 patients. These patients received several different chemotherapy combinations, including bleomycin, methotrexate, cisplatin (BMP), ifosfamide, paclitaxel, cisplatin (ITP), or paclitaxel/carboplatin. These 10 patients, drawn from a total cohort of 59 patients who presented with locally advanced or metastatic penile carcinoma, had a complete (4) or partial response (1) or stable disease (5) after chemotherapy; the remaining 49 patients remained unresectable after chemotherapy or had progressive disease. The 5-year survival for these 10 patients was 40%, with a median survival of 26 months. Notably, there were 3 patients with pathologic complete response (pN0), all of whom received ITP. All patients with 3 or more positive lymph nodes found at consolidative surgical resection after neoadjuvant chemotherapy ultimately died of their disease.

A notable phase II trial of chemotherapy, one of the few multi-institutional clinical trials ever conducted for penile carcinoma, was performed by the Southwest Oncology Group (SWOG), investigating a combination of cisplatin, methotrexate, and bleomycin (PMB) in 45 patients.[7] This study followed an earlier phase II SWOG trial of single-agent cisplatin for advanced disease, which reported poor response rates for cisplatin monotherapy.[8] There was a significant response rate to combination PMB chemotherapy, with an overall response rate of 33% and 5 complete responses. Similar to the retrospective analysis from Amsterdam, however, there was considerable toxicity with this regimen, with 5 treatment-related deaths and 6 grade 4 toxicities, and the investigators concluded that less toxic regimens were necessary.

More recently, a pilot study from Milan examined a combination regimen of paclitaxel, cisplatin, and 5-FU (TPF) in 6 patients, including neoadjuvant therapy in 2 patients, and in recurrent inguinal nodal disease after lymphadenectomy in 4, with consolidative lymphadenectomy planned in all patients.[9] Two patients completed 4 courses of TPF and had a pathologically confirmed complete response, and 3 others had significant tumor responses to TPF, indicating that TPF is very active in penile carcinoma, within the limitations of such a small study.

In a review by Culkin and Beer,[10] when combining the published literature of several cisplatin-based combination chemotherapy regimens, a response rate of 69% (24/35) was calculated in patients with unresectable nodal disease, highlighting the chemoresponsiveness of this disease. In summary, as advocated by the recent European Urology Association (EUA) practice guidelines,[11] neoadjuvant chemotherapy for locally advanced disease does demonstrate significant response when combination chemotherapy is used, and can allow subsequent surgical resection of previously unresectable disease in up to half of cases.[12] Surgical consolidation, however, is necessary to maximize long-term durable freedom of disease, even with dramatic clinical and radiographic responses to chemotherapy alone.

Adjuvant Chemotherapy

Despite aggressive surgery, the relapse rate and eventual cancer-related morbidity and mortality remain depressingly high for node-positive penile carcinoma. The 5-year survival for node-negative disease was 95% in a large retrospective single-institution review from India from 1962 to 1986, declining to 76% with positive inguinal lymph nodes, and no 5-year survivors when deep pelvic nodes were involved.[13] Therefore, multiple chemotherapy agents and combinations have been described in the adjuvant setting when positive lymph nodes are discovered after lymphadenectomy. The number of lymph nodes involved is an important predictor of recurrence, and the recent EUA guidelines advocate adjuvant chemotherapy for pN2-3 disease, but not for pN1 disease.[11]

The largest published series to date have come from the Milan group, where initially VBM was administered adjuvantly from 1979 to 1990, with improved long-term survival compared with historical controls.[5] Since 1991, cisplatin with 5-FU has been the primary adjuvant regimen given, with improved survival and lower toxicity.[11,12]

In another small retrospective review from Dresden, Germany, patients with penile carcinoma who received combination PMB chemotherapy were evaluated from 1996 to 2003.[14] This study represented a mixed cohort of 13 patients, including 8 patients receiving adjuvant therapy after lymphadenectomy and 5 patients with metastatic disease. Of the 8 patients receiving PMB in the adjuvant setting, 3 patients (38%) had a durable response, with no evidence of disease at a mean of 54 months. Although the patients with metastasis fared very poorly in this study, the investigators concluded that there was benefit in the adjuvant setting, but as with other studies of PMB, the toxicity is high.

Induction Chemotherapy for Metastatic Disease

Single-agent experience

Data on chemotherapy treatment of locally advanced or metastatic penile carcinoma is limited and difficult to generalize. Most of the available data are retrospective case series or studies with small numbers using mixed populations, including patients receiving chemotherapy in the neoadjuvant, adjuvant, and recurrent settings. In addition, many studies include patients whose regimens were also combined with radiation therapy or salvage surgery for cure.

Reports of the use of single-agent chemotherapy were scattered in the literature in penile cancer in the 1960s to 1980s. Reports using bleomycin, methotrexate, and cisplatin alone showed modest efficacy of short duration.

Experience with bleomycin was first reported by a Japanese group in 1969.[15] Biweekly intravenous or intramuscular bleomycin was delivered at 15 mg, and objective response was seen in 6 of 8 patients. One patient who showed complete response died of pneumonia while on treatment. Experience with bleomycin in combination with radiotherapy as a single agent, or in conjunction with vincristine and methotrexate, was also reported in 1983.[16] The investigators found improved response in patients with well-differentiated squamous cell carcinoma but also reported significant pulmonary toxicity, with pneumonitis in 3 and fibrotic changes in 6 of the 19 patients treated.

Single-agent cisplatin was used in 9 patients treated at the Memorial Sloan Kettering Cancer Center (MSKCC) in the 1970s.[17] Low (1.6–2.0 mg/kg) and high doses (3 mg/kg or 120 mg/m^2) of cisplatin were given every 21 days with an overall response rate of 33%, with 1 complete response lasting several months. An additional patient died 5 days following cisplatin administration. Permanent and transient renal insufficiency as well as tinnitus were observed. Before the availability of newer generation antiemetics, nausea and vomiting often delayed subsequent chemotherapy cycles.

The SWOG published their data on single agent cisplatin a decade later.[8] In this series of 26 patients, cisplatin at 50 mg/m^2 given weekly for 2 weeks on and 2 weeks off demonstrated little activity, with 4 partial responses lasting only 3 months. Toxicity included cytopenias, nausea, and vomiting. Entry criteria for the study included creatinine clearance greater than 60 mL/min. Following treatment 9 patients had a decline in creatinine clearance to less than 50 mL/min, and 2 patients had creatinine clearance less than 30 mL/min.

Success of single-agent high-dose methotrexate chemotherapy with leucovorin rescue was reported by Garnick and colleagues[18] in a patient who had disease progression while undergoing radiation treatment. Complete pathologic response was noted after 10 weekly cycles lasting for 9 months, when the patient suffered sudden infectious pulmonary death. Sklaroff and Yagoda[19] of MSKCC also reported on experience with high- and low-dose methotrexate. In this group of 8 patients, 5 had previously undergone radiotherapy or chemotherapy, and the overall response rate to methotrexate treatment was 38%. Five patients were treated with high-dose chemotherapy, of whom 2 achieved partial remission lasting as long as 11 months. The remaining 3 patients were given low-dose therapy, with 1 short-lived partial response.

In 1984 Ahmed and colleagues[20] published the MSKCC experience of all men presenting with penile carcinoma since 1975 who treated with single-agent methotrexate, cisplatin, or bleomycin. Sixty-one percent of patients treated with methotrexate achieved response, which lasted for greater than 12 months in 2 patients. Responses were also seen in 3 patients who had prior cisplatin therapy. Of 12 patients thought to have received adequate cisplatin treatment, 1 achieved a complete response lasting 7 months and 2 had brief partial responses. Of the 14 men treated with bleomycin, 3 responses were seen, but unfortunately 1 developed treatment-related pulmonary fibrosis and died.

COMBINATION CHEMOTHERAPY

Similar to experience with other solid tumor malignancies, penile cancer investigators began to have success treating patients with cytotoxic combinations with backbone agents such as methotrexate and bleomycin based on previous success, as well as combinations used for other squamous cell carcinoma sites.

The first group to report on their experience with combination 5-fluorouracil and cisplatin were Hussein and colleagues in 1990.[21] Five men with recurrent or unresectable squamous cell carcinoma of the penis and 1 of the urethra were treated with cisplatin day 1 followed by 5-fluorouracil infusions on days 2 to 6 (Table 1). The patient with urethral squamous cell carcinoma achieved clinical complete response after 2 cycles of therapy. Microscopic disease was found at lymphadenectomy, and local recurrence 12 months later was treated successfully with chemoradiotherapy and the patient had a durable clinical complete response for more than 32 months. The 5 patients with penile squamous cell carcinoma had partial responses. One patient underwent inguinal dissection for cure followed by adjuvant radiotherapy. He succumbed 18 months later to local recurrence. The remaining patients were thought to be unresectable and underwent local radiation therapy, with median duration of overall survival of 15 months. Toxicities were reportedly mild and consisted of mucositis, nausea and vomiting, and renal insufficiency.

Shammus and colleagues[22] reported on a series of 8 patients, 6 with initial surgery for cure with subsequent recurrence, 1 with regional lymph node, and 1 with regional lymph node and lung metastasis treated with combination cisplatin and 5-fluorouracil, with a slightly modified dose and schedule of 5-fluorouracil than reported in the Hussein series. None of the patients with recurrent disease responded to chemotherapy. Both patients with response had partial response that was durable after either surgery or radiotherapy, and were reportedly tumor free at 32 and 57 months.

In the largest published prospective study to date on advanced penile carcinoma, the SWOG investigated the multiday regimen of cisplatin, methotrexate, and bleomycin in men with locally advanced or metastatic disease, and reported an excellent response rate of 32% with chemotherapy only.[7] However, the 28% grade 4 and 5 toxicity rate precluded general adoption of this regimen. Toxicities included cytopenias, infection, pulmonary and gastrointestinal toxicity, as well as renal insufficiency. The routine integration of granulocyte growth factor into chemotherapy regimens with toxicity in this range was not available during the accrual period of 1986 to 1994.

Additional retrospective experiences with cisplatin, methotrexate, and bleomycin were

Table 1
Cisplatin combinations in locally advanced and metastatic disease

Regimen	N	Response	Responder Survival	Treatment-related Deaths	References
Cisplatin 5-Fluorouracil	6	1 complete 5 partial	6 to 32 mo	0	Hussein et al[21]
Cisplatin 5-Fluorouracil	8	2 partial	32 and 57 mo	0	Shammas et al[22]
Cisplatin Methotrexate Bleomycin (CMB)	14	2 complete 8 partial 3 minor	6 to 24 mo (median = 10 mo)	0	Dexeus et al[23]
Cisplatin Methotrexate Bleomycin (CMB)	45	5 complete 8 partial	9 to 57 mo (median = 28 wk)	5	Haas et al[7]
Cisplatin Methotrexate Bleomycin (CMB)	13	3 adjuvant without recurrence	N/A	1	Hakenberg et al[14]
Cisplatin Irinotecan	28	2 complete 6 partial	N/A		Theodore et al[24]
Cisplatin Gemcitabine (GC)	2	2 partial	11 mo		Power et al[25]

reported by Hakenberg and colleagues[14] and Dexeus and colleagues.[23] Dexeus and colleagues reported on 12 men with penile squamous cell carcinoma and 2 men with other genitourinary squamous cell malignancies who were treated with either an intravenous regimen (11 men), or intravenous methotrexate combined with intra-arterial cisplatin and bleomycin in 3 men with only unilateral unresectable inguinal lymphadenopathy.[23] Two of the 11 patients who received intravenous chemotherapy achieved a complete response, with 1 lasting longer than 24 months. All 3 patients who had combination intravenous/intra-arterial chemotherapy achieved partial response. The median duration of response was 6 months (range 4–24 months). Toxicities included cytopenias, infection, neutropenic fever, pulmonary and gastrointestinal toxicity, as well as renal insufficiency. The same doses and chemotherapy schedule were used in the series reported by Hakenberg and colleagues,[14] which comprised 8 patients treated adjuvantly, 2 with metastatic disease at presentation and 3 with recurrent disease after resection. In the 5 patients with measurable disease, initial stable disease or minimal response was demonstrated, followed by progression and death in all 5 after a mean of 5 months of treatment. Of the 8 patients who underwent this regimen in the adjuvant setting, 1 died from pulmonary fibrosis, which was thought to be treatment related, and 3 remain without evidence of disease.

In a phase II multicenter study, the European Organization for Research and Treatment of Cancer (EORTC) prospectively studied combination cisplatin and irinotecan in men with T3 or N1 or N2 disease for 4 cycles in the neoadjuvant setting or with 8 cycles in the locally advanced or metastatic setting.[24] All patients were chemotherapy naive, and this report therefore represents a more homogeneous population than reported in other studies of penile carcinoma. Of the 28 patients enrolled, 26 were evaluable with an overall response rate of 30.8%. Seven patients were treated neoadjuvantly. Two clinical complete responses were seen, 1 in each of the neoadjuvant and distant disease groups. Furthermore, 3 patients were pathologically disease free at surgery following neoadjuvant chemotherapy. One patient in the neoadjuvant group had a partial response, as did 5 with advanced disease. Toxicity was as expected with these agents, notably 3 episodes of grade 3 diarrhea, and 2 of grade 4 neutropenic fever. Grade 4 events also included 8 episodes of granulocytopenia, 1 of each hemoglobin and thrombocytopenia, and 1 each of myocardial infarction and pulmonary

embolus. No treatment-related deaths were reported.

The combination of cisplatin and gemcitabine, an accepted standard of care for bladder cancer, was studied in patients with penile squamous cell carcinoma.[25] In this small series of 2 case reports, cisplatin and gemcitabine at slightly higher doses than traditionally delivered for bladder carcinoma were given every 21 days. After 3 cycles both patients demonstrated partial response that was sustained through 6 cycles. At 12 months, 1 patient had relapsed disease and the other remained disease free. The regimen was reportedly well tolerated, with 1 patient experiencing tinnitus necessitating change to carboplatin.

TAXANE COMBINATIONS

Taxanes are another active class of agents with known activity in other squamous cell carcinomas such as lung, and are generally used as second-line therapy for patients with urothelial carcinoma. Like cisplatin, potentially irreversible neuropathy can be dose limiting and this class necessitates prophylaxis for hypersensitivity during infusion.

Four series of taxane combinations administered in the metastatic or recurrent setting have been reported, as shown in **Table 2**. Joerger and colleagues[26] noted a case of a 64-year-old man with unresectable nodal disease who had a partial response with paclitaxel and carboplatin allowing subsequent curative surgery and adjuvant radiotherapy. The use of carboplatin rather than cisplatin in this combination makes it potentially feasible for patients with impaired creatinine clearance. Furthermore this regimen is generally well tolerated; many medical oncologists are familiar with this combination as a result of its efficacy in other solid tumors.

Di Lorenzo and colleagues[27] reported a single-arm phase II study of paclitaxel alone in patients who had been previously treated with neoadjuvant cisplatin-based regimens. In addition, 17% had received previous radiotherapy and 25% had received adjuvant chemotherapy. In this group, paclitaxel dosed at 175 mg/m^2 at 3-week intervals demonstrated a modest partial response in 3 of 12 patients. One patient had grade 4 neutropenia, and grade 3 neutropenia, anemia, and thrombocytopenia were also seen in a minority of patients. Considering that this population had been pretreated with cisplatin, with some patients receiving cisplatin within 6 months or sooner of enrollment into this study, the combined 50% partial response and stable disease rate is promising.

Table 2
Taxane combinations in locally advanced and metastatic disease

Regimen	N	Response	Responder Survival	Treatment-related Deaths	References
Paclitaxel Carboplatin	1	1 partial	N/A	0	Joerger et al[26]
Paclitaxel	12	3 partial	Median 8 mo	0	Di Lorenzo et al[27]
Paclitaxel Cisplatin 5-Fluorouracil (TPF)	6	2 complete 1 partial 2 complete with rapid relapse[a]	>24 mo	0	Pizzocaro et al[9]
Paclitaxel or docetaxel Cisplatin 5-Fluorouracil	26	7 partial	Median 10.5 mo for all patients	0	Nicolai et al[28]

[a] Both refused >2 cycles of chemotherapy.

Pizzocaro and colleagues[9] performed a small prospective study of the 3-drug combination of paclitaxel, cisplatin, and 5-fluorouracil. They included 1 patient who had received docetaxel 75 mg/m^2 in addition to cisplatin and 5-fluorouracil for 7 cycles, and who showed clinical and pathologic complete response at the time of surgery, with reported survival of at least 25 months. Another patient who received 5 courses of the planned paclitaxel, cisplatin, and 5-fluorouracil treatment also attained pathologic complete response after a recurrence following initial surgery and radiotherapy. One patient with partial response could only tolerate 2 cycles because of gastrointestinal toxicity. Nevertheless, a dramatic partial response was achieved and 2 small lymph node metastases were pathologically noted. The patient was reportedly disease free at 46 months. Of the 3 remaining patients who died of disease, 2 tolerated only 2 cycles of chemotherapy and the third had a superficial surgical procedure after clinical response but recurred 4 months later with peritoneal carcinomatosis.

A single-institution Italian series was presented in abstract form at the 2010 American Society of Clinical Oncology Genitourinary Cancers Symposium.[28] Cisplatin, 5-fluorouracil, and either docetaxel or paclitaxel were given in the neoadjuvant, adjuvant, and metastatic settings. Of the 26 patients treated in this pilot study, 8 received paclitaxel, cisplatin, and 5-fluorouracil, and the remainder received docetaxel, cisplatin, and 5-fluorouracil. Eight patients were treated neoadjuvantly, with 6 experiencing partial remission, with 3 patients surviving after a median of 29 months. Of the 12 patients treated adjuvantly, 58.3% were alive at 16 months. Only 1 of the 6 patients with metastatic disease achieved partial response, which was of short duration.

TARGETED THERAPY

The last 10 years in oncology have been punctuated with the advent of targeted agents, which either alone (renal cell carcinoma) or combined with cytotoxic chemotherapy (breast, lung, and colorectal cancer) have truly advanced cancer care. Understanding of the up-regulation of epidermal growth factor receptor (EGFR) on other squamous cell malignancies, such as head and neck cancers, have led to success with the addition of agents targeted against this receptor in treating these cancers, improving response to radiotherapy and improving survival.[29]

Carthon and colleagues[30] presented their retrospective experience treating men with penile carcinoma at the MD Anderson Cancer Center with EGFR targeted agents alone or in combination with chemotherapy. All tumors were tested and found to express EGFR before treatment with erlotinib alone, cetuximab, or cetuximab in conjunction with cisplatin. The median time to disease progression ranged from 0.37 to 37.3+ months, and overall survival ranged from 2.87 to 48.03 months. Grade 1 acne is an expected toxicity of this class of drugs, and has been shown to be indicator of efficacy in the treatment of other solid tumors.[31,32] Grade 3 and 4 events of cellulitis, thrombocytopenia, and tumor hemorrhage were also reported.

URETHRAL CARCINOMA

The histology of urethral carcinoma varies based on the anatomic location of the lesion and the sex of the patient. For men, lesions in the proximal urethra are typically urothelial carcinoma, usually in the prostatic urethra, and are treated analogously to urothelial carcinoma of the bladder. Distal lesions are typically squamous cell carcinoma, and are treated similarly to penile squamous cell carcinoma. In women, most tumors are squamous cell histology, which are treated analogously to other squamous cell tumors of the genitalia. However, a distinct rare tumor can arise in the female urethra, clear cell adenocarcinoma, which may be derived from paraurethral ducts and can be found in urethral diverticulae.[33,34] This is a rare tumor that can be locally advanced at presentation with an aggressive phenotype, and the mainstay of treatment is surgical. For locally advanced tumors or positive surgical margins, neoadjuvant and adjuvant chemotherapy have been attempted without a clear consensus regimen.

SUMMARY

Carcinomas of the penis and urethra are uncommon in the Western world, and treatment algorithms are hampered by the lack of prospective data and rigorous clinical trials. The amalgamation of single-institution retrospective reviews indicate that multi-agent cisplatin-based chemotherapy has significant activity for penile carcinoma, and can be used in the neoadjuvant, adjuvant, and metastatic settings. The mainstay of curative therapy remains surgical, however, and the reports are consistent that for patients who do not respond or who do not undergo consolidative surgical resection, the prognosis is dismal.

REFERENCES

1. Jemal A, Siegel R, Ward E, et al. Cancer statistics, 2009. CA Cancer J Clin 2009;59:225.
2. Horenblas S, Van Tinteren H, Delemarre JF, et al. Squamous cell carcinoma of the penis: accuracy of tumor, nodes and metastasis classification system, and role of lymphangiography, computerized tomography scan and fine needle aspiration cytology. J Urol 1991;146:1279.
3. Ornellas AA, Seixas AL, Marota A, et al. Surgical treatment of invasive squamous cell carcinoma of the penis: retrospective analysis of 350 cases. J Urol 1994;151:1244.
4. Leijte JA, Kerst JM, Bais E, et al. Neoadjuvant chemotherapy in advanced penile carcinoma. Eur Urol 2007;52:488.
5. Pizzocaro G, Piva L. Adjuvant and neoadjuvant vincristine, bleomycin, and methotrexate for inguinal

6. metastases from squamous cell carcinoma of the penis. Acta Oncol 1988;27:823.
7. Bermejo C, Busby JE, Spiess PE, et al. Neoadjuvant chemotherapy followed by aggressive surgical consolidation for metastatic penile squamous cell carcinoma. J Urol 2007;177:1335.
8. Haas GP, Blumenstein BA, Gagliano RG, et al. Cisplatin, methotrexate and bleomycin for the treatment of carcinoma of the penis: a Southwest Oncology Group study. J Urol 1999;161:1823.
9. Gagliano RG, Blumenstein BA, Crawford ED, et al. cis-Diamminedichloroplatinum in the treatment of advanced epidermoid carcinoma of the penis: a Southwest Oncology Group Study. J Urol 1989; 141:66.
10. Pizzocaro G, Nicolai N, Milani A. Taxanes in combination with cisplatin and fluorouracil for advanced penile cancer: preliminary results. Eur Urol 2009; 55:546.
11. Culkin DJ, Beer TM. Advanced penile carcinoma. J Urol 2003;170:359.
12. Pizzocaro G, Algaba F, Horenblas S, et al. EAU Penile Cancer Guidelines 2009. Eur Urol 2010. [Epub ahead of print]. PMID: 20163910.
13. Pizzocaro G, Piva L, Bandieramonte G, et al. Up-to-date management of carcinoma of the penis. Eur Urol 1997;32:5.
14. Ravi R. Correlation between the extent of nodal involvement and survival following groin dissection for carcinoma of the penis. Br J Urol 1993; 72:817.
15. Hakenberg OW, Nippgen JB, Froehner M, et al. Cisplatin, methotrexate and bleomycin for treating advanced penile carcinoma. BJU Int 2006; 98:1225.
16. Ichikawa T, Nakano I, Hirokawa I. Bleomycin treatment of the tumors of penis and scrotum. J Urol 1969;102:699.
17. Maiche AG. Adjuvant treatment using bleomycin in squamous cell carcinoma of penis: study of 19 cases. Br J Urol 1983;55:542.
18. Sklaroff RB, Yagoda A. Cis-diamminedichloride platinum II (DDP) in the treatment of penile carcinoma. Cancer 1979;44:1563.
19. Garnick MB, Skarin AT, Steele GD Jr. Metastatic carcinoma of the penis: complete remission after high dose methotrexate chemotherapy. J Urol 1979;122:265.
20. Sklaroff RB, Yagoda A. Methotrexate in the treatment of penile carcinoma. Cancer 1980;45:214.
21. Ahmed T, Sklaroff R, Yagoda A. Sequential trials of methotrexate, cisplatin and bleomycin for penile cancer. J Urol 1984;132:465.
22. Hussein AM, Benedetto P, Sridhar KS. Chemotherapy with cisplatin and 5-fluorouracil for penile and urethral squamous cell carcinomas. Cancer 1990;65:433.

22. Shammas FV, Ous S, Fossa SD. Cisplatin and 5-fluo-rouracil in advanced cancer of the penis. J Urol 1992;147:630.

23. Dexeus FH, Logothetis CJ, Sella A, et al. Combination chemotherapy with methotrexate, bleomycin and cisplatin for advanced squamous cell carcinoma of the male genital tract. J Urol 1991;146:1284.

24. Theodore C, Skoneczna I, Bodrogi I, et al. A phase II multicentre study of irinotecan (CPT 11) in combination with cisplatin (CDDP) in metastatic or locally advanced penile carcinoma (EORTC PROTOCOL 30992). Ann Oncol 2008;19:1304.

25. Power DG, Galvin DJ, Cuffe S, et al. Cisplatin and gemcitabine in the management of metastatic penile cancer. Urol Oncol 2009;27:187.

26. Joerger M, Warzinek T, Klaeser B, et al. Major tumor regression after paclitaxel and carboplatin polyche-motherapy in a patient with advanced penile cancer. Urology 2004;63:778.

27. Di Lorenzo G, Carteni G, Autorino R, et al. Activity and toxicity of paclitaxel in pretreated metastatic penile cancer patients. Anticancer Drugs 2009;20:277.

28. Nicolai N, Necchi A, Piva L, et al. A combination of cisplatin and 5-fluorouracil plus a taxane for advanced squamous-cell carcinoma (SCC) of the penis: a single-institution series [abstract #255]. In: American Society of Clinical Oncology Genitourinary Cancers Symposium, San Francisco (CA), March 5–7, 2010.

29. Bonner JA, Harari PM, Giralt J, et al. Radiotherapy plus cetuximab for squamous-cell carcinoma of the head and neck. N Engl J Med 2006;354:567.

30. Carthon BC, Pettaway CA, Pagliaro LC. Epidermal growth factor receptor (EGFR) targeted therapy in advanced metastatic squamous cell carcinoma (AMSCC) of the penis [abstract #254]. In: American Society of Clinical Oncology Genitourinary Cancers Symposium, San Francisco (CA), March 5–7, 2010.

31. Bonner JA, Harari PM, Giralt J, et al. Radiotherapy plus cetuximab for locoregionally advanced head and neck cancer: 5-year survival data from a phase 3 randomised trial, and relation between cetuximab-induced rash and survival. Lancet Oncol 2010;11:21.

32. Jonker DJ, O'Callaghan CJ, Karapetis CS, et al. Cetuximab for the treatment of colorectal cancer. N Engl J Med 2007;357:2040.

33. Kawano K, Yano M, Kitahara S, et al. Clear cell adenocarcinoma of the female urethra showing strong immunostaining for prostate-specific antigen. BJU Int 2001;87:412.

34. Seballos RM, Rich RR. Clear cell adenocarcinoma arising from a urethral diverticulum. J Urol 1995; 153:1914.

Management of the Male Urethra After Cystectomy

Shawn E. White, MD, S. Bruce Malkowicz, MD*

KEYWORDS

- Cystectomy • Male urethra • Bladder cancer
- Urothelial carcinoma

Approximately 70,000 new cases of bladder cancer are diagnosed yearly, of which 52,000 are male patients. In 2009, there were approximately 14,000 deaths attributed to bladder cancer, 10,000 of which were men.[1] Approximately 40% to 45% of all cases are high-grade tumors with half of these being muscle-invasive tumors at the time of diagnosis.[2] These statistics demonstrate the large number of patients who may be candidates for radical cystectomy and urinary diversion. With the preponderance of men in this population, there is a need for clear management strategies regarding the retained urethra in those men undergoing radical cystectomy.[3] This article reviews the incidence of urothelial carcinoma in the retained urethra, risk factors for the development of urethral urothelial carcinoma, surveillance strategies, treatment modalities, and outcomes following intervention.

INCIDENCE

Several theories exist concerning the pathophysiology of urethral carcinoma following radical cystectomy. Given the field defect nature of urothelial carcinoma, urethral lesions may reflect metachronous occurrences of the primary disease. Such lesions may also represent a true recurrence of disease at the margin of resection or anastomosis in the case of orthotopic diversions. Lastly, these may be previously unrecognized areas of disease in the proximal urethra. Regardless of the true pathophysiology, the incidence of this entity has been reported as ranging from 0% to 18% in several series.[4,5] A 2002 meta-analysis combined several large series of patients undergoing radical cystectomy and reported a urethral recurrence rate of 8.1% in a pooled cohort of 3165 subjects.[6] A more recent analysis of urethral tumors following radical cystectomy from the University of Southern California reported an incidence of 4.4% in more than 1000 subjects. A preponderance of these subjects underwent some form of continent diversion with a large proportion receiving an orthotopic diversion.[7–9] A total of 42% of these subjects were diagnosed within 1 year of cystectomy with a median time to diagnosis of 18.5 months.

RISK FACTORS

Several clinic features have been associated with urethral urothelial carcinoma following radical cystectomy, including multifocal disease, carcinoma in situ, upper tract urothelial carcinoma, bladder neck involvement, and involvement of the prostatic urethra.[10–17] Although most of the aforementioned factors implied various degrees of risk within the literature, the involvement of the prostate had proven to be the most consistent risk factor noted across cystectomy series.[10] Furthermore, the degree of prostatic involvement has been shown to correlate with recurrence of urothelial carcinoma in the retained urethra.[18,19] In a 1990 series of 30 subjects with urothelial carcinoma of the prostate, there were no recurrences in those with mucosal involvement, there were recurrences in 25% of those with ductal involvement, and

Division of Urology, Department of Surgery, University of Pennsylvania School of Medicine, University of Pennsylvania Health System, 9 Penn Tower, 34th and Civic Boulevard, Philadelphia, PA 19104, USA
* Corresponding author.
E-mail address: Bruce.malkowicz@uphs.upenn.edu

Urol Clin N Am 37 (2010) 475–479
doi:10.1016/j.ucl.2010.04.008
0094-0143/10/$ – see front matter © 2010 Published by Elsevier Inc.

a recurrence rate of 67% in subjects with prostatic stromal involvement.[20] In another series of 436 subjects who underwent radical cystectomy, the 5-year urethral recurrence was 6% in subjects without prostatic involvement, 15% in subjects with mucosal involvement of the prostate, and 21% in those with stromal invasion of the prostate gland.[21]

As orthotopic neobladder substitution has become an option for many patients, the issue of recurrent urothelial carcinoma in the functional male urethra has been assessed in several series. Overall, the evidence points toward a protective effect of maintaining a functional urethra via orthotopic neobladder when compared with ileal conduit cutaneous diversion and the resulting dry urethra. The first complete report of this trend is from a 1996 series of 436 subjects and reported a urethral recurrence rate of 2.9% in subjects undergoing orthotopic neobladder substitution compared with 11.1% in those undergoing ileal conduit cutaneous diversion.[21] A more recent series reported a urethral recurrence rate of 0.5% of subjects undergoing orthotopic neobladder compared with 2.1% of those undergoing ileal conduit in a series of 415 subjects undergoing radical cystectomy.[22] Although these overall recurrence rates are lower, the trend toward lower recurrence rate in subjects undergoing orthotopic neobladder is consistently evident. Whether this is caused by patient selection, a systemic effect of continent diversion, excretion of protective substances from the bowel segment used in the diversion, or a protective effect of urine exposure to the retained urethra is unclear.

A cohort of 252 men undergoing orthotopic ileal neobladder was analyzed to determine if preoperative transurethral prostatic urethral biopsy was a predictor of final distal urethral margin status at the time of radical cystectomy. Although this is not a direct predictive model for urethral recurrence following cystectomy, it may affect the patients' candidacy for orthotopic bladder substitution. Positive transurethral biopsies of the prostatic urethra only correlated with frozen section urethral margin status at the time of cystectomy in 68% of cases. The negative predictive values for transurethral biopsies and intraoperative frozen section were 99.4% and 100%, respectively.[23] Overall, this data does not support the routine use of preoperative transurethral prostatic urethra biopsies to determine fitness for orthotopic neobladder.[23–26] This point is significant when discussing urethral recurrence following cystectomy because orthotopic neobladder has been associated with lower rates of urothelial carcinoma in the retained urethra.[22]

SURVEILLANCE

Screening strategies for patients following radical cystectomy include urethral cytology and endoscopic examination of the urethra. Symptomatic bleeding or urethral discharge are indications for urethroscopy and correlate with the presence of urothelial carcinoma in the retained urethra.[7,27] Cytology has been shown to be a reliable indicator of urethral urothelial carcinoma in patients who are symptomatic and asymptomatic. In a series of 24 subjects who underwent urethrectomy following cystectomy for urethral urothelial carcinoma, 17 (71%) were asymptomatic but had a positive urethral wash cytology, whereas 7 (29%) were not followed with urethral cytology and presented with symptomatic bleeding.[28] Another earlier series reported similar results. In a group of 47 subjects who underwent radical cystectomy, urethral urothelial carcinoma was diagnosed by screening cytology alone in 35% of these subjects, and 94% of all subjects diagnosed with urethral urothelial carcinoma in this group had a positive urethral cytology.[7] One series also reported a 12.5% false-positive rate for urethral cytology in screening subjects for recurrence following radical cystectomy.[29] These screening practices can be applied to patients with cutaneous diversions and a dry urethra, and those with orthotopic neobladders. However, patients with orthotopic neobladders and urethral urothelial carcinoma may also present simply with a change in voiding habits.[7] This data provides support for periodic cytology obtained by urethral washing as a minimum screening tool, with endoscopic evaluation of the urethra a useful addition particularly in patients who present with symptomatic bleeding or urethral discharge. In the case of these patients, urethrectomy should be strongly considered even in the absence of frank pathology. In the case of gross findings on cystoscopy or palpable disease, cross-sectional imaging should be obtained.

TREATMENT

The gold-standard therapy for urethral urothelial carcinoma following radical cystectomy is total urethrectomy. This procedure involves the complete excision of the urethra, including the urethral meatus.[30] A previously accepted method of treatment that advocated sparing the glanular urethra has been abandoned in light of various reports of significance recurrence rates. One such series reported a glanular urethral recurrence rate of 27% following subtotal urethrectomy in subjects who had previously undergone radical cystectomy.[31]

Because of the generally low rate of urethral recurrence, urethrectomy is not empirically performed at the time of cystoprostatectomy. This practice has been bolstered by anecdotal reports of increased incidence of pelvic abscesses and the general degree of added time and occasional difficulty that the procedure can bring to the cystoprostatectomy. Consideration for the inclusion of urethrectomy in the principle surgery may be considered in higher risk cases, such as those with prostatic stromal involvement. In such cases a 2-team approach, with 1 group concentrating on the cystectomy and the other on the urethrectomy, can be useful.

Preservation of sexual function following urethrectomy either at the time of radical cystectomy or for recurrent disease following cystectomy has been improved by an anatomic approach developed following elucidation of the course of the cavernous nerves; which is a discovery that has also improved functional outcomes following radical prostatectomy. The basic anatomic principle that the cavernous nerves course posterolateral to the membranous urethra facilitates a perineal dissection that allows these nerves to be spared. Early reports showed preserved potency in subjects undergoing this nerve-sparing approach to urethrectomy.[32]

Management decisions become more complex in patients with orthotopic neobladders. Total urethrectomy in patients with this type of diversion requires conversion to cutaneous incontinent diversion, which can be a major technical undertaking.[33] Although eradication of recurrent disease remains the goal, several attempts at intravesical or intraurethral instillation therapy have been made with varying results. In a series of 371 subjects who underwent ileal orthotopic neobladder, 4% experienced recurrent urethral urothelial carcinoma. Some of these subjects received intraurethral bacille Calmette-Guérin (BCG) therapy using a standardized delivery protocol with a modified Foley catheter and higher concentration of BCG than intravesical therapy for bladder carcinoma. A total of 83% of the subjects who had CIS responded to BCG without recurrence, but all subjects with papillary or invasive disease failed intraurethral therapy.[34] Another series of 516 subjects reported successful treatment of recurrent urethral CIS in 10 subjects with orthotopic neobladder.[35,36]

OUTCOMES

Urethral urothelial carcinoma following radical cystectomy is associated with a poor overall and disease-specific survival.[37] In a large, previously mentioned series, the median survival in subjects with recurrent disease in the urethra following cystectomy was 28 months.[7] The most significant predicting factor for survival in this series was stage of urethral urothelial carcinoma at the time of diagnosis. Invasive disease was associated with a worse overall survival than superficial disease or CIS. Another large series from the SEER database analyzed over 2400 subjects who underwent radical cystectomy. A total of 195 of these subjects underwent urethrectomy either concurrently or as a salvage procedure following recurrence. Survival was slightly higher in subjects who underwent urethrectomy at the time of cystectomy; however, these results did not reach significance.[38] One area of controversy in the literature is the best predictor of survival following urethrectomy. The aforementioned series showed an association between urethral stage at recurrence and mortality. However, some series have failed to demonstrate this association but have asserted that the most significant predictor of survival is initial bladder pathologic stage. In a series of 24 men who underwent urethrectomy reported in 2003, 58% of subjects were alive with no evidence of disease at a mean follow-up time of 27.7 months, 21% were alive with disease, and 12.5% had died of disease. Cystectomy pathology was the only significant predictor of disease-free survival in these subjects.[28]

SUMMARY

With more than 52,000 new cases of bladder cancer diagnosed in men and 10,000 deaths from bladder cancer in 2009, clear management strategies for the male urethra in these patients are useful. This issue becomes particularly relevant when surgeons and patients are faced with making an informed decision concerning urinary diversion in those undergoing radical cystectomy. The incidence of urethral urothelial carcinoma following radical cystectomy has been reported as 0.0% to 18.0%, with a large meta-analysis reporting an 8.1% rate.

Clinical features associated with urethral urothelial carcinoma following radical cystectomy include multifocal disease; carcinoma in situ; upper tract urothelial carcinoma; bladder neck involvement; and involvement of the prostatic urethra, with prostatic urethra involvement being the most consistent factor across series. A lower rate of urethral urothelial carcinoma following cystectomy has been consistently demonstrated in patients undergoing orthotopic neobladder when compared with ileal conduit urinary diversion.

This frequency of 3.0% to 4.5% indicates careful patient selection and probably some undefined protective effect of orthotopic bladder substitution on the retained urethra. When selecting patients to undergo orthotopic neobladder, preoperative transurethral biopsies of the prostatic urethra do not correlate precisely with urethral frozen margin status at the time of cystectomy. They are still of value in discerning candidates for orthotopic diversion compared with cutaneous continent or standard ileal loop diversion and are worthwhile especially in patients with a history of high-risk nonmuscle invasive disease that has not responded to intravesical therapy.

When considering surveillance strategies, urethral cytology has been shown to correlate with the presence of urethral urothelial carcinoma in the retained urethra. The frequency of cytology is an issue of authority opinion and generally performed more often in the early postoperative period or in high-risk patients. Urethroscopy is also reliable in detecting recurrent disease and is an adjunct in patients who are cytology positive and those presenting with symptomatic bleeding or discharge. Patients with an orthotopic neobladder should have their cytology evaluated and attention should be given to a change in voiding habits.

The gold-standard treatment for patients with urothelial carcinoma following cystectomy is a total urethrectomy. An anatomic approach to nerve-sparing urethrectomy can improve functional outcomes following urethrectomy performed following cystectomy or at the time of cystectomy. The role of intraurethral BCG is less well defined but some data suggest this as an effective therapy, particularly in patients who have not developed invasive disease or those with CIS.

Overall and disease-specific survival in patients with urethral urothelial carcinoma following cystectomy is poor. Mean survival has been reported as 28 months, with urethral stage and final cystectomy pathology both postulated as predictors of survival.

REFERENCES

1. Jemel A, Siegel R, Ward E, et al. Cancer Statistics, 2009. CA Cancer J Clin 2009;59:225–49.
2. Thorstenson A, Larsson H, Wijkstrom H, et al. Bladder cancer characteristics in a population based study of newly detected tumors. J Urol 2003;169:864A.
3. Spiess PE, Kassouf W, Brown G, et al. Immediate versus staged urethrectomy in patients at high risk of urethral recurrence: is there a benefit to either approach? Urology 2006;67(3):466–71.
4. Hickey DP, Soloway MS, Murphy WM. Selective urethrectomy following cystoprostatectomy for bladder cancer. J Urol 1986;136(4):828–30.
5. Tobisu K, Tanaka Y, Mizutani T, et al. Transitional cell carcinoma of the urethra in men following cystectomy for bladder cancer: multivariate analysis for risk factors. J Urol 1991;146(6):1551–3 [discussion: 1553–4].
6. Stenzl A, Bartsch G, Rogatsch H. The remnant urothelium after reconstructive bladder surgery. Eur Urol 2002;41(2):124–31.
7. Clark PE, Stein JP, Groshen SG, et al. The management of urethral transitional cell carcinoma after radical cystectomy for invasive bladder cancer. J Urol 2004;172(4 Pt 1):1342–7.
8. Skinner DG, Stein JP, Lieskovsky G, et al. 25-year experience in the management of invasive bladder cancer by radical cystectomy. Eur Urol 1998; 33(Suppl 4):25–6.
9. Stein JP, Clark P, Miranda G, et al. Urethral tumor recurrence following cystectomy and urinary diversion: clinical and pathological characteristics in 768 male patients. J Urol 2005;173(4):1163–8.
10. Sherwood JB, Sagalowsky AI. The diagnosis and treatment of urethral recurrence after radical cystectomy. Urol Oncol 2006;24(4):356–61.
11. Ayyathurai R, Gomez P, Luongo T, et al. Prostatic involvement by urothelial carcinoma of the bladder: clinicopathological features and outcome after radical cystectomy. BJU Int 2007;100(5):1021–5.
12. Saad M, Abdel-Rahim M, Abol-Enein H, et al. Concomitant pathology in the prostate in cystoprostatectomy specimens: a prospective study and review. BJU Int 2008;102(11):1544–50.
13. Barbisan F, Mazzucchelli R, Scarpelli M, et al. Urothelial and incidental prostate carcinoma in prostates from cystoprostatectomies for bladder cancer: is there a relationship between urothelial and prostate cancer? BJU Int 2009;103(8):1058–63.
14. Cho KS, Seo JW, Park SJ, et al. The risk factor for urethral recurrence after radical cystectomy in patients with transitional cell carcinoma of the bladder. Urol Int 2009;82(3):306–11.
15. Mazzucchelli R, Barbisan F, Santinelli A, et al. Prediction of prostatic involvement by urothelial carcinoma in radical cystoprostatectomy for bladder cancer. Urology 2009;74(2):385–90.
16. Beahrs JR, Fleming TR, Zincke H. Risk of local urethral recurrence after radical cystectomy for bladder cancer. J Urol 1984;131(2):264–6.
17. Tongaonkar HB, Dalal AV, Kulkarni JN, et al. Urethral recurrences following radical cystectomy for invasive transitional cell carcinoma of the bladder. Br J Urol 1993;72(6):910–4.
18. Lerner SP, Shen S. Pathologic assessment and clinical significance of prostatic involvement by

transitional cell carcinoma and prostate cancer. Urol Oncol 2008;26(5):481–5.

19. Shen SS, Lerner SP, Muezzinoglu B, et al. Prostatic involvement by transitional cell carcinoma in patients with bladder cancer and its prognostic significance. Hum Pathol 2006;37(6):726–34.

20. Hardeman SW, Soloway MS. Urethral recurrence following radical cystectomy. J Urol 1990;144(3):666–9.

21. Freeman JA, Tarter TA, Esrig D, et al. Urethral recurrence in patients with orthotopic ileal neobladders. J Urol 1996;156(5):1615–9.

22. Hassan JM, Cookson MS, Smith JA Jr, et al. Urethral recurrence in patients following orthotopic urinary diversion. J Urol 2004;172(4 Pt 1):1338–41.

23. Kassouf W, Spiess PE, Brown GA, et al. Prostatic urethral biopsy has limited usefulness in counseling patients regarding final urethral margin status during orthotopic neobladder reconstruction. J Urol 2008; 180(1):164–7 [discussion: 167].

24. Liedberg F, Anderson H, Blackberg M, et al. Prospective study of transitional cell carcinoma in the prostatic urethra and prostate in the cystoprostatectomy specimen. Scand J Urol Nephrol 2007; 41(4):290–6.

25. Lebret T, Herve JM, Barre P, et al. Urethral recurrence of transitional cell carcinoma of the bladder. Predictive value of preoperative latero-montanal biopsies and urethral frozen sections during prostatocystectomy. Eur Urol 1998;33(2):170–4.

26. Tobisu K, Kanai Y, Sakamoto M, et al. Involvement of the anterior urethra in male patients with transitional cell-carcinoma of the bladder undergoing radical cystectomy with simultaneous urethrectomy. Jpn J Clin Oncol 1997;27(6):406–9.

27. Slaton JW, Swanson DA, Grossman HB, et al. A stage specific approach to tumor surveillance after radical cystectomy for transitional cell carcinoma of the bladder. J Urol 1999;162(3 Pt 1):710–4.

28. Lin DW, Herr HW, Dalbagni G. Value of urethral wash cytology in the retained male urethra after radical cystoprostatectomy. J Urol 2003;169(3):961–3.

29. Wolinska WH, Melamed MR, Schellhammer PF, et al. Urethral cytology following cystectomy for bladder carcinoma. Am J Surg Pathol 1977;1(3):225–34.

30. Levinson AK, Johnson DE, Wishnow KI. Indications for urethrectomy in an era of continent urinary diversion. J Urol 1990;144(1):73–5.

31. Schellhammer PF, Whitmore WF Jr. Urethral meatal carcinoma following cystourethrectomy for bladder carcinoma. J Urol 1976;115:61–4.

32. Brendler CB, Schlegel PN, Walsh PC. Urethrectomy with preservation of potency. J Urol 1990;144(2 Pt 1): 270–3.

33. Bell CR, Gujral S, Collins CM, et al. The fate of the urethra after definitive treatment of invasive transitional cell carcinoma of the urinary bladder. BJU Int 1999;83(6):607–12.

34. Varol C, Thalmann GN, Burkhard FC, et al. Treatment of urethral recurrence following radical cystectomy and ileal bladder substitution. J Urol 2004;172(3): 937–42.

35. Huguet J, Palou J, Serrallach M, et al. Management of urethral recurrence in patients with Studer ileal neobladder. Eur Urol 2003;43(5):495–8.

36. Witjes JA, Debruyne FM, van der Meijden AP. Treatment of carcinoma in situ of the urethra with intraurethral instillations of bacillus Calmette-Guerin. Case report and review of literature. Eur Urol 1991;20(2): 170–2.

37. Cheville JC, Dundore PA, Bostwick DG, et al. Transitional cell carcinoma of the prostate: clinicopathologic study of 50 cases. Cancer 1998;82(4):703–7.

38. Nelles JL, Konety BR, Saigal C, et al. Urethrectomy following cystectomy for bladder cancer in men: practice patterns and impact on survival. J Urol 2008;180(5):1933–6 [discussion: 1936–7].

Index

Note: Page numbers of article titles are in **boldface** type.

Moving?

Make sure your subscription moves with you!

To notify us of your new address, find your **Clinics Account Number** (located on your mailing label above your name), and contact customer service at:

Email: journalscustomerservice-usa@elsevier.com

800-654-2452 (subscribers in the U.S. & Canada)
314-447-8871 (subscribers outside of the U.S. & Canada)

Fax number: 314-447-8029

Elsevier Health Sciences Division
Subscription Customer Service
3251 Riverport Lane
Maryland Heights, MO 63043

*To ensure uninterrupted delivery of your subscription, please notify us at least 4 weeks in advance of move.

Printed and bound by CPI Group (UK) Ltd, Croydon, CR0 4YY

14/10/2024

01773707-0001